Exploring Body-Mind Interactions and Their Impact on Well-Being:

Holistic Practices

Charlène Clonts
https://orcid.org/0000-0003-4228-4868
Kyushu University, Japan

Lorenzo Cardilli
University of Udine, Italy

Yoshihara Kazufumi
https://orcid.org/0000-0001-6499-3900
Kyushu University, Japan

IGI Global
Scientific Publishing
Publishing Tomorrow's Research Today

Vice President of Editorial	Melissa Wagner
Director of Acquisitions	Mikaela Felty
Director of Book Development	Jocelynn Hessler
Production Manager	Mike Brehm
Cover Design	Jose Rosado

Published in the United States of America by
IGI Global Scientific Publishing
701 East Chocolate Avenue
Hershey, PA, 17033, USA
Tel: 717-533-8845 | Fax: 717-533-7115
Website: https://www.igi-global.com E-mail: cust@igi-global.com

Library of Congress Cataloging-in-Publication Data

Names: Clonts, Charlène, 1982- editor. | Cardilli, Lorenzo editor. | Kazufumi, Yoshihara, 1966- editor.
Title: Exploring body-mind interactions and their impact on well-being : holistic practices / edited by Charlène Clonts, Lorenzo Cardilli, Yoshihara Kazufumi.
Description: Hershey, PA : IGI Global Scientific Publishing, [2026] | Includes bibliographical references and index. | Summary: "This book delves into the intricate relationships between body-mind practices and well-being, drawing from a diverse range of interdisciplinary perspectives"-- Provided by publisher.
Identifiers: LCCN 2025031536 (print) | LCCN 2025031537 (ebook) | ISBN 9798337335216 hardcover | ISBN 9798337335223 paperback | ISBN 9798337335230 ebook
Subjects: LCSH: Mind and body--Case studies. | Well-being--Case studies.
Classification: LCC BF161 .E97 2026 (print) | LCC BF161 (ebook)
LC record available at https://lccn.loc.gov/2025031536
LC ebook record available at https://lccn.loc.gov/2025031537

British Cataloguing in Publication Data
A Cataloguing in Publication record for this book is available from the British Library.

Table of Contents

Detailed Table of Contents

Fanon's time at Saint-Alban hospital, under the mentorship of Francesc Tosquelles, significantly influenced his thought. They saw psychiatry as aiming to dissolve pathological personality reconstructions caused by neurological shocks, using shock therapies, various psychotherapies, and socialtherapy within a hospital microcosm. Fanon applied this model to his analysis of the anticolonial liberation struggle, viewing it as a form of socialtherapy that dissolves pathological identities created by colonisation and prepares for a new decolonised world. Fanon's work at the Blida-Joinville hospital in Algeria continued Saint-Alban though his experiments there led him to a new form of ethnopsychiatry, emphasising the importance of cultural context in understanding mental illness. He later took some distance from Tosquelles, but his thought and practice would certainly not have developed in the same way without the experience he gained in Saint-Alban during the year and a half he spent there with him.

Stress triggers mind-body symptoms by activating the autonomic nervous system through the brain. Neuroimaging studies have identified the anterior cingulate cortex (ACC) and the insular cortex as being central to this interaction. Abnormalities in these regions have been linked to stress-related disorders such as depression, irritable bowel syndrome, and chronic pain. Recent research shows that modern psychotherapy and traditional body-mind practices can improve symptoms by modulating these neural pathways. For example, active listening activates the brain's reward system and insula. Additionally, a 12-week yoga intervention significantly improved mood and psychological symptoms such as depression and anxiety. Practices like mindfulness meditation also alter neural activity and brain volume in the ACC and insula. In conclusion, the ACC and insular cortex are crucial for body-mind interaction. Interventions targeting these pathways can improve health. Brain imaging research is essential for developing objective biomarkers and personalized treatments for stress-related conditions.

After fourteen years of wandering across Asia, Alexandra David-Neel became the first Western woman to enter the forbidden city of Lhasa in 1924. To get there, the explorer passed herself off as an old Tibetan beggar, a metamorphosis that was not only physical but also spiritual, marking her identity and enabling her to transcend cultural boundaries. The body certainly affects the mind by transforming its identity, but the mind also affects the body. The Buddhist explorer's walk was close to a physical feat, as her body was constantly tested by hunger and cold. The mind can also plunge the body into a state of half-dream, leading the explorer to have hallucination and mystical apparition. Therefore, the experience of the environment takes on a magical dimension that can be apprehended through the motif of walking, whose writing is marked by hesitation and exaggeration. This paper will consider Alexandra David-Neel's walk as an artistic and spiritual performance through an itinerary influenced by divine apparitions and natural events interpreted as prodigies.

In Western culture, war trauma is generally looked at as a syndrome (PTSD) and mostly treated pharmaceutically. However, war affects the human soul in a variety of ways, and holistic approaches have therefore been practised since ancient times in different cultures, aimed at maintaining the well-being of veterans. In Japanese culture, Bushido, Zen, as well as the tea ceremony or the "swordsmanship" and other forms of ethical education have been traditionally practiced as effective ways of keeping the human in harmonic homeostasis with nature, especially under stressful or potentially traumatic circumstances. This chapter considers the case of Italian WW2 veteran Mario Rigoni Stern: to overcome his war trauma, he undertook holistic healing based on storytelling and reconnecting with the sacred dimension of nature. The author will claim that Rigoni Stern's holistic way of healing war trauma can be understood from a transcultural perspective that blends the Western cognitive theories of emotional intelligence and adaptive storytelling with the Eastern traditions of Bushido and Zen.

The escalation of collective traumata, hegemonic oppression, and growing limitations on civil rights continue to exacerbate the precarious mental well-being of marginalised communities. The systemic mutism to which these groups are subjected makes it imperative to investigate the potential of the arts to heal traumatised and subaltern subjects. Ekphrasis, among the various media and rhetorical devices employed in the Humanities, appears to be a congenial dialogical instrument for researching this topic. This chapter aims to disentangle ekphrasis from its classical representational understanding as a means for translating a (visual) medium into another (verbal) (Heffernan, 1993). Drawing on the theories of Melanie Klein, Silvan S. Tomkins (1962-1991), W.J.T. Mitchell (1994), and Elena Ferrante's poetics ekphrasis is reevaluated—using Ferrante's Troubling Love (1992) as a case study—as a powerful tool for subaltern groups to become aware of their status and traumata, thereby opening a path towards psychological recovery.

This chapter investigates the method applied in the project "The Legacy of the Second World War in the Memory of the Third Generation," which collects a corpus of video interviews with Italian people born between the 1960s and the 1980s. The interviews are dialogues developed according to the Socratic dialeghestai, which is based on listening and understanding and is aimed at developing a critical reflection that starts with the recollections of the past to reach our contemporaneity. This chapter investigates how this methodology produces well-being in the witnesses in connection with the pleasure of remembering their childhood and grandparents. Eventually, it is claimed that the interviewees' well-being partially derives from aesthetic pleasure and, by referring to Fischer-Lichte's aesthetics, the interviewer is defined as a maieutic director.

The chapter studies the transformative aesthetics of Ghérasim Luca, a Francophone poet and visual artist, whose practice, allegedly obsessive, mobilizes the body as

embodied artistic practices—such as walking, photography, and storytelling—can function as epistemic methods. The embodied research presented in this chapter demonstrates a methodology in which practice and theory are entangled. Rather than separating artistic creation, daily life, and scientific inquiry, this chapter advances an integrated mode of embodied research in which the human being as a whole is situated at the center of epistemic practices.

The expression "every cloud has a silver lining" focuses on identifying a positive aspect in a gloomy or negative situation. Traumatic events can have long-lasting and adverse impacts, but some individuals may experience growth. The personal growth aftermath of adverse or traumatic events is referred to as adversarial growth. While experiencing trauma, cultivating gratitude may help to foster a positive outlook. This research analysed the role of gratitude on adversarial growth following chronic illness in India. A survey method was employed to collect responses from individuals who have experienced chronic illness in the last year. An updated version of SLQ-38 and GQ-6 was employed to measure constructs. A total of 368 respondents filled out the survey, and PLS-SEM on SmartPLS was employed to analyse the data. The findings of the study established a positive and significant association between gratitude and adversarial growth. In conclusion, theoretical contributions, interventional implications and future directions were discussed.

Ritual recitation, central to many religious traditions, is increasingly recognized as a promising mind-body intervention for trauma recovery. Trauma often disrupts the nervous system, leaving survivors in cycles of emotional dysregulation, hyperarousal, and loss of meaning. While conventional trauma therapies offer significant support, they may not fully address all the dimensions of trauma recovery. In this context, mantra-based meditation (MBM) emerges as a culturally grounded, low-cost practice that supports healing across physiological, cognitive, emotional, and spiritual dimensions. This chapter employs a theoretical approach and synthesizes existing research and conceptualizes the role of ritual recitation in trauma recovery. It further explores the neural mechanisms underlying mantra recitation and understands the integration of recitation-based interventions into trauma therapy. By bridging psychological, spiritual, cultural, and religious perspectives, this chapter positions ritual recitation as a holistic tool for fostering mental well-being in trauma survivors.

This study investigates art therapy as a culturally embedded, non-pharmacological approach to mental well-being in contemporary Japan. It examines how visual and plastic art practices function within therapeutic contexts, contributing to identity formation, emotional expression, and social inclusion. Emphasising the embodied and relational dimensions of art therapy, the research highlights its potential to foster psychophysical transformation through sensory, symbolic, and intersubjective experiences. Adopting an interdisciplinary approach, it explores how local traditions, institutional structures, and socio-cultural values shape access to art-therapeutic practices – particularly concerning social anxiety disorder, one of Japan's most prevalent and socially debated mental health conditions. Fieldwork was conducted at two art therapy ateliers selected for their engagement with this issue. The methodology combines socio-cultural analysis with qualitative tools, including on-site visits, semi-structured interviews, and a visual research component featuring therapeutic artworks.

This article explores the potential therapeutic effects of heterolingual literature in the context of bibliotherapy closely linked to cognitive behavourial therapy, through a close reading of Sekiguchi Ryōko's exophonic essay Nagori (2018). According to Sekiguchi, French people are as sensitive as Japanese people to the unique sensation of nagori, but lack a word to express it. Althought this essay is mainly written in French, Sekiguchi decided to use the Japanese word "nagori" as the title of her book, along with many other Japanese words within the text. This literary practice is called heterolingualism, and I argue that it impacts the body and the mind of the readers. Studies in neurosciences have called attention to the fact that there are strong relationships between word and face processing. The readers' interactions with a written text mirrors the dynamics between body and language that heterolingualism enhances as it provides more scope for cultural and emotional awareness.

Preface

BODY-MIND PRACTICES AND THE ECOLOGIES OF WELL-BEING

Conceptual Overview and Editorial Rationale

This book, *Exploring Body-Mind Interactions and Their Impact on Well-Being: Holistic Practices*, proposes a practice-led account of body-mind interactions. Rather than treating health as a set of symptoms to manage or the arts as objects to contemplate, it focuses on methods—repeatable, situated practices that reorganize how bodies feel, how minds mean, and how communities care. Listening, voicing, walking, cutting, collaging, drawing, reading, and dialoguing are not ancillary techniques; they are media through which perception stabilizes, affect regulates, and meaning returns—often by indirection and in company. The fourfold architecture of this volume—theoretical foundations, narratives and literature, cultural perspectives, and applications—was designed to carry readers from conceptual baselines to portable practices adaptable in classrooms, clinics, studios, and civic spaces, in line with the running order established for the present volume.

We adopt a concise, plural understanding of well-being. Following the WHO Glossary (2021), well-being is a state experienced by individuals and communities, shaped by intersectional factors—environment, social relationships, and inner phenomena—where purpose, contribution, meaning, and perceived quality of life are central; and arts can address well-being issues (WHO, 67th Synthesis Report, 2019). Complementing this, the OECD Guidelines (2013)—in line with expert consensus (e.g., Dolan & White 2007; Sen, Stiglitz, & Fitoussi 2009; ONS 2011; Takahashi 2022)—define well-being as "good mental states, including all of the various evaluations, positive and negative, that people make of their lives, and the affective reactions of people to their experiences." Operationally, the book treats well-being as well-becoming: a dynamic, practice-based process that reorganizes body-mind relations *with and through* culture. We further specify ecologies of well-being as the *relational networks*—somatic, affective, social, cultural, and environmental—through which well-being is generated, sustained, or disrupted, and within which arts-based practices function as ecological interventions.

At the origin of this book is a four-day international conference held at Kyushu University during the Asia Week (*Body-Mind Interactions in Arts, Health, Literatures, and Sciences: Asian and Indo-Oceanian Perspectives*, 4-8 November 2024, Fukuoka, Japan), which we convened as an early milestone of the cross-disciplinary Well-Being with Arts (WBA) research project (Leader: Charlène Clonts) with a four-year grant from Q-AOS, the Institute for Asian and Oceanian Studies. This academic meeting gathered researchers and practitioners around two intersecting axes: first, body-mind practices and holistic theories—with attention to Asian and Indo-Oceanian traditions, and to transcultural circulations—and second, the experience of arts (performance, sound, text, visual arts, arts of balance, *Ways*) understood in their performative and transformative dimensions within social, material, and natural environments. The present volume acknowledges that origin while welcoming additional authors whose work extends and deepens the themes launched there.

Amid post-pandemic isolation, social anxiety, eco-distress, and the need for low-barrier, somatically literate interventions, the book argues for practice ecologies: situated, repeatable exercises—attentional, somatic, narrative, creative—through which persons and communities cultivate regulation, meaning, and care.

Why This Topic Matters Today

The present moment is marked by converging pressures: long recoveries from pandemic-era isolation; rising social anxiety and withdrawal; renewed attention to trauma, eco-anxiety, and care; and a growing demand for interventions that are culturally responsive, low-barrier, and somatically literate. The conference's guiding framework emphasized interventional research on arts of balance and mindful, holistic practices; a rebalancing of subjective and objective conceptions of well-being from classical philosophy through contemporary social science; and transcultural dialogues that honor both difference and shared capacities to foster healing. It also called for bridges between biomedical/neuroscientific accounts of regulation and the practical wisdom embedded in ancient medicine, rituals, and embodied arts, echoing recent syntheses that urge more cross-cultural work and better taxonomies. These priorities shape the book's stance throughout.

What follows, then, is not a single method but a family of practice ecologies: autonomic-informed voice and breath; creative and movement-based sessions and ateliers; environmentally situated forms of ethical action; attentional grammars in listening, reading, and making. The book's wager is modest and demanding: no erasure of difficulty is promised; instead, it offers methods by which difficulty can be lived otherwise and relation renewed, and portable exercises that readers can test in their own settings while attending to cultural and environmental fit.

Intended Readership and Applications

Thus, this volume is written for scholars and students in medical humanities, cultural studies, psychology, music and performance studies, literary studies, anthropology, and public health; for artists, curators, educators, and therapists designing holistic and low-threshold interventions; and for practitioners in community, health, and educational settings who need rigorously framed, adaptable practices. Its four-part design supports multiple entry paths—foundations for conceptual bearings; narrative and cultural casework for forms that do what they discuss; and application chapters for immediately transferable protocols—while preserving a coherent through-line for readers who prefer to read the book end-to-end.

STATE OF THE ART IN BODY-MIND INTERACTIONS AND HOLISTIC WELL-BEING

Theoretical Landscape of Holism and Body-Mind Integration

The intellectual terrain traversed by this volume sits at the intersection of several converging scholarly traditions, each of which has independently arrived at the conclusion that human well-being cannot be adequately understood through reductive, symptom-focused frameworks alone. The concept of holism—understood as the principle that the body, mind, and spirit constitute an integrated, irreducible whole—has deep historical roots, traceable in Western medicine to Hippocratic thought around 300 BCE, which already recognized that weather, nutrition, emotional factors, and environmental conditions all contribute to human health (He, 2019). Yet holism is equally central to non-Western medical traditions: in Traditional Chinese Medicine (TCM), for instance, holism is not merely a philosophical orientation but the operative logic of diagnosis and treatment, premised on the understanding that "the body and mind are a unified system connected intimately and complexly to social, political-economic and biological systems" (He, 2019). Contemporary definitions of holistic health extend this understanding further, adding spiritual and emotional components to the physical, mental, and social dimensions already recognized by the World Health Organization's foundational 1948 definition (Labbé et al., 2019).

The present volume inherits and extends this long genealogy while situating it within contemporary interdisciplinary research, especially in Health Humanities.

What distinguishes the current moment is not the novelty of holistic thinking per se, but rather the renewed urgency with which scholars, clinicians, and practitioners are demanding that holistic frameworks be operationalized—made portable, culturally responsive, and empirically accountable—across diverse settings. As Frisch and Rabinowitsch's integrative literature review demonstrates, the terms "holistic nursing", "integrative health care", and "integrative nursing" share considerable philosophical overlap, all converging on the notion of "whole person care" that acknowledges body-mind-spirit as an integrated unit (Frisch & Rabinowitsch, 2019). Yet the same review reveals persistent conceptual ambiguity: the relationship between these terms remains contested, and their practical implementation is shaped by the cultural contexts in which care is delivered (Frisch & Rabinowitsch, 2019). This volume takes that ambiguity seriously, treating it not as a problem to be resolved by definitional fiat but as a productive tension that different contributions address from different disciplinary vantage points—from neuroscientific accounts of interoception and autonomic regulation, to cultural laboratories of haptic poetics, listening-led musicianship, and gratitude practice, and finally to implementable protocols of mantra-based meditation, atelier art therapy, bibliotherapy, and movement-based creative practice.

Challenges in Operationalizing Holism in Contemporary Practice

One of the central challenges facing any volume committed to holistic practice is the gap between conceptual aspiration and institutional reality. Bryk et al.'s scoping review of holism in palliative care practice found that, despite holism being widely invoked as an overarching theoretical framework, "the literature revealed a focus on curative and biomedical approaches to disease management with holistic aspects acknowledged, but not in the forefront of core service delivery" (Bryk et al., 2022). Holism, in other words, tends to function as an adjunct rather than a foundation—acknowledged in principle, marginalized in practice. This finding resonates with Dooris et al.'s analysis of well-being programs in public health, which demonstrated that programs may "superficially appear to be holistic by addressing multiple health-related issues, but in reality operate in a disconnected and essentially reductionist way" (Dooris et al., 2017). The tension between holistic aspiration and reductionist institutional design is not merely a technical problem; it reflects deeper epistemological commitments embedded in biomedical systems that privilege measurable, discrete outcomes over the relational, processual, and meaning-laden dimensions of healing (Baars & Hamre, 2017).

Baars and Hamre's critical narrative review of whole medical systems (WMS) versus conventional biomedicine identifies the structural sources of this tension with particular clarity (Baars & Hamre, 2017). They argue that the integration of WMS and conventional medicine requires not only legal frameworks and quality standards but also resolution of "unresolved ontological, epistemological, and methodological issues" (Baars & Hamre, 2017). Specifically, WMS conceptualizes the human being as a "wholeness and complexity" characterized by "emergent, nonlinear dynamic, and epigenetic properties" and "the ability of self-organization and adaptation as a network system", while conventional biomedicine tends toward atomistic, reductionist models of disease causation (Baars & Hamre, 2017). The present volume does not adjudicate this debate but rather demonstrates, through its practice-led contributions, that the two orientations can be held in productive dialogue—that rigorous, repeatable exercises can be designed that honor complexity without abandoning accountability.

The tension between reductionism and holism is not unique to medicine. As Hickford et al. note in the context of agricultural science, "singular reductionism can result in key relationships and linkages being missed, whereas holism can ignore the need to identify how confounding factors can affect the outcomes derived from complex systems" (2025). Their argument that science "comprises a more fluid and complex mission" (Hickford et al., 2025) rather than a simple dichotomy between reductionism and holism applies with equal force to the health and humanities practices assembled in this volume: the contributions that follow do not choose between rigor and wholeness but seek methodological approaches adequate to both. This dual commitment—to empirical accountability and to the irreducible complexity of lived experience—is what distinguishes the present volume's practice-led approach from both purely biomedical and purely humanistic accounts of well-being.

Mind-Body Practices: A Rapidly Expanding Field

The scholarly and clinical landscape of mind-body practices has expanded dramatically in recent decades, generating a substantial evidence base that this volume both draws upon and extends. Zhang et al.'s bibliometric analysis of "global research trends in mind-body therapies", covering 29.710 articles published between 1999 and 2024, documents the field's extraordinary growth and identifies its current hotspots: the promotion and application of mind-body therapies across diverse disease conditions, with particular attention to inflammatory interventions and higher-level research assessment methods (Zhang et al., 2025). The most widely studied practices include meditation, yoga, tai chi, qigong, and various relaxation techniques, with common research keywords clustering around quality of life, depression, and pain (Zhang et al., 2025)—precisely the domains of suffering that this volume's practice ecologies seek to address.

Mind-body interventions (MBIs) are broadly defined as practices designed to work on both physical and mental levels "in such a way as to enhance the mind's positive impact on the body" (Cozzolino et al., 2021). They encompass ancient practices for self-care and well-being such as meditation, yoga, and tai chi, as well as more contemporary practices including hypnosis, autogenic training, mindfulness, biofeedback, guided imagery, arts therapy, and relaxation training (Cozzolino et al., 2021). Park's review of mind-body complementary and alternative medicine (CAM) interventions in clinical health psychology notes that these modalities are the most commonly used CAM approaches in the United States, with deep breathing, meditation, and yoga leading in prevalence, and that their preventive use—oriented toward promoting a general state of health and well-being rather than treating specific diseases—is increasing (Park, 2012). This preventive, health-promoting orientation is central to the present volume's stance: rather than positioning humanities, arts-based and embodied practices as supplements to biomedical treatment, the contributions assembled here propose them as primary media through which perception stabilizes, affect regulates, and meaning returns.

The evidence base for mind-body practices spans an impressive range of clinical populations and conditions. Systematic reviews and meta-analyses have documented beneficial effects of yoga, mindfulness, tai chi, and qigong for menopausal symptoms (Innes et al., 2010), anxiety disorders (Sarris et al., 2012), chronic pain in older adults (Morone & Greco, 2007), fibromyalgia (Steen et al., 2024), fear of cancer recurrence (Hall et al., 2018), cancer-related distress (Chaoul et al., 2014), traumatic brain injury (Hernández et al., 2016), and people living with HIV (Ramirez-Garcìa et al., 2019). School-based MBIs have shown promise for reducing stress and promoting overall well-being in children and adolescents (Cozzolino et al., 2021), while mind-body approaches have been proposed as low-cost adjunctive therapies for cardiovascular disorders (Prasad, 2016), and as components of palliative care for children (Giacomelli et al., 2024). Kanherkar et al.'s review of the epigenetic mechanisms of integrative medicine provides a molecular-level account of how holistic practices affect gene expression and epigenetic state, offering a biological grounding for the observed health benefits of these practices (Kanherkar et al., 2017). Taken together, this evidence base confirms that mind-body practices are not merely cultural or aesthetic phenomena but interventions that operate at the interface of somatic regulation and meaning-making, engaging the body's self-organizing capacities in ways that purely cognitive or pharmacological approaches cannot.

Notwithstanding this growing evidence base, important methodological challenges remain. Many studies in the field suffer from small sample sizes, lack of control groups, high risk of bias, and insufficient attention to long-term outcomes and underlying mechanisms (Ramirez-Garcìa et al., 2019; Innes et al., 2010; Giacomelli et al., 2024). Ramirez-García et al.'s scoping review of mind-body practices for people living with HIV found that "almost half of the studies in this review were at high risk of bias" and called for "more rigorous studies" to confirm promising results (Ramirez-Garcìa et al., 2019). Nelson et al.'s systematic review of pre-surgical mind-body therapies similarly concluded that "the quality of evidence for the efficacy of mind-body therapies for improving post-surgical outcomes is limited" (Nelson et al., 2013). These methodological limitations underscore the importance of the present volume's commitment to specifying mechanisms, contexts, and ethical guardrails alongside practical protocols—ensuring that practice can travel responsibly across diverse settings.

Political and Historical Dimensions of Embodiment

A defining feature of this volume's theoretical orientation is its insistence that embodiment must be understood not only in neurophysiological but also in political and historical terms. The body is not merely a biological substrate for mental processes; it is the site where social structures, historical forces, and cultural meanings are inscribed, contested, and potentially transformed. This insight—central to the phenomenological and critical psychiatric traditions that inform the volume's theoretical foundations—has been elaborated with particular force in recent scholarship on Frantz Fanon's psychiatric writings.

Fanon's project of disalienation—understood by Shatz as "the careful dismantling of psychological obstacles to an unfettered experience of selfhood that opens onto a broader project for the mental well-being of oppressed communities" (Summers, 2025)—has been recognized as a foundational contribution to critical phenomenology and to the psychoaffective dimensions of social and political psychology (Abi-Ghannam et al., 2023). As Zahavi and Loidolt demonstrate in their survey of phenomenological psychiatry, Fanon is part of a long history of critical approaches in psychopathology and psychiatry that has "firm roots in the phenomenological tradition" and that "keeps up its critical work today" (Zahavi & Loidolt, 2021). His clinical innovations at Blida-Joinville, where he reorganized social therapy programs to fit the cultural morphology of his Algerian patients, after realizing that he had "misrecognized" them by expecting them to respond to European sociality in the therapeutic setting (Summers, 2025), anticipate our book's broader commitment to culturally responsive practice. Luxon argues that Fanon's innovations with the institutional form of the psychiatric hospital serve to "intervene differently in psychic conflict", offering "different ways to diagnose and respond to patients, along with different strategies for managing psychic disintegration in colonial contexts" (Luxon, 2021)—a rethinking of the relation between material and imagined worlds that resonates with our understanding of humanities, arts-based and embodied practices as transitional spaces where perception, affect, and social meanings are reorganized.

Burman's reading of Fanon similarly emphasizes that "resistance and transformation are simultaneously intrapersonal, interpersonal, and sociopolitical" (Burman, 2016), a claim that resonates with the book's insistence that body-mind practices are always already embedded in social, material, and political environments. Gregson's recent analysis further clarifies that for Fanon, freedom is best understood as "self-constitution", for which "certain forms of recognition serve a necessary albeit subordinate function" (Gregson, 2025)—a formulation that illustrates the reparative dimensions of the ekphrastic and dialogic practices theorized in the second part of our volume, where subjects move from paranoid to reparative positions and the access to a reenchanted world through affect-driven encounters with images, voices, and memories. The genealogy of critical psychiatry that Fanon's work inaugurates has been further elaborated in recent scholarship: Balibrea's work identifies a shared "genealogy of radical psychiatry" emerging at the end of the Second World War, premised on phenomenological approaches to "socially inflicted mental pathologies of exile and displacement" (Balibrea, 2025), while Auguste et al.'s recovery of Louis Mars' contributions to ethnopsychiatry demonstrates that the field's founding gesture—asserting that "non-Western culture should be intimately considered, rather than stigmatized, in treating people around the world" (Auguste et al., 2023)—was itself a decolonial intervention that has been largely erased from the disciplinary canon. These genealogies enrich our transcultural orientation by demonstrating how body-mind thought travels across clinical, aesthetic, and political domains, and how the insights of critical psychiatry remain urgently relevant to contemporary practice.

Neuroscientific and Somatic Dimensions of Body-Mind Regulation

This particular transcultural engagement with neuroscientific and somatic accounts of regulation reflects a broader scholarly movement toward bridging biomedical and humanistic frameworks. Baars and Hamre note that future research must address "the mechanisms of placebo, context, or meaning effects" as well as "process aspects, such as the emergence of new meanings and understanding during or after treatment" (Baars & Hamre, 2017)—precisely the kinds of effects that humanities, arts-based and embodied practices are well positioned to generate. The neuroscientific literature on mind-body practices has identified several key mechanisms through which these practices produce their effects: vagal-mediated parasympathetic activation, heart rate variability (HRV) increases, fronto-limbic modulation, and neuroplasticity-based changes in cortical structure and function

(Zhang et al., 2025; Kanherkar et al., 2017). Zhang et al. note that "contemporary MBT encompass three core modalities: (1) Cognitive Optimization Therapies (e.g., meditation, positive psychology), utilizing neuroplasticity-enhancing training to improve executive function through cognitive reframing and attentional control; (2) Dynamic Somatic Therapies (yoga, tai chi, qigong), achieving psychophysiological equilibrium via biomechanical alignment and synchronized breath-energy modulation; (3) Deep Relaxation Modalities (breathwork, hypnotherapy), attenuating stress" (Zhang et al., 2025).

The role of interoception—the brain's representation of the body's internal state—is increasingly recognized as central to the regulation of affect, attention, and autonomic function. The anterior cingulate and insular cortices function as hubs integrating interoception, affect, and autonomic control, and functional connectivity analyses show how emotional states couple with sympathetic responses (Zhang et al., 2025; Kanherkar et al., 2017). This neuroscientific understanding of body-mind regulation provides a biological grounding for the book's practice-led claims: the voice and breath practices, movement-based sessions, and attentional exercises assembled in its chapters are not merely cultural or aesthetic phenomena but interventions that engage the body's self-organizing capacities at the level of neural architecture. Hanna's account of somatic psychotherapy similarly emphasizes that somatic approaches work either "top down"—from mind to body—or "bottom up"—from body to psychological states—and that different lineages and cultural traditions have developed distinct approaches to this bidirectional relationship (Hanna, 2026). The volume's contributions span both orientations, from the cognitive and narrative approaches of bibliotherapy and oral history to the somatic and movement-based approaches of mantra meditation, Art-Yoga, and atelier-based art making.

The visual perspective literature provides a further neuroscientific grounding for our engagement with ekphrasis and autobiographical memory. Küçüktaş and Jacques's review of behavioral and neuroimaging findings demonstrates that "shifting from an own eyes to an observer-like perspective is an efficient way of regulating the affect elicited by emotional autobiographical memories" (Küçüktaş & Jacques, 2022), and that such shifts alter emotional experience by changing the retrieval orientation and the episodic details that are reconstructed. This finding provides a neuroscientific basis for understanding how encounters with images—mirrors, photographs, paintings, garments—can reorganize the affective charge of autobiographical memory, enabling the movement from paranoid to reparative positions that the volume's literary and narrative chapters trace in their respective textual and performative contexts.

Patterson's philosophical analysis of holistic health care, drawing on quantum theory, argues that holism involves "a willingness to use a wide range of interventions… an emphasis on a more participatory relationship between doctor and patient; and an awareness of the impact of the 'health' of the practitioner on the patient" (Patterson, 1998). This participatory, relational dimension of holistic practice is central to the present volume: some of the practices and protocols described in its chapters are not administered to passive recipients but co-created with and by participants, in ways that honor the practitioner's own embodied presence as a therapeutic resource. Freysteinson et al.'s identification of holistic nursing research priorities for 2023-2026 similarly emphasizes "person-centered, philosophical, theoretical, and practice knowledge that positively transforms human health", with particular attention to "the interrelationship of person-environment-health-healing" (Freysteinson et al., 2023)—a formulation that resonates with our attention to environmentally situated forms of ethical action and community care.

Cultural Responsiveness and Transcultural Dimensions of Well-Being

A defining feature of our book is its commitment to transcultural dialogue—its insistence that body-mind practices cannot be understood, evaluated, or transmitted without attention to the cultural contexts in which they are embedded. This commitment is theoretically grounded in a substantial body of scholarship on transcultural care and culturally responsive practice. Leininger's Theory of Culture Care Diversity and Universality, whose historical overview and contemporary applications are documented by McFarland and Wehbe-Alamah, provides one foundational framework: it holds that culturally congruent care—care that fits the cultural beliefs, norms, and practices of those receiving it—is essential to meaningful health outcomes (McFarland & Wehbe-Alamah, 2019). The theory's "Sunrise Enabler" model maps the multiple dimensions of cultural context that shape care, from kinship and social factors to religious and philosophical orientations, and its influence has extended well beyond nursing into interdisciplinary health practice (McFarland & Wehbe-Alamah, 2019).

The importance of cultural responsiveness is underscored by evidence from multiple contexts. In Aboriginal and Torres Strait Islander health in Australia, Luke et al. found that despite strong governmental rhetoric placing importance on "a holistic concept of health, capacity building, cultural competence and partnership", these principles were "not consistently embedded" in evaluation practice (Luke et al., 2020). The holistic concept of health operative in these communities—defined by the National Aboriginal Community Controlled Health Organization (NACCHO) as encompassing "not just the physical well-being of an individual but... the social, emotional and cultural well-being of the whole Community"—was frequently reduced in practice to "dominant social determinants, or individualized mental health measures" (Luke et al., 2020). Similarly, Carey's analysis of Indigenous well-being definitions reveals that "the indices of well-being that are important to the Government may not always be important to Indigenous Australians", pointing to a fundamental political tension between externally imposed frameworks and community-defined conceptions of flourishing (Carey, 2013).

These findings have direct implications for our present approach. The conference from which this book emerged explicitly foregrounded Asian and Indo-Oceanian perspectives in dialogue with European's, recognizing that transcultural circulation of body-mind practices requires not only translation but genuine epistemological humility. Ohajunwa et al.'s ethnographic study of healthcare practices in a South African Indigenous community illustrates what is at stake: in the Bomvana community, "well-being within the African Indigenous cosmos is about connection and balanced relationships between people, nature, and the divine", a conception that cannot be reduced to biomedical or even standard psychosocial frameworks (Ohajunwa et al., 2022). Their idea of "transformational engagement"—a "transcultural movement between the past and the present, between Western and African Indigenous practices"—offers a model for the kind of dialogue this volume seeks to facilitate (Ohajunwa et al., 2022). Likewise, McKelvie-Sebileau et al.'s work in Aotearoa New Zealand demonstrates that Systems Thinking approaches, when combined with Mātauranga Māori (Indigenous knowledge), can create synergies that are "an effective way to approach public health issues that emerge from complex adaptive systems" (McKelvie-Sebileau et al., 2022), suggesting that holistic frameworks from different traditions can be brought into productive conversation without either being subordinated to the other.

The transcultural dimension of holistic practice also encompasses the integration of spiritual and ritual dimensions of healing that biomedical frameworks have historically marginalized. Parks's analysis of African American folk beliefs demonstrates that spirituality, ritual, the power of words, and dreams function as culturally specific healing resources that can be productively incorporated into therapeutic practice (Parks, 2003). He's examination of TCM from a holistic medicine perspective similarly argues that "the future architecture of modern holistic medicine should incorporate the thinking modes, clinical experience, treatment methods of traditional Chinese medicine" (He, 2019), while O'Brien and Charura's study of transculturally informed therapeutic practice with refugees emphasizes the need to incorporate "spiritual or religious support from faith leaders" and "community-based organizations" as part of a "holistic constellation of care" (O'Brien & Charura, 2024). Beneduce's critique of global mental health discourse further cautions against "reproducing and globalizing Western hegemonic values concerning health, illness, and healing" (Beneduce, 2019), urging attention to the "political meaning of suffering and symptoms" and to the epistemological resources embedded in local healing knowledge—a caution that our transcultural orientation takes seriously throughout.

The volume's attention to non-Western social and cultural contexts—in its chapters on art therapy and social anxiety in contemporary Japan, and on the Well-Being with Arts project's implementation in Fukuoka (Japan), then in Istanbul (Turkey); but also, in its chapters on mindful practices in India—reflects a broader scholarly recognition that body-mind practices must be adapted to local cultural codes and sociopolitical constraints. This recognition is supported by the broader literature on culturally responsive practice: Mukherjee's argument that "a humanistic and imaginative engagement with the psychic lives of the dispossessed is key to an adapted psychoanalysis for the poor" (Mukherjee, 2021) resonates with our insistence that well-being practices must be designed with and for specific communities, rather than imported wholesale from other cultural contexts.

Narrative, Literature, and Embodied Method

The volume's second part proceeds from the conviction that narrative is not only what we tell but what we do: a set of embodied operations—moving, seeing, handling, voicing—through which sense and self are re-composed. This conviction is grounded in a substantial body of scholarship on the therapeutic dimensions of narrative, memory, and embodied attention. The role of visual art and narrative perspectives in autobiographical memory retrieval is particularly relevant here: Küçüktaş and Jacques's review demonstrates that shifting visual perspective during memory retrieval "is an efficient way of regulating the affect elicited by emotional autobiographical memories" (Küçüktaş & Jacques, 2022), and that such shifts alter emotional experience by changing the retrieval orientation and the episodic details that are reconstructed. This finding provides a neuroscientific grounding for the reparative function of ekphrastic and dialogic practices: the act of looking at an image, creating one, or narrating a memory from an autoethnographical standpoint can reorganize the affective charge of autobiographical experience, enabling movements from vigilance to reparative poise that literary and narrative forms are uniquely positioned to facilitate.

For this reason, the emergence of a new standpoint may at times require a geographical shift, where movement through space supports movement in thought. Accordingly, the therapeutic dimensions of walking as embodied practice have been acknowledged across multiple scholarly traditions. Somatic psychotherapy, as Hanna notes, encompasses approaches that begin with the body and its effects on psychological states (Hanna, 2026), and ambulatory practices have been integrated into community-level practice in ways that honor both ecological and social dimensions of well-being (Boetto, 2024). Our book's engagement with walking as artistic and spiritual performance, and with place-based practices of ecological and ethical repair, extends this somatic tradition into the domains of literary and cultural analysis, demonstrating that the body's movement through space is always already a reorganization of attention, identity, and relation.

This emphasis on embodied reconfiguration also underpins the dialogic dimensions of well-being, where structured conversation becomes another medium for meaning-making, self-knowledge, and catharsis—an insight supported by a substantial evidence base. For instance, Parks's analysis of African American folk beliefs demonstrates that the power of words functions as a culturally specific healing resource (Parks, 2003), while O'Brien and Charura's study of transculturally informed therapeutic practice emphasizes the importance of "universally understood emotions, cultural strengths, preferences for therapy" in any dialogic encounter with embodied trauma (O'Brien & Charura, 2024). The volume's relation to oral history as a performed event that fosters meaning-making and re-enchantment extends these insights into the domain of collective memory and transgenerational transmission, proposing that the interview—constructed through trust, non-judgmental listening, and open-ended co-narration—can function as a portable protocol for dialogic well-being.

Cultural Forms as Technologies of Attention

The third part of our book gathers contributions that argue, from diverse disciplinary vantage points, that cultural forms can be built as technologies of attention—manual, musical, narrative, mindful—each offering a way to practice well-being rather than merely describe it. This argument resonates with the broader literature on mind-body practices as methods of presence and self-cultivation. Cozzolino et al.'s review of school-based MBIs notes that such interventions are effective: meditation, yoga, and tai chi, but also "hypnosis, autogenic training, mindfulness, biofeedback, guided imagery, arts therapy, relaxation training, and psychological therapies" (Cozzolino et al., 2021)—a list that encompasses many of the practices theorized in the cultural perspectives section of our book. The inclusion of arts therapy in this taxonomy is significant: it signals a growing recognition that creative and aesthetic practices are not merely adjuncts to mind-body care but are themselves methods of body-mind regulation, capable of producing measurable changes in affect, attention, and autonomic function.

This continuity between creative practices and affect-focused techniques provides the backdrop for our engagement with mindful and gratitude practices, whose qualitative and quantitative evidences for their effects on adversarial growth and resilience are particularly relevant to the volume's third part. Prasad's review of mind-body therapies for cardiovascular disorders notes that "practicing 'heartfelt' emotions including gratitude and compassion" may be "novel low-cost approaches to reduce morbidity and mortality" (Prasad, 2016), while the broader literature on positive psychology has documented robust associations between mindfulness, gratitude and multiple dimensions of well-being, including improved personal relationships, greater appreciation for life, and enhanced personal inner strength. The volume's studies of mindful practices supply rigorous empirical support for these claims while remaining embedded in a broader holistic framework that honors the complexity of lived experience.

Such evidence-based demonstrations of relational, affective care find an institutional counterpart in Rosa et al.'s synthesis of nursing theory and the United Nations Sustainable Development Goals, which shows that holistic, caring frameworks can be operationalized across diverse institutional and cultural contexts, from educational settings to clinical practice to policy advocacy (Rosa et al., 2020). Their argument that "we can always promote greater wholeness and soundness in any given setting through our authentic presence, deep listening, holistic skill set, and clear intentionality" (Rosa et al., 2020) articulates the practical ethos that animates our book. At the same time, Boetto's EcoSocial Work model demonstrates that "nature-based therapeutic interventions, such as 'walk and talk' counselling, animal-assisted therapy, and nature mindfulness" can be efficiently integrated (Boetto, 2024), while Rihtman et al.'s occupational therapy research raises important questions about the institutional conditions that enable or constrain holistic practice, finding that practitioners often know "what needs to happen to improve social-emotional outcomes" but are prevented from acting on this knowledge by service structures "not geared to supporting social-emotional needs" (Rihtman et al., 2022). This finding underscores the importance of our commitment to portable, adaptable practices that can be implemented across diverse settings without requiring institutional transformation as a precondition for their use.

Furthermore, all aesthetic experiences—especially those grounded on performative elements—can potentially trigger a body–mind reconnection, and not just those specifically designed for therapeutic use. As Fischer-Lichte (2008) claims, the traditional aesthetics of representation can be fully integrated with an aesthetic of performance, since an "absolute opposition between 'presence' and 'representation' is not sustainable." Her aesthetics of performance is based on a "radical concept of presence" that collapses the body–mind dichotomy: "In the aesthetic state alone body and mind, the sensual nature of man and his reason, the material and the formal instinct reconcile and are at peace" (Fischer-Lichte, 2008). Such a conception foregrounds the transformative power of performative aesthetic experience, which enables the experiencer to access a reenchanted and yet everyday world.

Well-Being in the Post-Pandemic Context

The present moment's particular urgency—marked by long recoveries from pandemic-era isolation, rising social anxiety, and renewed attention to trauma and eco-anxiety—provides the immediate social context for this publication. Maxwell and Radford's analysis of Long Covid and nursing theory highlights the need for "holistic models" that move beyond diagnosis toward comprehensive, person-centered care (Maxwell & Radford, 2021). They invoke Leininger's argument that "transcultural nursing is directed toward holistic, congruent (appropriate), and beneficial health care" as a framework for addressing the complex, multidimensional needs of Long Covid patients (Maxwell & Radford, 2021), whose conditions resist purely biomedical management. The pandemic has, in this sense, made visible the limitations of reductionist approaches and created new demand for the kind of integrative, culturally responsive, somatically literate interventions this volume proposes.

Similarly, Freysteinson et al. note that holistic nursing principles—including "cultural sensitivity, promotion of well-being/well-becoming"—could be incorporated into disaster planning and pandemic response to "help mitigate the vulnerability of climate change-related disasters" (Freysteinson et al., 2023). Their idea of "well-becoming"—health understood not as a static state but as an ongoing, dynamic process of becoming—captures something essential about the orientation of this volume: the contributions assembled here do not promise the elimination of difficulty but rather the cultivation of capacities for ongoing self-organization, meaning-making, and community care (Freysteinson et al., 2023). This orientation echoes Baars and Hamre's characterization of whole medical systems as premised on "the ability of self-organization and adaptation as a network system" (Baars & Hamre, 2017), and with the broader literature on mind-body practices as methods of building resilience and adversarial growth in the face of chronic illness, trauma, and social adversity (Ramirez-Garcìa et al., 2019; Prasad, 2016; Hall et al., 2018).

It is precisely this evidence of adaptability and resilience-building that fuels the rising demand for low-barrier, scalable interventions across multiple clinical and community contexts. Park notes that mind-body CAM modalities are increasingly used not to treat current problems or diseases, but "to prevent disease or promote a general state of health and well-being" (Park, 2012), while Shen's analysis of yoga and meditation in prison settings demonstrates that mind-body practices can be implemented in even the most constrained institutional environments, with "overall positive outcomes" for the mental health of incarcerated individuals and prison personnel (Shen, 2024). These findings underscore our claim that holistic practices are not slogans but methods by which difficulty can be lived with differently and relation can be renewed—and that their implementation requires attention to cultural and environmental fit rather than one-size-fits-all protocols.

The Stakes of Practice-Led Scholarship in the Health Humanities

The scholarly landscape surveyed above converges on a set of shared convictions that this volume both inherits and advances: that human well-being is irreducibly holistic; that effective interventions must be culturally responsive, somatically informed, and relationally embedded; that the gap between holistic aspiration and reductionist institutional practice must be actively bridged through rigorous, portable methodologies; and that transcultural dialogue between traditions is not a luxury but a necessity for any practice ecology adequate to the present moment. The evidence base for mind-body practices has grown substantially in recent decades (Zhang et al., 2025), yet methodological challenges remain (Ramirez-Garcìa et al., 2019; Nelson et al., 2013), and the integration of situated embodied experiences, arts-based, literary, and narrative practices into this evidence base is still in its early stages. The present volume contributes to this integration by proposing a family of practice ecologies—autonomic-informed voice and breath; creative and movement-based sessions and ateliers; environmentally situated forms of ethical action; attentional grammars in listening, reading, and making—each analyzed in specific cultural and environmental contexts, or proposing practices that readers can adapt to their own settings.

SYNOPSIS OF CHAPTERS AND THEIR CONTRIBUTIONS

Part I – Theoretical Foundations of Body-Mind Interactions

Part I lays the conceptual ground for the volume. It situates embodiment in historical and political time—showing how bodies become sites where alienation is produced and freedom reclaimed—and then turns to contemporary sciences of interoception, affect, and autonomic regulation to clarify how mind and body co-modulate in practice. Read together, its two chapters argue that any credible account of well-being must be both structural and somatic: attentive to institutions, histories, and culture, and equally precise about mechanisms that make change felt and measurable.

In "Fanon and Tosquelles: Disalienation, Psychiatry, and Colonial Histories", Jean Khalfa places embodiment within political and historical time. Tracking how Frantz Fanon's psychiatric writings—shaped by his dialogue with Francesc Tosquelles—forge a link between alienation, freedom, and the body, the chapter moves between phenomenology (body schema, mirror stage), psychopathology (pathologies of identification), and decolonial struggle. It shows how Fanon's analyses of the colonial situation prefigure social therapy as a process of disalienation, and revisits his clinical innovations at Blida-Joinville alongside his attention to cultural frames in therapy—anticipating later ethnopsychiatry and institutional critique. In doing so, it anchors the volume's transcultural orientation and demonstrates how body–mind thought travels across clinical, aesthetic, and political domains.

"Neural Basis of Body–Mind Interaction and Body–Mind Practice", by Kazufumi Yoshihara, then asks how such situated processes register in the organism. Using bronchial asthma as a paradigmatic psychosomatic condition, the chapter integrates epidemiology, stress physiology, and brain imaging to show how early-life adversity, anxiety/depression, and traits such as alexithymia modulate inflammation, airway hyperresponsiveness, and symptom trajectories. Central to the account are the anterior cingulate and insular cortices as hubs of interoception, affect, and autonomic control; functional connectivity analyses illuminate couplings between emotional states (e.g., fear) and sympathetic responses. The chapter closes by outlining psychological (active listening, CBT, mindfulness) and somatic (yoga, qigong) approaches, proposing neuroplasticity-based hypotheses for improvements in psychosomatic care.

Taken together, these chapters establish a double commitment: to the conditions that generate alienation or care, and to the mechanisms by which practice makes change both felt and measurable. If Part I maps the ground, Part II—"More than Words": Healing, Literature, and Narratives—walks it, showing how writing, memory, performance, and dialogue operate as methods that transform attention and stance from within lived experience. Here, literature and narrative are not decorative surfaces but staged events—on the page, on the path, at the table—where meaning is co-produced by bodies, images, and voices in relation.

Part II – "More than Words": Healing, Literature and Narratives

This part treats narrative as embodied method: not only what is told, but what bodies *do*—moving, seeing, handling, voicing—to reorganize attention, identity, and relation. Four trajectories structure the arc: walking as artistic-spiritual performance; dwelling and repair after catastrophe; looking as a reparative encounter; and dialogue as a performed event of meaning-making.

We begin in motion with Oriane Chevalier, who reads Alexandra David-Néel's travelogues and correspondence to show how walking functions as artistic and spiritual practice, where techniques such as *tummo* and *lung-gom* serve both as survival strategies and modalities of self-transformation. Chevalier traces how mobility and metamorphosis—along with a poetics of performance (disguise, "passing")—generate a holistic sense of well-being that unsettles hard borders between hallucination, mystical vision, and embodied attention. By revisiting gendered Orientalism, Chevalier highlights anti-colonial and feminist inflections that complicate Western imaginaries while disseminating Buddhist and Tibetan practices; in this light, walking becomes a re-enchantment of the world, where art, spirituality, and corporeality converge in an ecology of resilience.

From pilgrimage the focus turns to dwelling after rupture with Gianluca Cinelli, who reads Mario Rigoni Stern through embodied-mind theory and transcultural care. Cinelli reframes war trauma as a disruption across body, mind, and environment, and recovery as holistic re-attunement. Western cognitive/clinical traditions (PTSD, art therapy, mind-body interventions) converse here with Zen and Bushidō ethics (no-mind, *wabi/sabi*, present awareness) and Shintō conceptions of nature's sacred immanence. In Cinelli's account, ethical compensation, memorial work, and a *vita activa*—gardening, walking, even ritualized, ecologically framed hunting—operate as practices of homeostasis and moral repair; storytelling moves in parallel, translating experience into meaning while preserving complexity and responsibility.

Having seen how place-based practices sustain repair, attention shifts to images as sites of encounter with Alessandro Toma, who recasts ekphrasis beyond representation as an affect-driven meeting—*gaze object*—capable of moving subjects from paranoid to depressive/reparative positions (Kleinian psychoanalysis). Through Elena Ferrante's *Troubling Love*, Toma shows how mirrors, paintings, photographs, and garments stage incremental encounters with transgenerational trauma and hegemonic scripts; guided by Tomkins' affects (hope, fear, joy), the culminating "joy" moment sutures split self-states into a new awareness that supports mental well-being. Methodologically, Toma braids affect theory, psychoanalysis, ekphrasis studies, and Gramscian hegemony to demonstrate how imagery and voice co-produce reparative meaning for subaltern subjects.

From image-events to voice-events, Patrizia Piredda draws on the MemoGen oral-history project (Italy, launched 2024) to stage dialogue as a maieutic encounter capable of inducing subjective well-being as participants recount the Second World War through transgenerational memory. Piredda situates well-being within a philosophical lineage (eudaimonia; Delphic maxims) and develops an aesthetics of performance for the interview, informed by Portelli's oral-history praxis and Fischer-Lichte's notion of re-enchantment. Built on trust, non-judgmental listening, and open-ended co-narration, the interview becomes an event that fosters meaning-making, self-knowledge, and often catharsis; close readings of field testimonies, together with Dewey's aesthetics of experience, clarify a reproducible arc for dialogic well-being: amazement → storytelling/critique → closure.

Altogether, these movements present narrative as a toolkit of practices: the step that steadies attention, the dwelling that roots memory in place, the image that invites a reparative gaze, the conversation that performs meaning in common. With this toolkit in hand, the volume turns next to cultural laboratories—arts and practices that design the very conditions of attention and relation they teach.

Part III – Cultural Perspectives on Body-Mind Interactions

This part turns to the cultural laboratories where practices are designed, repeated, and refined. Here, artists and researcher-practitioners do not merely *represent* body-mind interaction; they *engineer* conditions of attention and relation—the cut that reorganizes a gaze, the near-silent sonority that trains listening, the walked trace that reopens family speech, the measured exercise through which gratitude thickens into resilience. Read together, these contributions show how cultural forms become methods, making well-being learnable, repeatable, and shareable across differing milieus.

We begin with Charlène Clonts, who reconceives Ghérasim Luca's cutting–assembling praxis—*cubomanies*, Objectively Offered Objects (O.O.O.), handmade albums, collaborative "patchworks"—as a haptic poetics that transmutes fragmentation into mobile relationality. Through close readings, Clonts shows how serial gestures (cut, paste, collage) unsettle fixed identities and canonical iconographies (including colonial photographs), opening transitional spaces where perception, affect, and social meanings are reorganized. The essay advances an ethics of recycling and reconfiguration—material, semiotic, interpersonal—yielding a non-institutional model of self-care: not by smoothing anxiety but by inhabiting it creatively, so that viewers and readers co-produce rhythmic, tactile forms of attention and agency. In this sense, Luca's work offers a transformative aesthetics of well-being grounded in craft, repetition/variation, and interactive offering.

Where the manic hand teaches the eye to feel again, Stefano Lombardi Vallauri turns to the ear. Proposing music as a physical-psycho-spiritual praxis, he traces how Scelsi, Nono, Guaccero, Sciarrino, and Buccino train perception and presence: from Scelsi's magnified micro-events and Nono's late, listening-led extemporaneity, to Guaccero's *azione sacra* that shifts spectators from representation to exercise; from Sciarrino's liminal sound/noise ecologies to Buccino's *HN (hic et nunc)* action-notation and performer embodiment. The result is music not as sign or style but as method—a school of attentiveness where performance becomes vehicle and ethos is reorganized through iterative, here-and-now engagement.

From scores in sound to a path on the ground, Julie-Marie Duro-Sasaki explores how walking another's traces and composing fictional postcards can lower the heat around silence so that truth can be approached without harm. Grounded in somaesthetics (Shusterman) and Deweyan inquiry, her autoethnographic project—*Looking for my Japanese Family* (2014–2019)—is treated as research-in-the-arts. She theorizes footstepping (walking in another's traces) and novelistic fiction (the curated detour of the *I am a cloud* postcards) as embodied, affective methods that open a speakable space around inherited opacity, catalyze relational repair, and produce epistemic intimacy without forcing premature disclosure. Here, fiction is not retreat but mediation—a device that turns opacity into shared intelligibility and enables new dialogue within the kin network.

The sequence concludes with the contribution of Poonam Khurana, Deepika Chhikara, and Renuka Kapoor, who provide a quantitative perspective. Their study—"Silver Lining": Gratitude and Adversarial Growth in Chronic Illness—asks whether a simple, everyday gratitude practice can support broad-based growth after illness. Working with a cohort of adults in India who had experienced chronic illness in the preceding year ($N = 368$), the authors show that gratitude, measured using the GQ-6 scale, significantly predicts all five dimensions of adversarial growth: improved personal relationships, greater appreciation for life, shifts in life philosophy, positive influence on others, and strengthened inner resilience. The statistical associations ($\beta = .41–.68$, with moderate explanatory power across domains) suggest that even low-intensity practices—such as gratitude lists or expressive exercises—may offer accessible, scalable forms of support. The study also notes its methodological strengths (including structural validity checks) and limitations (self-report measures, sampling frame), ultimately providing an empirical anchor for the volume's practice-led claims about affect regulation and resilience.

Viewed together, these perspectives show how manual, musical, narrative, and mindful forms can be built as technologies of attention, offering ways to practice well-being rather than merely describe it. With this ensemble of practices in place, the volume turns in the final part from cultural laboratories to applications, translating insight into accessible protocols for clinics, classrooms, studios, and community spaces.

Part IV – Art as a Medium for Healing. Practical Applications and Future Directions

The final part of the volume turns from cultural laboratories to applied practice, gathering contributions that translate the book's core wager—*practice changes well-being*—into methods that can be taught, adapted, and responsibly implemented. Here, voice and breath, gesture and material, reading and language, movement and imagery become modalities through which care is enacted. Application does not imply simplification: each contribution specifies its mechanisms, contexts, and ethical guardrails so that practices may travel with integrity across settings.

We begin with Aira Dutta and Kirti Tyagi, who synthesize theoretical and emerging empirical work on mantra-based meditation for trauma recovery. Their contribution details how vagal-mediated parasympathetic activation, increases in heart-rate variability, and fronto-limbic modulation can reduce hyperarousal, support emotional regulation, and foster meaning-making—framed through polyvagal theory's understanding of safety and engagement. Clinically, mantra-based meditation is presented as low-cost, portable, and culturally grounded, and as particularly useful when early-stage verbal processing risks retraumatization. Dutta and Tyagi close with ethical considerations—cultural context, spiritual bypass—and outline a research agenda for rigorous, trauma-informed trials.

From cadence and sound, the focus shifts to gesture and material in shared spaces that welcome those who hesitate to speak. In her qualitative study of the Tokyo Soteria Art Circle and Kokorokaradaart (Kyoto), Sofia Rossatelli shows how embodied art-making—ink that stains, collage that resists, chalk that flows—can anchor regulation and identity work for people navigating social anxiety, *taijin kyōfushō*, stigma, and withdrawal. Testimonies and artworks reveal processes of body-mind regulation, identity re-authoring (signatures, authorship), and gradual reintegration into social life, from returning to work to exhibiting publicly. Rossatelli situates these practices within Japanese sociocultural dynamics (*tatemae/honne*, *amae*, *kachigumi/makegumi*) and current policy shifts, positioning atelier-based art therapy as a non-pharmacological, relational, culturally consonant avenue toward well-being.

The sequence then turns to a quieter medium: reading. Anna Bourges-Celaries asks whether curated, heterolingual texts can extend bibliotherapy by giving readers new words—and therefore new handles—for previously unnamed feelings, especially in alexithymic (emotional blindness) contexts. Drawing on affective neuroscience (distributed representations for emotion words; adjacency of lexical and affective systems), she argues that heterolingual, exophonic literature—exemplified by Sekiguchi Ryōko's *Nagori*—provides lexical attractors (e.g., *hashiri*, *sakari*, *nagori*) that help readers categorize and articulate subtle affective states. Bourges-Celaries outlines practical parameters for such interventions (text curation, linguistic fit, interdisciplinary facilitation, group formats) and cautions against over-matching narratives to readers' experiences. Her contribution expands the volume's repertoire of arts-and-language-based modalities for body-mind care.

From words that catch feelings, we return to bodies that move together. Positioned at the intersection of arts practice and analysis, mental health, and education, Charlène Clonts presents the framework developed within the Well-Being with Arts (WBA) project—including Art-Yoga—piloted in Japan and Turkey. Integrating insights from psychology, neuroscience, and arts studies, she argues that creativity, movement, rhythm, music, and poetic imagery catalyze emotional regulation and relational attunement. She illustrates the efficiency of the framework by exposing the results of a case study in Istanbul. It combines quantitative mood measures (e.g., POMS) with qualitative interviews, demonstrating reductions in tension, anxiety, and fatigue while attending to local cultural codes and sociopolitical constraints. The chapter mobilizes enactive cognition and autopoiesis to theorize how aesthetic movement practices "self-organize" across perception, action, and meaning, and revisits classical yogic practices to situate contemporary mindful movement within longer genealogies.

Across these contributions, application means design: the tempo of a mantra, the materials of an atelier, the lexicon of a reading list, the arc of breath and step in an Art-Yoga session. Each approach is teachable and adaptable; together they reinforce the book's central claim that holistic practices are not abstractions but methods, offering readers principles and protocols for cultivating ecologies of well-being that honor physiology, story, and place.

CONTRIBUTIONS TO THE HEALTH HUMANITIES FIELD

To conclude our preface, this volume establishes the arts as practice ecologies—not static objects but repeatable processes through which perception, affect, and meaning are reorganized. The chapters show how well-designed practices, sometimes seemingly small—the cut, the step, the breath, the vowel, the near-silent sonority—can be taught and learned in ways that co-regulate physiology and sense. They also bind felt change to mechanism and milieu: autonomic and attentional accounts of voice and breath sit beside environmental and narrative repair; studio testimonies sit beside cultural analyses of stigma and self; sonic micro-events sit beside ethical claims about presence. What emerges is a set of transferable protocols—portable, evaluable, and adaptable across education, health, and community practice—guided by cultural responsiveness and clear ethical guardrails. Looking ahead, the work continues: integrating new domains (e.g., performance and body/technology), strengthening trial designs and mixed-methods evaluation, and extending partnerships seeded by the conference.

The claim is modest and demanding in equal measure: that listening, voicing, walking, cutting, collaging, drawing, reading, and dialoguing are not ancillary techniques but primary media through which bodies, minds, and communities reorganize their capacities for health, meaning, and care. If a mindful exercise steadies a morning; if a cut surface reopens a conversation long deferred; if a studio restores a path to companionship or work; if listening slows time until patience returns—then the wager of holistic practices has, in some measure, been won.

Charlène Clonts and Lorenzo Cardilli

REFERENCES

Abi-Ghannam, G., Perkins, K., & Fine, M. (2023). The comrade on the crossroads of scholarship and struggle: Troubling the exile of Frantz Fanon from social and political psychology. *Social and Personality Psychology Compass, 17*(2). Advance online publication. DOI: 10.1111/spc3.12727

Auguste, E., Beauliere, G., Jenson, D., LeBrun, J., & Blanc, J. (2023). La lutte continue: Louis Mars and the genesis of ethnopsychiatry. *The American Psychologist, 78*(4), 469–483. DOI: 10.1037/amp0001097 PMID: 37384501

Baars, E., & Hamre, H. J. (2017). Whole Medical Systems versus the System of Conventional Biomedicine: A Critical, Narrative Review of Similarities, Differences, and Factors That Promote the Integration Process. *Evidence-Based Complementary and Alternative Medicine : eCAM, 2017*(1), 469–483. DOI: 10.1155/2017/4904930 PMID: 28785290

Balibrea, M. (2025). 'Pourquoi pas Solanes?' Retracing genealogies of critical psychiatry through the emergence of mass exile and displacement as mental pathologies. *History of Psychiatry, 36*(1-3), 71–86. DOI: 10.1177/0957154x251316112 PMID: 40119677

Beneduce, R. (2019). "Madness and Despair are a Force": Global Mental Health, and How People and Cultures Challenge the Hegemony of Western Psychiatry. *Culture, Medicine and Psychiatry, 43*(4), 710–723. DOI: 10.1007/s11013-019-09658-1 PMID: 31729692

Boetto, H. (2024). Promoting sustainable development in the Australian Murray-Darling basin: Envisioning an EcoSocial work approach. *Sustainable Development, 33*(1), 904–915. DOI: 10.1002/sd.3158

Bryk, A., Roberts, G., Hudson, P., Harms, L., & Gerdtz, M. (2022). The concept of holism applied in recent palliative care practice: A scoping review. *Palliative Medicine, 37*(1), 26–39. DOI: 10.1177/02692163221129999 PMID: 36333861

Burman, E. (2016). Fanon, Foucault, feminisms: Psychoeducation, theoretical psychology, and political change. *Theory & Psychology, 26*(6), 706–730. DOI: 10.1177/0959354316653484

Carey, T. (2013). Defining Australian Indigenous Wellbeing: Do weReallyWant the Answer? Implications for Policy and Practice. *Psychotherapy and Politics International, 11*(3), 182–194. DOI: 10.1002/ppi.1305

Chaoul, A., Milbury, K., Sood, A., Prinsloo, S., & Cohen, L. (2014). Mind-Body Practices in Cancer Care. *Current Oncology Reports*, *16*(12). Advance online publication. DOI: 10.1007/s11912-014-0417-x PMID: 25325936

Cozzolino, M., Vivo, D., & Celia, G. (2021). School-Based Mind–Body Interventions: A Research Review. *Human Arenas*, *5*(2), 262–278. DOI: 10.1007/s42087-020-00163-1

Dolan, P., & White, M. P. (2007). How can measures of subjective well-being be used to inform public policy? *Perspectives on Psychological Science*, *2*(1), 71–85. DOI: 10.1111/j.1745-6916.2007.00030.x PMID: 26151920

Dooris, M., Farrier, A., & Froggett, L. (2017). Wellbeing: The challenge of 'operationalising' an holistic concept within a reductionist public health programme. *Perspectives in Public Health*, *138*(2), 93–99. DOI: 10.1177/1757913917711204 PMID: 28574301

Fischer-Lichte, E. (2008). *The Transformative Power of Performance. A new aesthetics* (S. I. Jain, Trans.). Routledge. (Original work published 2004).

Freysteinson, W., Hines, M., Wardell, D., Friesen, M., Conrad, S., Zahourek, R., Gallo, A.-M., & Prather, J. (2023). Identifying Holistic Nursing Research Priorities for 2023–2026. *Journal of Holistic Nursing*, *42*(2), 182–201. DOI: 10.1177/08980101231213725 PMID: 37968961

Frisch, N., & Rabinowitsch, D. (2019). What's in a Definition? Holistic Nursing, Integrative Health Care, and Integrative Nursing: Report of an Integrated Literature Review. *Journal of Holistic Nursing*, *37*(3), 260–272. DOI: 10.1177/0898010119860685 PMID: 31257971

Giacomelli, L., Papa, S., Vecchi, L., Mercante, A., & Benini, F. (2024). Unravelling the role of mind–body therapies in paediatric palliative care: A narrative review. *Acta Paediatrica (Oslo, Norway)*, *113*(5), 881–891. DOI: 10.1111/apa.17097 PMID: 38197439

Gregson, W. (2025). The "Recognition Trap": Self-Constitution, Culture, and Mutual Recognition in Fanon's Project of Freedom. *Political Theory*, *53*(5), 599–626. DOI: 10.1177/00905917251321287

Hall, D., Luberto, C., Philpotts, L., Song, R., Park, E., & Yeh, G. (2018). Mind-body interventions for fear of cancer recurrence: A systematic review and meta-analysis. *Psycho-Oncology*, *27*(11), 2546–2558. DOI: 10.1002/pon.4757 PMID: 29744965

Hanna, E. (2026). Somatic psychotherapy. In L. Hoffman, L. X. Vallejos, D. Hocoy, P. Tummala-Narra, & E. M. DeRobertis (Eds.), APA handbook of humanistic and existential psychology: Clinical and social applications (pp. 315–334). American Psychological Association. DOI: 10.1037/0000432-016

He, K. (2019). Modern holistic medicine from the perspective of traditional chinese medicine. *International Journal of Complementary & Alternative Medicine*, *12*(3), 115–120. DOI: 10.15406/ijcam.2019.12.00459

Hernández, T., Brenner, L., Walter, K., Bormann, J., & Johansson, B. (2016). Complementary and alternative medicine (CAM) following traumatic brain injury (TBI): Opportunities and challenges. *Brain Research*, *1640*, 139–151. DOI: 10.1016/j.brainres.2016.01.025 PMID: 26806403

Hickford, J., Goldson, S., Caradus, J., & Rowarth, J. (2025). Reductionist science in agriculture and horticulture. *New Zealand Journal of Agricultural Research*, *68*(5), 829–838. DOI: 10.1080/00288233.2023.2294783

Innes, K., Selfe, T., & Vishnu, A. (2010). Mind-body therapies for menopausal symptoms: A systematic review. *Maturitas*, *66*(2), 135–149. DOI: 10.1016/j.maturitas.2010.01.016 PMID: 20167444

Kanherkar, R., Stair, S., Bhatia-Dey, N., Mills, P., Chopra, D., & Csòka, A. (2017). Epigenetic Mechanisms of Integrative Medicine. Evidence-Based Complementary and Alternative Medicine, 2017(1). DOI: 10.1155/2017/4365429

Küçüktaş, S., & Jacques, P. (2022). How shifting visual perspective during autobiographical memory retrieval influences emotion: A change in retrieval orientation. *Frontiers in Human Neuroscience*, *16*. Advance online publication. DOI: 10.3389/fnhum.2022.928583 PMID: 36226260

Labbé, E., Naylor, P., & Huennekens, A. (2019). Mindfulness, spirituality, and exercise performance. In Anshel, M. H., Petruzzello, S. J., & Labbé, E. E. (Eds.), *APA handbook of sport and exercise psychology: Exercise psychology* (pp. 409–428). American Psychological Association. DOI: 10.1037/0000124-021

Luke, J., Ferdinand, A., Paradies, Y., Chamravi, D., & Kelaher, M. (2020). Walking the talk: Evaluating the alignment between Australian governments' stated principles for working in Aboriginal and Torres Strait Islander health contexts and health evaluation practice. *BMC Public Health*, *20*(1). Advance online publication. DOI: 10.1186/s12889-020-09983-w PMID: 33272249

Luxon, N. (2021). Fanon's Psychiatric Hospital as a Waystation to Freedom. *Theory, Culture & Society*, *38*(5), 93–113. DOI: 10.1177/0263276420981612

Maxwell, E., & Radford, M. (2021). Long Covid and the ghost of nursing theory. *Journal of Research in Nursing : JRN, 26*(5), 362–366. DOI: 10.1177/17449871211037473 PMID: 35251264

McFarland, M., & Wehbe-Alamah, H. (2019). Leininger's Theory of Culture Care Diversity and Universality: An Overview With a Historical Retrospective and a View Toward the Future. *Journal of Transcultural Nursing, 30*(6), 540–557. DOI: 10.1177/1043659619867134 PMID: 31409201

McKelvie-Sebileau, P., Pekepo, C., Rees, D., Swinburn, B., Gerritsen, S., & Tipene-Leach, D. (2022). Applying the complementary knowledge bases of System Dynamics and Indigenous knowledge in public health research in Aotearoa, New Zealand. *Alternative an International Journal of Indigenous Peoples, 18*(4), 576–585. DOI: 10.1177/11771801221119266

Morone, N., & Greco, C. (2007). Mind–Body Interventions for Chronic Pain in Older Adults: A Structured Review. *Pain Medicine, 8*(4), 359–375. DOI: 10.1111/j.1526-4637.2007.00312.x PMID: 17610459

Mukherjee, A. (2021). Unseen City. *The Psychic Lives of the Urban Poor*. Cambridge University Press. DOI: 10.1017/9781009042680

Nelson, E., Dowsey, M., Knowles, S., Castle, D., Salzberg, M., Monshat, K., & Choong, P. (2013). Systematic review of the efficacy of pre-surgical mind-body based therapies on post-operative outcome measures. *Complementary Therapies in Medicine, 21*(6), 697–711. DOI: 10.1016/j.ctim.2013.08.020 PMID: 24280480

O'Brien, C., & Charura, D. (2024). Advancing transculturally informed, humanistic therapeutic practice for refugees and asylum seekers presenting with embodied trauma. *Counselling & Psychotherapy Research, 24*(4), 1612–1631. DOI: 10.1002/capr.12808

Office for National Statistics. (2011). *Measuring what matters: National Statistician's reflections on the National Debate on Measuring National Well-being*. Office for National Statistics.

Ohajunwa, C., Mji, G., & Chimbala-Kalenga, R. (2022). Encouraging reciprocal healthcare practice within a South African Indigenous community. *AlterNative: An International Journal of Indigenous Peoples, 18*(1), 141–146. DOI: 10.1177/11771801221085631

Organisation for Economic Co-operation and Development. (2013). *OECD guidelines on measuring subjective well-being*. OECD Publishing. DOI: 10.1787/9789264191655-

Park, C. (2012). Mind-Body CAM Interventions: Current Status and Considerations for Integration Into Clinical Health Psychology. *Journal of Clinical Psychology, 69*(1), 45–63. DOI: 10.1002/jclp.21910 PMID: 22936306

Parks, F. (2003). The Role of African American Folk Beliefs in the Modern Therapeutic Process. *Clinical Psychology: a Publication of the Division of Clinical Psychology of the American Psychological Association, 10*(4), 456–467. DOI: 10.1093/clipsy/bpg046

Patterson, E. (1998). The philosophy and physics of holistic health care: Spiritual healing as a workable interpretation. *Journal of Advanced Nursing, 27*(2), 287–293. DOI: 10.1046/j.1365-2648.1998.00533.x PMID: 9515638

Prasad, K. (2016). Viewpoint: Role of Mind–body Therapies in the Management of Cardiovascular Disorders. *European Cardiology Review, 11*(2), 111. DOI: 10.15420/ecr.2016:17:2 PMID: 30310456

Ramirez-Garcìa, P., Gagnon, M., Colson, S., Côté, J., Flores-Aranda, J., & Dupont, M. (2019). Mind-body practices for people living with HIV: A systematic scoping review. *BMC Complementary and Alternative Medicine, 19*(1). Advance online publication. DOI: 10.1186/s12906-019-2502-z PMID: 31185970

Rihtman, T., Gadsby, N., & Porter, J. (2022). Supporting the social-emotional needs of children and young people with developmental coordination disorder: Occupational therapists' perceptions of practice in England. *British Journal of Occupational Therapy, 85*(9), 653–661. DOI: 10.1177/03080226211054383 PMID: 40336656

Rosa, W., Dossey, B., Koithan, M., Kreitzer, M., Manjrekar, P., Meleis, A., & Watson, J. (2020). Nursing Theory in the Quest for the Sustainable Development Goals. *Nursing Science Quarterly, 33*(2), 178–182. DOI: 10.1177/0894318420903495 PMID: 32180518

Sarris, J., Moylan, S., Camfield, D., Pase, M., Mischoulon, D., Berk, M., & Schweitzer, I. (2012). Complementary Medicine, Exercise, Meditation, Diet, and Lifestyle Modification for Anxiety Disorders: A Review of Current Evidence. *Evidence-Based Complementary and Alternative Medicine : eCAM, 2012*, 1–20. DOI: 10.1155/2012/809653 PMID: 22969831

Sen, A., Stiglitz, J. E., & Fitoussi, J.-P. (2009). *Report by the Commission on the Measurement of Economic Performance and Social Progress*. Commission on the Measurement of Economic Performance and Social Progress.

Shen, A. (2024). Mental Health and Yoga in Prisons. *Journal of Criminal Law, 88*(4), 258–281. DOI: 10.1177/00220183241265170

Steen, J., Kannan, V., Zaidi, A., Cramer, H., & Ng, J. (2024). Mind-body therapy for treating fibromyalgia: A systematic review. *Pain Medicine*, *25*(12), 703–737. DOI: 10.1093/pm/pnae076 PMID: 39093008

Summers, S. (2025). Book Review: The Rebel's Clinic: The Revolutionary Lives of Frantz Fanon; Frantz Fanon: Combat Breathing; How We Walk: Frantz Fanon and the Politics of the Body. *Journal of Asian and African Studies*, *60*(8), 5442–5451. DOI: 10.1177/00219096251337931

Takahashi, T., Asano, S., Uchida, Y., Takemura, K., Fukushima, S., Matsushita, K., & Okuda, N. (2022). Effects of forests and forest-related activities on the subjective well-being of residents in a Japanese watershed: An econometric analysis through the capability approach. *Forest Policy and Economics*, *139*, 102723. DOI: 10.1016/j.forpol.2022.102723

World Health Organization. (2021). *Health promotion glossary of terms 2021*. World Health Organization.

Zahavi, D., & Loidolt, S. (2021). Critical phenomenology and psychiatry. *Continental Philosophy Review*, *55*(1), 55–75. DOI: 10.1007/s11007-021-09553-w

Zhang, Y., Li, W., Xu, S., Li, S., Sun, Z., Zhang, M., Zuo, Y., & Chen, S. (2025). Global research trends in mind body therapies: A bibliometric analysis. *Journal of Translational Medicine*, *23*(1). Advance online publication. DOI: 10.1186/s12967-025-06389-3 PMID: 40128872

Chapter 1
Fanon and Tosquelles

Jean Khalfa
http://orcid.org/0000-0002-5815-1085
Trinity College, University of Cambridge, UK

ABSTRACT

Fanon's time at Saint-Alban hospital, under the mentorship of Francesc Tosquelles, significantly influenced his thought. They saw psychiatry as aiming to dissolve pathological personality reconstructions caused by neurological shocks, using shock therapies, various psychotherapies, and socialtherapy within a hospital microcosm. Fanon applied this model to his analysis of the anticolonial liberation struggle, viewing it as a form of socialtherapy that dissolves pathological identities created by colonisation and prepares for a new decolonised world. Fanon's work at the Blida-Joinville hospital in Algeria continued Saint-Alban though his experiments there led him to a new form of ethnopsychiatry, emphasising the importance of cultural context in understanding mental illness. He later took some distance from Tosquelles, but his thought and practice would certainly not have developed in the same way without the experience he gained in Saint-Alban during the year and a half he spent there with him.

INTRODUCTION

When Frantz Fanon resigned his position at Blida's psychiatric hospital, he famously wrote to the Governor General of Algeria that he could no longer work as a psychiatrist in a country run on principles that generated madness:

> *Madness is one of the ways that humans have of losing their freedom. And I can say that, placed at this junction, I have measured with terror the extent of the alienation of this country's inhabitants. (Letter sent in December 1956, Fanon, 2020b, p. 296)*

DOI: 10.4018/979-8-3373-3521-6.ch001

This was no exaggeration for him. Fanon's descriptions of the colonial system and the difficulties of escaping its effects in the postcolonial period are deeply determined by his psychiatric thought and practice, which were revolutionary too. My purpose here is to explain the links between Fanon's conceptions of disalienation in psychiatry and history, and to do so by looking at the pivotal moment when, after he wrote his first book, in 1952 and before he engaged in his Algerian trajectory in 1954, he trained with Francesc Tosquelles. Tosquelles was a Catalan psychiatrist whose remarkable work has been recently republished and celebrated in major exhibitions in Toulouse, Barcelona, Madrid and New York (Guerra & Masó, 2021; Tosquelles, 2021).

Most people today know Fanon through *Black Skin, White Masks* (BSWM), *Peau noire, masques blancs*, published in 1952, and written while he was finishing his psychiatric studies in Lyon. Its very title shows that it is about a negative experience, a troubled form of identity consciousness. At first sight this is different from the other books Fanon published in his lifetime, such as his 1959 book titled *Year V of the Algerian Revolution* (*L'An V de la Révolution Algérienne*, oddly known in English as *A Dying Colonialism*). This book is a sociological study of the transformations of the Algerian society caused by the very unfolding of the independence struggle. Another major book by Fanon was *The Wretched of the Earth* (WE), *Les Damnés de la terre*, published at the end of 1961. At that time, the psychiatrist—ambassador at large for sub-Saharan Africa of the Provisional Government of the Algerian Republic, tasked with obtaining recognition and funding from newly independent countries—was dying of leukemia. These books appear essentially historical and political and their scope is increasingly wide, from Algeria in 1959, to the totality of Africa in 1961, or even the totality of the earth as the final title suggests.

In BSWM the discussion is based on a phenomenological narrative about the alienation of the black man in the French Caribbean island of Martinique, who thinks he is essentially white, and who *desires* whiteness. But it is also about the moment when, having experienced the racist gaze in the metropole he proclaims a reactive but symmetrical *identity* in the form of *négritude*, a term another great Martiniquais writer, Aimé Césaire, had invented in his famous poem of 1939, *Notebook of a return to the native land* (*Cahier d'un retour au pays natal*). As a reaction to a pathologically constructed identity this identity too is invented: the native land of Césaire's poem turns out to be the African soil where he had never set foot, a myth, rather than his own birthplace, a volcanic Caribbean island, the reality of which is described physically and mentally as corrupt, with its poverty, fragmentation and lack of any cultural and historical depth. Césaire invented the term "négritude" in the late 30s, but the theme of a return to Africa and the idea of an inherent value in *identité nègre* had already been explored at length in the various black journals published in the 20s and 30s in Paris (such as *Les Continents*, *La*

Dépêche Africaine, or, in the early 30s, *Le Cri des nègres*, and *La Revue du monde noir*, see Khalfa 2009). Both Césaire and his friend Leopold Sedar Senghor claimed to have simply named a notion developed by the American writers and thinkers of the Harlem Renaissance. So there was nothing spontaneous or natural in this *prise de conscience*, an "awakening" which was then continued after WWII in the journal *Présence Africaine*, to which Fanon subscribed, but rather a progressive construction linked to a number of historical circumstances. Fanon went so far as parodying the metaphysical style of Césaire's text on negritude in BSWM. I insist on this idea of a historicity of forms of consciousness in the young Fanon as it was developed in parallel in his dissertation for the PhD in psychiatry, which deals with a specific illness but is also an epistemology of psychiatric concepts. For Fanon the psychiatric syndromes invented in the 19th century have nothing natural either. His whole project there was to inject temporality, he says, in the modes of understanding madness.

Now, what I aim to show is that Fanon's phenomenological descriptions of contradictory processes of identification which involve wearing masks, white or black, are not confined to his first book. He conceptualizes the experience of identity as alienation, in the strong sense, that is, not just as an illusion, but as a real psychopathology, in all of his works. It is in fact difficult to understand the *Wretched of the Earth*, published ten years and a whole, turbulent life later, in 1961, without referring to it. After his death, and in the context of decolonization, his last book was translated and published everywhere and debated, often negatively by communist thinkers because class was not a salient concept in it and it dismissed the revolutionary potential of the working class in colonised countries. At that time BSWM, with its focus on alienation and psychopathology, was neglected, even though a whole chapter of the WE is dedicated to psychopathology and includes authentic psychiatric case notes. In the 90s the opposite happened, his early work was read again and the anticolonial work was somewhat forgotten, perhaps because he was read as an advocate of a decolonization process that had blatantly failed and because people were now much more interested in hybridity and identity politics than in national consciousness. Twenty years ago, it seemed to me that this division was arbitrary and the title *Alienation and Freedom* immediately came to my mind for the publication of all his unpublished or lost works covering his whole writing life, I was preparing with Robert JC Young, because I thought that Fanon's professional reflection on alienation and its contexts, as a psychiatrist and phenomenologist, was a dominant thread of all his work. It was essential to have that in mind in order to understand his conception of the decolonizing struggle, which Fanon presented as a form of socialtherapy. He warned about the difficulties of a postcolonial future in societies that would not have undergone such a therapy, which to me is the main point of his final book.

So there is an underlying continuity in Fanon's oeuvre, but it should not be seen simply as a mechanical transposition of psychiatry to history, and this is where the fifteen months Fanon spent in Saint Alban with Tosquelles, after finishing his PhD and before he went to Algeria, play a pivotal role. I will now consider the two main phases of his work, BSWM and WE, in detailed reference to his psychiatric work, keeping in mind what our edition of Fanon's lost or forgotten texts allowed us to see. His remarks in this domain are really what gives depth and originality to his political thought, rather than just being signs of a parallel professional interest.

Psychiatry in Fanon's Early Texts

Let me first clarify how important the relationship of the psychiatric to the historical and sociological was in Fanon's first book, that is before he met Tosquelles. I will look at 3 major notions: corporeal schema, mirror image and pathologies of freedom, each corresponding to a major influence on Fanon, those of Maurice Merleau-Ponty, Jacques Lacan and Günther Anders.

In BSWM, the effect of the racist gaze upon the body of the person who is the object of this gaze is clearly defined as alienation in medical terms. In his detailed description of the lived experience of a man subjected to a racist slur, Fanon speaks of a disintegration of the body schema (*schéma corporel*), transposing a well-known concept in the French psychiatry of the time:

> *'Dirty nigger!' Or simply, 'Look, a Negro!'*
>
> *I came into the world anxious to uncover a meaning in things, my soul desirous to be the origin of the world and here I am an object among other objects."*
>
> *As a result, the body schema [emphasis added], attacked in several places, collapsed, giving way to an epidermal racial schema. In the train, it was a question of being aware of my body, no longer in the third person but in triple. In the train, instead of one seat, they left me two or three: I was taking up room. I approached the Other ... and the Other, evasive, hostile, but not opaque, transparent and absent, vanished. Nausea. [...]*
>
> *Disoriented, incapable of confronting the Other, the white man, who had no scruples about imprisoning me, I transported myself on that particular day far, very far, from my self, and gave myself up as an object. What did this mean to me? Peeling, stripping my skin, causing a hemorrhage that left congealed black blood all over my body. Yet, this reconsideration of myself, this thematization, was not my idea. I wanted quite simply to be a man among men.*
>
> *I arrive slowly in the world; sudden emergences are no longer my habit. I crawl along. The white gaze, the only valid one, is already dissecting me. I am fixed [emphasis added]. (Fanon, 1958, pp. 89, 92 and 95)*

The concept of body schema or corporal schema was invented by the psychiatrist Jean Lhermitte, a specialist of pathologies concerning the image of the body, and Fanon probably encountered it first via the teaching of Maurice Merleau-Ponty in Lyon, while he was a student. The notion of the body schema designates the constitutive capacity of living beings such as humans to move in the physical world on the basis of projects and combined representations of space and time and not just as a reaction in mechanical ways. In *La Structure du Comportement* Merleau-Ponty opposed "behaviour" and "conduct" and systematically questioned behaviourism using this notion. It is sufficient to think of the implicit knowledge mobilised in any movement we make, even simply walking or entering a room: knowledge about the physical characteristics of the spatial context, about the relationship of each muscle involved to this context and to other *relevantly mobilised* muscles, all this in relation to the specific situation, which includes a number of evolving expectations and purposes, all very hard to plan in advance, before experiencing them. The complexity of situated physical movement is crucial for Fanon, who referred to psychosomatic medicine in all his works, from both philosophical and psychotherapeutical perspectives. Complex situated physical movements reflect the capacity to act and experience oneself within space and time *as the seat or the origin of an individual spontaneity or freedom*, and not as a purely physical object, a thing. But within the racist encounter Fanon says that this mode of being disintegrates and the objects of the racist gaze, the persons who are "*racialisées*", as he writes, because there is nothing natural in "race", are now unable to perceive themselves in the first person. Rather, they experience themselves in the "third person", neither as a self or an alter ego, but as objects of a gaze that sees in them only fixed traits, in other words as things among things, as objects "taking up room" in public spaces such as a train carriage.[1] Persons who are racialized experience themselves no longer as indeterminate singular beings, having to deal with an unpredictable present and aiming to a future, but through all the racial categories inherited from history, which characterize the human as a thing: skin colour, of course, but also many other features (teeth, chest, sexual organ etc.). Historicity he says, borrowing a term from Karl Jaspers, bears on the individual like an unbearable weight, a monumental press that would flatten him or her to a skin.

Fanon was an early reader of Jacques Lacan, and borrowed from him the famous description of the mirror stage. He uses it in the same way to analyse the pathologies of the image of the self in the context of racism. The individual seems to be brought back to a stage prior to this stage of development, when the face in the mirror is not yet perceived as a recognizable unity, *un visage*, and is not yet associated to a name and leading to the symbolic domain of an abstract self, but rather as a set of coexisting physical elements. Chapter V of BSWM, "The lived experience of the Black Man", contains descriptions of this lived experience, this *Erlebnis* to use the phenomenological term, in the first person, and then moves on to a psychiatric analysis in the third person, a constant rhetorical structure of the book.[2]

Fanon wrote this book while working on his PhD in psychiatry, which contains a chapter on Lacan, focusing on the opposition between a definition of madness as a pathology of freedom, Henri Ey's position, and the position of Lacan who saw it as the upper limit of creative freedom (Lacan was close to Breton and Surrealism). Fanon sided with Ey on this issue, in the end, but used Lacan extensively elsewhere. Now this psychiatric discussion on alienation and freedom, which is at the heart of his doctoral dissertation, in particular in relationship to artistic creativity and the apparent kinship of Surrealist art with the art produced by mentally ill patients, this discussion also surfaces in BSWM when Fanon studies a reaction to the regression of the self that is induced by the colonial context. This reaction consists, for an individual, in claiming a reactive identity, in this case *negritude* and, like wearing a "white" mask, that too is a "pathology of freedom". While the descriptions of the decomposition of the corporal schema and the collapse of the image of the self were grounded on Fanon's psychiatric readings and research, the strange idea of a pathology proper to freedom is grounded on a philosophical reflection that several thinkers who were important for Fanon refer to at the time: Ey, Lacan, Sartre and unknown to Fanon yet, Tosquelles. This reflection is contained in texts where Günther Anders defines pathologies of freedom as pathological forms of identification. In BSWM this takes the form of a mysterious allusion to the notion of a pathology of identity in the context of the discussion of negritude:

> *A few years ago, the Association of Overseas Students in Lyon asked me to respond to an article that literally likened jazz to cannibalism irrupting into the modern world. Knowing full well where I was going, I rejected the article's premise and asked the defender of European purity to cure himself of a spasm that had nothing cultural about it. Some men want to fill the world with their being [Certains hommes veulent enfler le monde de leur être].*
>
> *One German philosopher described the process as the pathology of freedom. In the case in point, I didn't have to defend black music against white music; rather, I had to help my brother get rid of an unhealthy attitude.*
>
> *The problem considered here is located in temporality. Disalienation will be for those Whites and Blacks who have refused to let themselves be locked in the substantialized Tower of the Past. For many other black men disalienation will come from refusing to consider their reality as definitive.*
>
> *I am a man, and I have to rework the world's past from the very beginning. I am not just responsible for the slave revolt in Saint Domingue. (Fanon, 1958, p. 155)*

This German philosopher was Günther Anders, who published in 1935 and 1936 in *Recherches Philosophiques* the text of two lectures, the first on freedom and the second on pathologies of freedom, which Fanon read and referred to.[3]

Anders' 1935 lectures clearly influenced Sartre, who himself published in the 1936 issue of *Recherches Philosophiques* his *Transcendance of the Ego*, a sharp critique of the substantialism of the self, which was to have a significant impact on Merleau-Ponty, on Fanon of course, who quotes it, and on Deleuze, who refers to it from his first to his last published text. Anders' text is a phenomenological analysis of what he calls "pathologies of identification". In the earlier text, *Une Interprétation de l'a posteriori* (translated by Emmanuel Lévinas), Anders defined freedom ontologically rather than ethically, as a *distance* from what he called *material a priori*: the structures and the circumstances that determine animal existence. Animals, who live within the horizons of these material *a priori*, do not need to learn or invent the world, which is always already given, in the form of material determinations to which their instincts are attuned by nature. The world offered to the animal is by definition adequate to its needs and the animal is *fixed* in this reciprocal relation to the world as a well named *milieu*. Whatever remains exterior to an animal's anticipations simply escapes its apprehension. Humans, by contrast, are not fixed. While the animal lives in a world of material *a priori* the whole of the human world is an *a posteriori* that must be constantly interpreted. This human freedom is on the one hand nothing else than "the negation of a certain degree of integration", writes Anders, but it is also the condition of possibility of the *theorein*, the theoretical relationship to a world now at a distance. He wrote that "the starting point of the problem of freedom is in the fact that man, a foreigner to the world, is detached from it and abandoned to himself" (Anders, 1935, p. 70). While Andersian freedom is a detachment or a foreignness to the world as a given *milieu*, Fanon will use the term *fixed* to describe the racialised condition and the colonial situation that necessarily begets it, on the model of an internment, forcing upon the human precisely a *milieu*.

Now, Anders described phenomenologically this human ontological freedom of detachment or *worldlessness,* as the experience of an abandonment, of a radical solitude. This sense of the contingence of human existence can in turn produce pathologies of compensation, which are analysed in the second article, the one that Fanon quotes more directly. He was influenced in that by Ey, who went as far as defining psychiatry as a pathology of freedom, in the active sense of a medicine of freedom. For Anders, human beings discover their freedom through reflection, that is the capacity of abstracting from the world, and therefore through an act of freedom, but paradoxically what they discover is that they are not in fact absolutely free since they have not caused or determined themselves to be so: they are "just" born so. The human experience of freedom is one of pure contingence and this realisation is a shock which produces what he calls an ontological *shame*, a shame of the origin, which is commonly counterbalanced by the development of the private sphere, primarily that of the family, which is nothing else than a variety of forms of dissimulation of the subject's purely contingent origin. Reading this text Fanon marked the following passage: "The thousand forms of hypocrisy, of disguise, of comedy positively exemplify what shame and disgust prove negatively: the instability of man in relation to himself, his vagueness. The ego succeeds only temporarily in abandoning its existence precisely as such, and thus in taking the form of an other, and in making itself, so to speak, the occasion and the material for multiple personifications. The provisional itself is conclusive: among all species, man is the one with the least character" (Anders, 1937, p. 33).

However, for Fanon, the *privacy* or opacity that envelops and shelters the individual is negated by racist systems where the other, in her or his materiality is constantly subjected to the coloniser's analytical gaze, made to stand in pure visibility or publicness. Fanon often described the condition of the racialised subject in objectifying medical terms as a being-given-to-observation.

Anders considered the recourse to familial lineage and belonging as the general condition under which most humans compensate their ontological shame, but he goes further and diagnoses two *pathologies of identification* which may derive from this ontological shame. One is *nihilism* or the disgust with oneself as being just this or that, as purely contingent, and the other is a thirst for power and pride (*orgueil*). Though for him nihilism is closer to the truth of the human condition, it is actually when writing on the thirst for power that Anders speaks of a serious pathology of freedom. The historical context for this pathology of identification when men want to take their revenge from the world by equating and absorbing the whole world within their own self, now raised to the glory of a statue, as he describes it, is not named but it is clear, it is Nazism. Anders sees in this pathology "one of the radical dangers than man can face" (Anders, 1937, p. 39). Fanon, who had fought in the Free French Forces and read this a few years later, was very much aware of the historical context of Anders's reflection of course, but he appropriated his concepts and transposed them to a very different reality: first the inferiority complex of the colonised who have been forced to constantly feel their contingence, but in material conditions without a possible escape in the private sphere. Consciousness as opacity is constantly denied to them by the structural and material conditions of their existence. Secondly, the reaction of those who, at a later stage of history put on a white mask or, conversely, an African mask, as in the negritude movements, both reactions erecting a statue to an impossible or lost identity. Fanon wrote three plays while he was working on his PhD dissertation and on his first book. Of the two that survived, *L'Œil se noie* and *Les Mains parallèles*, each portrays one of the two pathologies, respectively the nihilistic and the promethean. Several passages in the *Wretched of the Earth* warn about pitfalls of national consciousness and the risk of regression into the imaginary and the reinvention of the statues that had been toppled.

So, in Fanon's early work, the dislocations of the body schema, the destruction of the image of the self or loss of one's face, and, as a reaction, the pathologies of identification that are ways of negating one's freedom, these three factors lead to the famous conclusion of his first book, which is a prayer to the body and a resolution to refuse all identities, seen as pathological reifications of freedom. If there is one principle in Fanon's ethics, it consists in never renouncing freedom by embracing an identity:

> *Sartre has shown that the past, along the line of an inauthentic position, catches on and "takes" into a mass, and, when solidly structured, then gives form to the individual. This is the past transmuted into a thing of value. But, I can also revise my past, prize it, or condemn it, through my successive decisions. [...]*
> *One duty alone: That of not renouncing my freedom through my decisions.*
> *I have no wish to be the victim of the Ruse of a black world.*
> *My life should not be devoted to drawing up the balance sheet of Negro values. (Fanon, 1958 pp. 157–158)*[4]

Another way to describe Fanon's ethics would be to say that it aims to create the conditions for the existence of a human world through "a permanent tension of freedom" (a permanent tension which he calls "vigilance" in many later texts). In all of that Fanon's perspective is Sartrian: in addition to the *Transcendance of the ego*, two other major reference in the book are Sartre's *Reflections on the Jewish question*, which poses identity as created by the gaze of the other, and *Black Orpheus*, which considers negritude, or the claim of a black identity, as the minor moment in a dialectic of liberation which will finally result in the negation of identities and the birth of what Fanon calls several times a "new humanism". But these famous philosophical and, as we will see, political views were initially grounded on the clinical, psychiatric and to some degree psychoanalytical descriptions of the alienation produced by the racializing gaze on the body which was essential, according to Fanon, to the colonial system.

Now, seeing our current historical and political phase one would be tempted to agree with Fanon, when he says in his PhD that history could be defined as the working out of collective psychopathological complexes:

> *The occasion will arise, in a work that I have been undertaking for a long time, to tackle the problem of history from a psychoanalytic and ontological angle. [That is to say the perspectives of Lacan and Anders]. In it, I will show that history is only the systematic valorization of collective complexes. (Fanon, 2020b, p. 94)*

To some extent he carried out this programme, for instance in Chapter VI of BSWM, on *The Black Man and Psychopathology*.

But is it legitimate to transpose an array of psychiatric concepts, such as body schema or mirror stage, meant to describe the development of the individual, and possible pathologies in this development, to a historical, social and cultural reality such as the colonial situation? The same could be said of the subsequent books, in particular his final descriptions of the revolutionary struggle as in itself a condition for disalienation, a process of *désintoxication*, a detoxifying process, as he wrote at the end of the famous chapter on violence in the *Wretched of the Earth*.

Also, beyond the epistemological question of the value of analogy in the philosophy of history, isn't there here the risk of a simplistic application of psychopathology to history that would negate a priori this possibility of freedom which Fanon held so dear? In other words does he not fall into both reductionism and self-contradiction?

It is unlikely that Fanon would have found enlightening the speculations at the beginning of the war in Ukraine about the supposed madness of the Russian president due to his Covid confinement, but he would have been interested in what the grand narratives of national identity used to justify the war tell us about the pathological nature of our historical situation at the level of the individuals that are targeted by these narratives. The same thing could be said of the idea of a mechanical link between colonial socio-historical contexts and politically or religiously justified mass killings. In reality Fanon ended up developing a much more complex thought than his initial view, a political thought, even if, given the consistence and relevance of his analyses and declarations on colonial alienation as a mental pathology, there was clearly for him something much deeper here than a mere analogy, assuming that there is ever such thing as a "mere" analogy in the history of thought. The interest of all the psychiatric texts we published is precisely to show, I think, how his thought complexified into a political theory, and at the heart of that was his encounter with Tosquelles.

Tosquelles and Fanon

Like Tosquelles the Catalan, who had fought against fascism during the Spanish civil war, Fanon came from a country where you had to think of yourself as other or wear a mask. At the age of 17, he had fled the island of Martinique under the Pétainist regime and joined the Free French Forces, also participating in a war against fascism. Conceptually, they shared a common understanding of psychiatry. In his PhD Fanon had empirically demonstrated, in the context of specific neuropsychiatric pathologies, the gap between the organic and the mental. In it, claiming the influence of Lacan, he defended the idea of a social genesis of the forms that mental illnesses take. These views were similar to those that Tosquelles had held since the 1940s. In addition to his medical thesis, before meeting Tosquelles Fanon had published two studies in *Esprit*, one on the unexplained pathologies of immigrant workers that doctors attributed to a mental "constitution" of the natives, a "North African syndrome", and the other on the "lived experience of the Negro", impregnated with the ideas of Günther Anders, Sartre and Merleau-Ponty on the corporeality essential to any free human existence, which was destroyed by the ordeal of the racist gaze, as we have just seen. This notion of *lived experience*, *Erlebnis*, was essential for Tosquelles. He too referred to it in 1945–1946 in relation to Anders: "The notion of *Erlebnis*, as defined by Stern [...] goes beyond thought and knowledge and includes all experience, including its organic aspect."[5]

The rejection of mental *constitutionalism* and the sustained attention to the total, and therefore also corporeal, situation of the human being within society are essential themes of Tosquelles' anthropology and form the basis of his clinic. This common network of thought probably explains why the psychiatrist Paul Balvet, whom Fanon saw regularly at the Vinatier clinic in Lyon, had directed the young Martinican towards the remote Lozère hospital where surrealist figures such as Paul and Nusch Éluard, or Tristan Tzara had been hidden during the war, and where Tosquelles had started to revolutionize psychotherapy.[6] It is Balvet who had called Tosquelles to Saint Alban, from the concentration camp where he was kept with Spanish refugees in the South of France.

What Saint-Alban, a psychiatric hospital that was totally integrated in its rural and urban environments, was to bring to Fanon, was not only the techniques and requirements of socialtherapy, a clinical practice corresponding to his conception of the complexity of the individual's mind, but also a cultural perspective. For Tosquelles the disease had to be studied and treated in its geographical and social "sector," and taking into account its conceptualization by the patients themselves. This apprenticeship allowed Fanon to extend the psychopathology of the experience of racism analysed in his first book, in the very specific context of the French Caribbean, towards a much more general description of alienations in any colonial environment and by consequence towards a political theory of historical disalienation. It seems that he also acquired something of the *simultaneously* experimental and reflexive ("paranoid-critical") style of Tosquelles, who emphasized that one essentially learns by failure and by transforming oneself through contact with others, in short that the work of psychiatrists was also their own socialtherapy: "He was moving towards a place where the psychiatrists' concerns in practice converged in the irrevocable resolution to arrange the proper field of their work through collective labour" said Tosquelles (1975a, p. 10) about Fanon, in one of the several articles he wrote on him after Fanon's death.[7] In November 1953, not long after his internship at Saint-Alban, Fanon was appointed to the psychiatric hospital of Blida-Joinville, in Algeria, reformed it and developed Tosquellian socialtherapy there until 1956 while becoming involved in the Algerian liberation struggle. In developing these new mental health approaches, Fanon was also led to make some pioneering work in ethnopsychiatry. However, as Tosquelles noted in one of his texts on Fanon, he did not suffer from "normopathy": at the end of his Algerian period, he started to differ sharply from him on a point of theory: the question of violence induced by any psychiatric institution, reformed or not. Later, during his last period of practice as a psychiatrist, in a recently independent Tunisia, Fanon also defended an alternative model of the clinic, replacing the occupational therapy microcosm with a psychiatric day center inserted in the city. So let me now point out some significant aspects of this influence of the Saint Alban period, with Tosquelles, on Fanon's later work. Among the large amount of psychiatric material which I hope I have made accessible through more than a hundred pages of footnotes and explanations, and a long introduction, I will stress two crucial examples: first the parallelism between Fanon's conception of "socialtherapy" in the clinical context and his view on the liberation struggle as a therapy for society. It is always about dissolving fixed, reified identities and creating a new type of political personhood. Secondly I will consider his critique of the dominant ethnopsychiatry of his time as essentially linked to colonialism and to a fixist or "constitutionalist" idea of personality.

What is socialtherapy, how can alienation be cured, in a strictly psychiatric sense for Fanon and Tosquelles and how can that be transposed onto the collective historical sphere? In his 1975 homage, Tosquelles said that Fanon had come to Saint Alban to escape from a psychiatry modelled on the classifications of "the anatomo-pathophysiological object which is the foundation of medicine in general and fragments into specialisations without end or measure" (Tosquelles, 1975a, p. 10). The singular patient disappeared under such a reductionist, mechanistic approach. Tosquelles and Fanon shared an ideal of therapy, which was based on the very different model of mental life and mental illness that had been proposed by the major French psychiatrist of that time, Henri Ey.

Ey thought that serious mental illness derived from a neurological shock, which was followed by a pathological reconstruction of personality. But because there is a fundamental gap between the neurological plane and the psychiatric one, which Ey called *écart organo-clinique*, these reconstructions of personality can take different forms, which we categorise as various mental illnesses. Fanon wrote his medical PhD on a neurological degenerescence, Friedreich's disease, which is often *but not always* accompanied by religious delirium, and he did that precisely to study this gap between the organic and the mental and to show how much the social environment (or disturbances in it) determined the forms that illness could take. Pathological forms of personality were therefore for him as much determined by the organogenesis and the psychogenesis of the illness in the individual as by its sociogenesis (a view he derived from reading Lacan's doctoral dissertation, which, as we have seen, Tosquelles had printed by patients in Saint Alban's psychiatric hospital as part of work therapy).

Now, Fanon and Tosquelles published several joint papers where they defined the therapy they proposed as reversing this pathological process: it was first necessary to dissolve the pathological reconstructions of personality that had followed the organic shock. For that they practiced and experimented with what was then called shock therapies: electroshocks, insulin comas or sleep cures (hypnotherapy). Then a long work or reconstruction of personality could start, which they based on psychotherapies, individual or in group, (they experimented in particular with drama therapy), and, crucially, what they called socialtherapy, which consisted in constructing within the hospital a microcosm within which the patients would regain autonomy and agency, by working, running cultural societies, publishing a newspaper (in which Fanon wrote a number of significant editorials), managing a sports club etc. This revolutionized the traditional model of the psychiatric hospital where patients had been essentially passive and where, as was well documented, their pathologies only worsened, their behaviour becoming mechanical or subject to bursts of delirium or so called "agitation", to which nurses and doctors reacted with essentially repressive methods. Their new therapeutical model generated the antipsychiatry of the 60s and 70s. There is a line that goes from Tosquelles to Fanon and Oury and then Guattari. The catalogue of the *Déconniatrie* exhibition illustrates this history very well, starting from Catalan anarchist communes.

Anticolonial Struggle and Disalienation

Fanon spent 15 months with Tosquelles, in this very remote and rural environment in the South of France, from April 1952 to August 1953. Tosquelles later noted that Fanon's insistence on the fact that in colonized countries the revolution and the formation of a new national consciousness would come from the peasant class, rather than the proletariat, probably came from his lived experience both in Martinique and around the Saint Alban Hospital. And indeed, Fanon's clinical training at Saint Alban leads to the model he used for his analysis of the anticolonial liberation struggle.

Like the reification of behaviour produced by the neurological illness, the initial shock of colonization has generated, he argues, a rigidification of attitudes: the cultural heritage has become ossified and it has produced pathological personalities characterized by compensatory behaviour. In the first chapter of the *Wretched of the Earth*, "On violence," he describes it at length, identifying two main forms: criminal behaviour on the one hand, religious fervour on the other. These are explosions of violence either within society or within the mind, a violence which is always the substitute of the physical freedom rendered impossible in the compartmented colonial world, compared to an internment, whether it takes the form of the plantation system or of apartheid, with its more or less rigid varieties, all obstacles to the essential freedom of the body, which, as we have seen, produce a disintegration of the body schema.

The start of the liberation struggle introduces a counter shock and as in a shock therapy, it dissolves the pathological identities produced by the colonial organization of society, through the ferocious repression it elicits. No one can have illusions then and wear a white mask. However, Fanon was a pragmatist and insisted that such transformation can only happen if the historical circumstances make it possible, otherwise the uprising is doomed to failure (as in Madagascar after WWII).

Then, as it unfolds, the liberation struggle operates like a therapy for society, and it does so in two ways. First a collective subject is born, which realizes it has autonomy. The model here is the Algerian liberation struggle: when the police was overwhelmed and the French army intervened, the war became total, involved the whole society in supporting the fighters, transforming, for each individual, particular attitudes to objects, to the social structure, to gender roles etc. All of Fanon's sociological analyses need to be reread from this perspective. In Tunis Fanon taught a course on sociology and *Year V of the Algerian Revolution* is subtitled "sociologie d'une revolution". Secondly the struggle also prepares for Fanon a new decolonized world in that taking part in the shared struggle detoxifies, he says, from the cult of the leader. This is why he was suspicious of an independence simply given by the colonizers, side-stepping the revolutionary struggle. A new bourgeoisie would step in their shoes and use identitarian ideologies to ground their power. Nothing would change or things would become even worse. This neocolonial danger is in fact the main subject of the *Wretched of the Earth*, and Fanon was quite forceful in his calls to vigilance:

> *At the individual level, violence detoxifies. [...] Even if the armed struggle has been symbolic, and even if they have been demobilized by rapid decolonization, the people have time to realize that the liberation was the achievement of each and every one and no special merit should go to the leader. Violence hoists the people up to the level of the leader. Hence their aggressive tendency to distrust the system of protocol that young governments are quick to establish. When they have used violence to achieve national liberation, the masses allow nobody to come forward as "liberator". [...] The praxis which pitched them into a desperate man-to-man struggle has given the masses a ravenous taste for the tangible. Any attempt at mystification in the long term becomes virtually impossible. (Fanon, 2004, pp. 51–52)*

I hope it is now clear how strong the influence of Fanon's psychiatric thought and practice was on his political analysis of the liberation struggle. I would now like to briefly mention the reverse relation: the influence of his political experience and failures upon his psychiatric thought, and his attempt to develop a non-colonial form of ethnopsychiatry.

A Revolutionary Form of Ethnopsychiatry

When Fanon arrived in the psychiatric hospital at Blida-Joinville in Algeria in November 1953, equipped with his experience of socialtherapy, he immediately set out to transform the hospital, and in doing so he created a unique experimental situation that had a decisive impact on the evolution of his scientific thought. Patients had been separated along ethnic lines between "Europeans" and "Indigenous", with Fanon being given two wards, one of European women, the other of Indigenous men. This was in line with the racist doctrine of the "Algiers school of psychiatry" which thought that since the indigenous populations were mentally retarded, by *constitution*, they could not be treated in the same way as the Europeans in a psychiatric hospital. The founder of that school, Antoine Porot, had designed the hospital, which was built in the thirties. I reproduced its blueprint and Porot's justifications of it in our edition of Fanon's psychiatric writings. Now it turned out that while Tosquellian socialtherapy worked wonders with the European women, it was a complete failure with the Algerian men. Fanon and his intern, Jacques Azoulay, who wrote his PhD on this subject, published an important study on this failure and the lessons to be drawn from it. The singularity of the colonial situation gave them a unique chance to reflect in greater depth upon the process of socialtherapy itself and Tosquelles stressed much later on the importance of this work to understand Fanon's political thought.

It was clear to them that if the film club, the music society and the hospital newspaper (all of which were run by patients) could have a therapeutic function, it was not simply due to the films, music or texts in themselves, but because they were instruments through which the patients could re-learn to impart meaning to the constitutive elements of an environment: "Film ought not remain a succession of images with a sonorous accompaniment: it must become the unfolding of a life, of a history. Therefore, the film committee, by choosing the films, by commenting upon them in a special chronicle of the journal, gives to the cinematographic fact its true meaning," they wrote (Fanon, 2020b, p. 25). There are echoes here of the passages in BSWM where the self experiences its freedom through the constitution of the world as a meaningful totality. This worked in the European ward and soon Fanon was able to discard straightjackets and other instruments of restraint. But these reforms failed with the Algerian men, who remained stuck within their cycle of indifference, withdrawal and agitation, with their correlate of psychiatric internment and repression. Was it due to some constitutional racial features? Fanon, who had already debunked constitutionalist bias in his earlier work could not believe that. The situation of segregation they were faced with in fact was not in itself the solution psychiatrists like Porot had circularly manufactured. But it revealed an important dimension: the cognitive work of assigning meaning within ordinary existence can only be carried out within certain frames of reference, and these are not universal but culturally determined. This dimension was clearly manifested by the contrast between two groups in a segregated society in relation to responses to therapeutical methods. "Could our judgement have been more impaired than when we proposed to implement a Western-based socialtherapy program in a ward of mentally ill Muslim men?" asked Fanon and Azoulay. "How is a structural analysis possible if we bracket out the geographical, historical, cultural and social frameworks?" (Fanon, 2020b, p. 25). From then on Fanon could explain how the colonial medical system was geared to produce, within psychiatry, precisely the realities which were then used to justify the colonial enterprise, in a vicious circle. The solution was to change the cultural framework under which therapy was taking place, and Fanon and his interns developed new social therapeutical methods and even new cognition tests that brought within the therapeutical community a consciousness of the importance of taking into account local cultural and social dimensions in devising treatments. There are several fascinating texts on that, in particular on the local conceptualisations of mental illness through religious practices of exorcism.

So Fanon became a pioneer of a new form of ethnopsychiatry because from the very outset he had refused substantialism and "constitutionalist" points of view which assigned mental illness differences to racial differences. This was already present in the early article he had written in Lyon on the inability of French medical doctors to see in psychosomatic symptoms presented by North African immigrant workers anything else than a sort of constitutive tendency to lie or to fantasize because they were blind to the structural impact of their social condition. But Saint-Alban and then Blida gave him the extraordinary opportunity to reveal the biases inherent to the dominant pseudo-scientific psychiatric constructions. There would be much more to say, but I hope I have given you a simple summary of the framework I proposed for the understanding of Fanon's political texts in a dialectical relationship with his epistemological and clinical texts.

To conclude I would just like to draw your attention to an anecdotal text that one might wrongly be tempted to skip, a series of editorials Fanon took the time to write in the inner journal of the Blida hospital just before he left Algeria, when he was fully involved in helping the Algerian National Liberation Front and the situation had become very dangerous for him. Oddly, given the circumstances, they are about the internal regulations that the nurses supervising the hospital's football club had just instituted. This code aimed to punish and discipline the behaviour of unruly patient players. You will find here a very precise description of how easily institutions of which the purpose is disalienation, or liberation, can produce disciplinary mechanisms that infantilise the patients in the processes that were precisely aimed to bring about their cure. This was probably inspired by an anecdote Tosquelles recounted much later, and often, to explain the birth of his psychiatric approach.

As a child he had observed a football match between patients and nurses in the psychiatric asylum of Reus, and noted that the referee penalised the patients much more often than the sane players. That was because the psychiatrists were scared of the mad, he said. Later Fanon discovered in Sartre's *Critique of Dialectical Reason*, of which he was one of the first readers, very similar analyses of the solidification of what should essentially be a process of liberation, of a group "in fusion". It is clear that this reflection on the dangers of a spontaneous deviation and corruption of the very institutions of which the aim was to cure madness as a pathology of freedom is at the heart of his worries about the nationalist parties and the new neo-colonial hierarchies he denounces in his final book. We are now moving away from phenomenology and psychiatry to a sociological and political critique of the operations of institutions, which is also reflected in his late psychiatric reflection and practice in the day clinic he created in Tunis. This is the line that Foucault will develop after Fanon when writing on asylums or the prison. But for Fanon none of this would make sense if it was not grounded on his early reflections and clinical practice on mental alienation.

REFERENCES

Anders, G. (1935–1936). [Günther Stern] (1935). Une interprétation de l'a posteriori. *Recherches Philosophiques, IV*, 65–80.

Anders, G. (1936–1937). [Günther Stern] (1937). Pathologie de la liberté. *Recherches Philosophiques, VI*, 22–54.

Cole, E. (1967). *House of Bondage*. Ridge Press/Random House.

Fanon, F. (2004). *The Wretched of the Earth* (Philcox, R., Trans.). Grove Press. (Original work published 1961)

Fanon, F. (2020). *The Psychiatric Writings from Alienation and Freedom* (Khalfa, J., & Young, R. J. C., Eds.). Bloomsbury Academic.

Guerra, C., & Masó, J. (Eds.). (2021). *La Déconniatrie: art, exil et psychiatrie autour de François Tosquelles*. Arcàdia.

Khalfa, J. (2009). Naissance de la négritude. *Les Temps Modernes, 656*(5), 38–63. DOI: 10.3917/ltm.656.0038

Lacan, J. (2001). *Autres écrits*. Le Seuil.

Macey, D. (2012). *Frantz Fanon: A Life*. Verso.

Peck, R. (2024a). *Ernest Cole, photographe*. Denoël.

Peck, R. (Director). (2024b). *Ernest Cole, photographe*. Velvet Film.

Tosquelles, F. (1975a). Frantz Fanon à Saint-Alban. *Sud/Nord, 22*(1), 9–14. .DOI: 10.3917/sn.022.0009

Tosquelles, F. (1975b). *Trait d'union, journal de Saint-Alban: éditoriaux, articles, notes, 1950–1962*. Éditions d'une.

Tosquelles, F. (1986). *Le Vécu de la fin du monde dans la folie: le témoignage de Gérard de Nerval*. Éditions de l'AREFPPI.

Tosquelles, F. (2021). *Soigner les institutions*, textes choisis et présentés par Joana Masó. L'Arachnéen/Arcàdia.

ENDNOTES

1 Ernest Cole's photographic work is perhaps the most extraordinary visual representation of such an experience of the human body by itself as superfluous in a racist context. See Cole (1967) and Raoul Peck's 2024 film and book *Ernest Cole, photographe.*

2 Lacan discussed the mirror stage in his encyclopaedia article "Les complexes familiaux dans la formation de l'individu" originally published in 1938 (see Lacan 2001). It echoes, on the preconceptual experience of the self, the lectures Alexandre Kojève gave in Paris between 1933 and 1938 on Hegel's *Phenomenology of the Spirit*, a work Fanon referred to at length. On Fanon and Lacan, see Jean Khalfa's introduction to Fanon (2020b) and Jean Khalfa and Stéphane Thibierge, The specular image in Fanon's psychiatric and political thought, in D. Hook & S. Richards (Eds.), *Fanon and Psychoanalysis*, forthcoming, Routledge, 2026.

3 These texts were signed Günther Stern as Anders used his birth name before WWII. Fanon's annotations are reproduced in Fanon 2020b.

4 Translation modified. See Khalfa, 2021.

5 Presentation to the Medico-Psychological Society made by the Saint-Alban group, reproduced in Tosquelles, 1986, p. 289.

6 In *Frantz Fanon: A Life* David Macey (2012) suggests that Fanon may have read Lacan's thesis on "Paranoid Psychosis in its Relation to Personality" in one of the handmade copies made in Saint-Alban on Tosquelles' initiative, and procured by Balvet. Lacan had indeed refused to allow it to be reprinted.

7 See Pierre Delion's remarks in his preface to Tosquelles' editorials in *Trait d'union, journal de Saint-Alban: éditoriaux, articles, notes, 1950-1962*, Paris, Éditions d'une, 2015, p. 8.

Chapter 2
Neural Basis of Body-Mind Interaction and Body-Mind Practice:
From Ancient Wisdom to Modern Neuroscience

Yoshihara Kazufumi
http://orcid.org/0000-0001-6499-3900
Division of Health Promotion and Development, Center for Health Sciences and Counseling, Kyushu University, Japan & Department of Psychosomatic Medicine, Kyushu University Hospital, Japan

ABSTRACT

Stress triggers mind-body symptoms by activating the autonomic nervous system through the brain. Neuroimaging studies have identified the anterior cingulate cortex (ACC) and the insular cortex as being central to this interaction. Abnormalities in these regions have been linked to stress-related disorders such as depression, irritable bowel syndrome, and chronic pain. Recent research shows that modern psychotherapy and traditional body-mind practices can improve symptoms by modulating these neural pathways. For example, active listening activates the brain's reward system and insula. Additionally, a 12-week yoga intervention significantly improved mood and psychological symptoms such as depression and anxiety. Practices like mindfulness meditation also alter neural activity and brain volume in the ACC and insula. In conclusion, the ACC and insular cortex are crucial for body-mind interaction. Interventions targeting these pathways can improve health. Brain imaging research is essential for developing objective biomarkers and personalized treatments for stress-related conditions.

DOI: 10.4018/979-8-3373-3521-6.ch002

1. INTRODUCTION

The idea that the mind and body influence each other has existed in various forms since ancient times. Words used to describe this interaction include "mind–body correlation" and the Japanese term "Shinshin-ichinyo," a Buddhist concept that the mind and body are one and inseparable. Physical symptoms appearing due to psychological factors have been proposed to be called "psychosomatic disorder" in Japan.

Mind–body correlation refers to the general concept that the mind (spirit, psychological state) and the body (physiological functions) influence each other. Mind–body correlation is the basic idea that the mind and body are not independent but are closely connected. For example, when a person feels stressed, the heart may race, or a stomachache may develop. This illustrates how the state of the mind affects the physiological functions of the body. Conversely, when the body is tired, a person may feel depressed or unmotivated—an example of how the state of the body affects the mind. Mind–body correlation is therefore a very important perspective when considering health, and it underscores the importance of maintaining a good balance between mental and physical health.

Shinshin-ichinyo is a Buddhist concept according to which the mind and body are one and inseparable. Rather than existing as separate entities, the mind and body form one continuous whole. This perspective encourages viewing the mind and body holistically, and it is linked to the promotion of harmony between the mind and body through practices such as qigong and yoga. In modern times, it is also related to the idea of holistic medicine.

Furthermore, the Japanese Society of Psychosomatic Medicine defines psychosomatic disorder as "a pathological condition in which psychosocial factors are closely involved in the onset and progression of a physical illness, and in which organic or functional disorders are recognized." In the narrow sense, psychosomatic disorder is a pathological manifestation of the mind–body correlation; it is not simply "in one's mind," but refers to a condition in which there is actually an abnormality in the body's organs or functions. Table 1 lists representative diseases that present as psychosomatic disorders. When a disorder is psychosomatic, this is indicated by adding the notation "(psychosomatic)" to the name of the disorder—for example, "bronchial asthma (psychosomatic)."

Table 1. Representative Diseases That Present as Psychosomatic Disorders

Category	Representative diseases
1. Respiratory diseases	Bronchial asthma, hyperventilation syndrome, nervous cough
2. Circulatory diseases	Essential hypertension, essential hypotension, orthostatic hypotension, some arrhythmias
3. Digestive diseases	Gastric and duodenal ulcers, chronic gastritis, functional dyspepsia, irritable bowel syndrome, ulcerative colitis, biliary dyskinesia, chronic pancreatitis, psychogenic vomiting, diffuse esophageal spasm, esophageal achalasia, aerophagia
4. Endocrine/metabolic diseases	Anorexia nervosa, bulimia, hyperthyroidism, simple obesity, diabetes
5. Nervous and muscular diseases	Tension headache, migraine, chronic pain, writer's cramp, spasmodic torticollis, autonomic imbalance
6. Other	Chronic rheumatoid arthritis, fibromyalgia, lower back pain, traumatic cervical syndrome, menopausal disorders, chronic urticaria, atopic dermatitis, alopecia areata, Meniere's syndrome, temporomandibular joint disorders

Note. Adapted from Japanese Society of Psychosomatic Medicine guidelines.

The terms "mind–body correlation," "Shinshin-ichinyo," and "psychosomatic disorder" each explain the interaction between the mind and body from a different perspective. Understanding this interaction and maintaining harmony between the mind and body is essential to living a healthy and fulfilling life. Methods for maintaining this harmony include psychotherapy that works on the mind and somatic practices that work on the body.

This chapter describes mind–body interactions and techniques for working with the mind and body, and examines the neural basis of these interactions.

2. MIND-BODY INTERACTION: EXPLORING THE RELATIONSHIP BETWEEN THE MIND AND THE BODY

This section provides an overview of the psychological and behavioral factors that affect the body, which are crucial for understanding mind–body interaction. First, it discusses how psychological states such as stress, anxiety, and depression contribute to the exacerbation of physical symptoms and disease progression, as well as how behavioral factors including lifestyle habits and medication adherence influence health outcomes. Using bronchial asthma as an example of a representative psychosomatic disorder, it explains the interrelationship between psychological states and physical symptoms revealed through epidemiological studies, and the pathophysiological mechanisms by which stress and childhood abuse affect inflammatory responses and airway hyperresponsiveness. Furthermore, it describes the mechanisms through which early-life stress and the interaction between chronic stress and infection induce chronic inflammation and hypersensitivity via the nervous, immune, and endocrine systems, incorporating findings from animal experimental studies.

2.1 Psychological Factors That Affect the Body

Stress may affect the progression, worsening, or delayed recovery of physical symptoms and physical illnesses. Stress includes life events (birth, marriage, divorce, relocation, employment, job change, further education, illness or death of a close relative, etc.) and stress in daily life (problems with interpersonal relationships at home, work, or school; chronic academic or occupational demands; etc.; Yoshihara & Sudo, 2016). The degree of an individual's reaction to these psychosocial stressors varies depending on personal factors such as the intensity and duration of the stress (e.g., conflict or overwork), personality traits (e.g., Type A behavior pattern, over-adaptation, and alexithymia), and coping behavior, as well as environmental factors such as the presence or absence of social support.

There is also a close relationship between psychological states (anxiety, anger, depression, etc.) and the worsening of physical symptoms and physical diseases (*Psychological factors affecting other medical conditions: Clinical features, assessment, and diagnosis*, 2025). Regarding anxiety, a meta-analysis of cardiovascular diseases has reported that increased anxiety is associated with increased mortality, myocardial infarction, and stroke. Regarding anger, it has been reported that anger is associated with increased risk of hypertension, peptic ulcer, and pain, and with increased arrhythmias, cardiovascular events such as myocardial infarction, and mortality from ischemic heart disease in patients with cardiovascular diseases. Anger is also associated with deterioration of the patient–physician relationship and decreased adherence to treatment. Depression has been reported to be a risk factor for cardiovascular diseases; to be associated with an increased risk of stroke; to be associated with hyperglycemia, complications, and mortality in patients with diabetes; to be associated with higher hospitalization and mortality in patients with end-stage renal disease; and to be associated with increased pain, fatigue, disability, and mortality in patients with rheumatoid arthritis.

2.2 Behavioral Factors That Affect the Body

Irregular sleep and eating patterns, lack of exercise or overexercise, smoking, excessive alcohol consumption, and excessive drug use can have an unfavorable effect on physical symptoms and physical illnesses. In addition, poor adherence to a physician's prescriptions or instructions can prevent appropriate treatment or management of physical symptoms or illnesses, significantly affecting treatment outcomes and disease progression. For example, irrational anxiety and fear regarding drugs and procedures (including steroid therapy), feelings of helplessness and depression regarding symptom control, and strong distrust of medical care or medical professionals are associated with decreased adherence (*Psychological factors affecting other medical conditions: Clinical features, assessment, and diagnosis*, 2025; Yoshihara, 2015; Yoshihara & Sudo, 2016).

2.3 Psychological Factors Influencing the Physical Symptoms of Psychosomatic Disorders

Although bronchial asthma is not primarily caused by psychological factors, it is one of the most common psychosomatic disorders and is greatly affected by them. Advances in asthma treatment and management methods, such as inhaled steroids, have improved control of asthma, and the number of asthma patients being treated for psychosomatic components has decreased. However, a search on PubMed for "asthma psychological" found 950 results from 1995 to 2004, but more than doubled to 2,359 results from 2005 to 2024. This shows that attention has been drawn once again to the importance of psychological factors in asthma patients, which may be related to the fact that basic research has revealed the mind–body correlation of asthma and its pathological mechanisms.

2.3.1 Psychosomatic Correlations of Bronchial Asthma in Epidemiological Studies

Epidemiological studies of bronchial asthma have reported that asthma patients frequently suffer from depression and anxiety disorders (Niti et al., 2007; Scott et al., 2007), and a relationship between bronchial asthma and psychological conditions has been noted.

Scott et al. (2007) conducted a survey of 85,088 people from 17 countries, including Japan, in the World Mental Health Survey. They found that the prevalence of major depressive disorder in asthma patients was about 5–10% in each country, and the prevalence of dysthymic disorder was higher in each country. The odds ratio (after adjusting for age and sex) for the presence or absence of major depressive disorder according to the presence or absence of asthma was 1.6 (95% CI = 1.4–1.8), the odds ratio for dysthymic disorder was 1.7 (95% CI = 1.4–2.1), and the odds ratio for depressive disorder was 1.6 (95% CI = 1.4–1.8). They also reported that the odds ratio for the presence or absence of generalized anxiety disorder based on the presence or absence of asthma was 1.7 (95% CI = 1.4–2.1), for agoraphobia or panic disorder the odds ratio was 1.7 (95% CI = 1.4–2.0), for social phobia the odds ratio was 1.3 (95% CI = 1.1–1.5), for post-traumatic stress disorder the odds ratio was 1.8 (95% CI = 1.4–2.3), and for combined anxiety disorders the odds ratio was 1.5 (95% CI = 1.4–1.7).

Ye et al. (2021) examined the prevalence of anxiety in people with asthma based on case-controlled studies, conducting a systematic review and meta-analysis using a random-effects model. The analysis included 19 studies involving a total of 106,813 participants. The results revealed that anxiety symptoms were prevalent in 32% of asthma patients (95% CI: 0.22–0.43), while anxiety disorders were prevalent in 24% of asthma patients (95% CI: 0.13–0.41). Compared with the control group without asthma, asthma patients were found to be at significantly higher risk of both anxiety symptoms (odds ratio = 1.89; 95% CI: 1.42–2.52; $p < .001$) and anxiety disorders (odds ratio = 2.08; 95% CI: 1.70–2.56; $p < .001$).

From these reports, a simple mind–body correlation model of bronchial asthma can be constructed in which "physical symptoms" and "psychological states (depression and anxiety)" are mutually related, as shown in Figure 1. Regarding the relationship between bronchial asthma and anxiety disorders, it is thought that asthma symptoms affect psychological states such as fear and catastrophic thinking, and that conversely, such psychological states affect asthma symptoms. It has been suggested that fear reactions caused by hypoxia and low carbon dioxide cause hypersensitivity of the brain's fear network, such as the amygdala (Katon et al., 2004).

Figure 1. A Simple Mind–body Model of Bronchial Asthma.

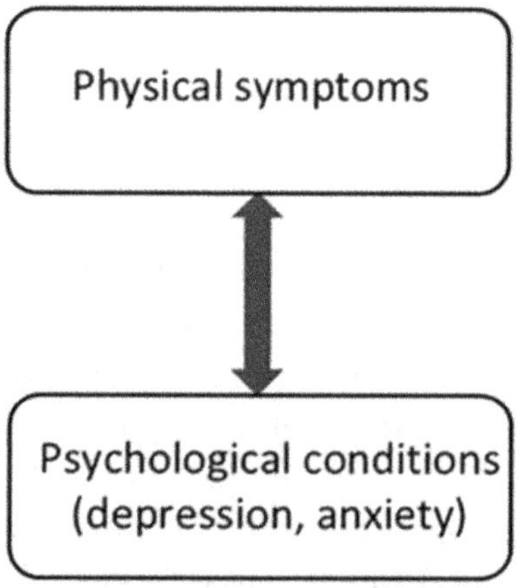

A simple mind–body correlation model in which physical symptoms and psychological states such as depression and anxiety are interrelated in bronchial asthma.

In addition, Nagano et al. (2010) reported that mothers who are in a chronic state of excessive stress or who tend to have an "inappropriate" parenting attitude, such as being overly involved with their children, affect the condition of their children's bronchial asthma. A self-administered questionnaire was administered to 274 mothers of children (ages 2–12) visiting a hospital for bronchial asthma; 223 (81%) participated in a follow-up survey one year later. The results showed that in children under 7 years of age, maternal chronic irritability and emotional suppression were associated with worsening of the children's bronchial asthma, while in children over age 7, an overly intrusive parenting attitude was associated with worsening.

In epidemiological studies it is difficult to clarify the pathological mechanisms by which psychosocial stress affects the nervous, immune, and endocrine systems in relation to the mind–body correlation of bronchial asthma. Nevertheless, these studies have revealed that asthma symptoms are related to psychological states such as depression and anxiety, and that psychological factors are related to the worsening of asthma symptoms. Future research is expected to further clarify psychosocial factors affecting bronchial asthma and to apply such knowledge to the prevention of its onset.

2.3.2 Mind-Body Correlation Model of Bronchial Asthma

The mind–body correlation of bronchial asthma and its pathological mechanisms are gradually becoming clearer through basic research including epidemiological surveys, animal experiments, and brain imaging studies. Regarding the relationship between stress and physical symptoms, it has been suggested that past abuse and stress from low socioeconomic status affect physical symptoms such as chronic inflammation and airway hyperresponsiveness in asthma patients. A systematic review by Saygideger et al. (2022) showed that childhood abuse may trigger epigenetic changes in asthma-related genes, activating pro-inflammatory pathways. Chen et al. (2003) reported that low-socioeconomic-status adolescents with asthma had significantly higher levels of Th2 inflammatory cytokines (IL-5) and Th1 cytokines (IFN-γ), as well as greater stress experience. These findings suggest that environmental stress at home may contribute to enhanced inflammatory responses and airway hyperresponsiveness.

Regarding the relationship between stress and psychological conditions, Han et al. (2022) demonstrated in a large UK cohort that a history of past abuse increased the risk of adult asthma, and that this effect was partly mediated by lifetime anxiety disorders (GAD) and major depressive disorder (MDD). Thus, increased depressive and anxiety symptoms may be one pathway through which abuse contributes to later asthma onset and exacerbation. Figure 2 shows a possible mind–body correlation model of bronchial asthma inferred from these studies.

Figure 2. Mind–body Correlation Model of Bronchial Asthma Inferred from Basic Research.

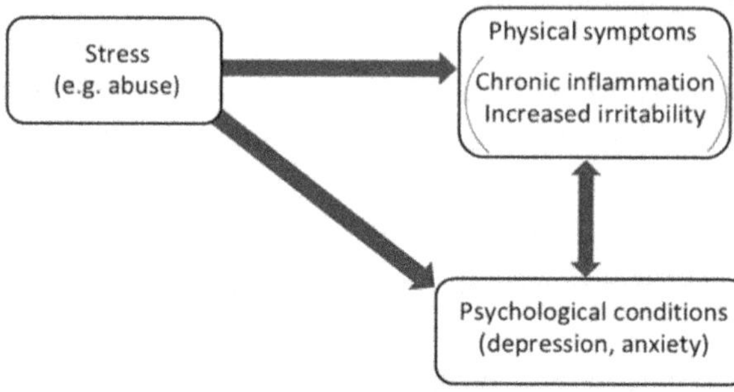

Stress, such as abuse, affects psychological states and physical symptoms, and those psychological states and physical symptoms mutually affect each other.

A high prevalence of alexithymia has been reported in asthma patients, and this has been shown to be associated with psychiatric comorbidities. Silvestro et al. (2023) reported that the prevalence of alexithymia was higher in asthma patients than in controls. Meanwhile, the correlation between child abuse and alexithymia was significant, as was the correlation between alexithymia and general psychopathology, suggesting that a history of abuse may also contribute to alexithymia in asthma patients (Kick et al., 2024). Alexithymia has also been reported to be associated with psychological conditions in asthma patients. Amore et al. (2013) reported that alexithymia was significantly associated with the severity of depression and anxiety symptoms. Furthermore, the review by Silvestro et al. (2023) suggested that the coexistence of asthma and alexithymia is associated with increased psychiatric comorbidities (e.g., depression and anxiety). Based on these findings, alexithymic tendencies in asthma patients appear likely to be associated with worsening depression and anxiety. When applying the above model to humans, it is necessary to take into account psychological characteristics such as alexithymia (Sifneos, 1973), as shown in Figure 3.

Figure 3. Example of a Mind–body Model of Human Bronchial Asthma.

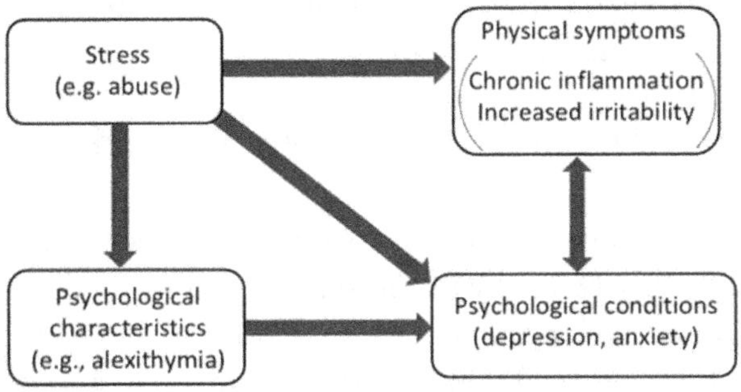

Stress, such as abuse, affects psychological traits such as alexithymia, psychological states, and physical symptoms; psychological traits affect psychological states; and psychological states and physical symptoms mutually affect each other.

Recently, psychosomatic disorders, which are considered multifactorial diseases, have been analyzed using structural equation modeling (covariance structure analysis). In structural equation modeling of functional dyspepsia, it has been shown that abuse, a past stressful experience, affects psychological characteristics such as alexithymia and physical symptoms; that psychological characteristics affect the psychological state; and that the psychological state and physical symptoms mutually affect each other (Jones et al., 2013). This model is highly similar to the mind–body correlation diagram shown in Figure 3. Therefore, performing a similar structural equation modeling analysis in bronchial asthma may clarify the relationships between various factors, and similar relationships may be observed in other psychosomatic disorders.

2.4 Psychological Factors That Influence Chronic Inflammation and Hyperresponsiveness

2.4.1 The Effects of Early Childhood Stress

Animal experiments are one method for elucidating the pathology related to chronic inflammation and hyperresponsiveness via the nervous system (dysregulation of the autonomic nervous system, etc.), immune system (dysregulation of cytokines, etc.), and endocrine system (hypothalamus–pituitary–adrenal axis, etc.). Chida et al. (2007) previously showed that mice exposed to psychological stress in early life had worse bronchial asthma that developed later in life (increased eosinophils in bronchoalveolar lavage fluid, increased airway hyperresponsiveness) compared with unexposed mice, and that the hypothalamus–pituitary–adrenal (HPA) axis was involved in the exacerbation. These results suggest that exposure to psychological stress during childhood is associated with exacerbation of chronic inflammation and increased airway hyperresponsiveness in adulthood in bronchial asthma via the nervous, immune, and endocrine systems.

2.4.2 Interaction Between Chronic Stress and Infection

Chronic fatigue syndrome (CFS), a disease characterized by prolonged periods of severe fatigue, is often associated with fibromyalgia (FM), a disease characterized by prolonged periods of severe pain across wide areas of the body. In addition, CFS is often associated with physical or psychological stress, such as overwork or over-exercise, prior to onset, and it has been reported that infection may be a trigger for the onset of CFS or FM (Clauw, 2014; Prins et al., 2006). Therefore, Chijiwa et al. (2015) investigated how physical symptoms (pain) and mental symptoms (depression and fatigue) change when rats are given poly I:C (polyinosinic-polycytidylic acid), a substance that induces inflammation similar to viral infection, in addition to chronic stress.

In an experiment with rats, it was found that chronic stress followed by an infection caused long-lasting symptoms of pain, depression, and fatigue. While rats with only an infection experienced temporary pain that resolved within a day, rats exposed to chronic stress before the infection developed delayed but persistent pain that continued for over 30 days. Similarly, this group also showed increased depressive-like behaviors 10 days after infection. Since stress or infection alone did not cause these prolonged effects, these results suggest that chronic stress before the onset of symptoms may be a pre-onset factor, and infection may be a triggering factor, causing prolonged pain, depression, and fatigue. In addition, it has been reported that the increase in glucocorticoid concentration due to stress aggravates inflammation caused by lipopolysaccharide (LPS) (Sorrells et al., 2009), suggesting that stress may cause chronic inflammation and increased tactile hypersensitivity via the HPA axis.

The results of this experiment revealed that although stress or infection alone does not cause the disease, the interaction between stress and infection causes long-lasting pain, depression, and fatigue. Furthermore, these symptoms could be suppressed by administering glucocorticoid receptor antagonists or minocycline (which suppresses microglial activity in the brain) in advance, suggesting that these symptoms are caused by the interaction between stress and infection, which causes chronic inflammation in the brain via the HPA axis and immune system. It has also been reported that when LPS is administered when glucocorticoid levels are elevated due to stress, inflammation is exacerbated compared with LPS administration without stress (Sorrells et al., 2009). In this way, the interaction between psychological factors and physical factors such as infection may cause CFS through the endocrine, immune, and nervous systems, and affect the subsequent course of the disease. In the future, elucidating these mechanisms is expected to be of great help in understanding the pathology of mind–body correlation in various stress-related diseases

3. THE NEURAL BASIS OF MIND-BODY INTERACTION: MIND-BODY CORRELATION REVEALED BY NEUROSCIENCE

The following reports have been published about brain regions related to psychiatric and physical symptoms. In particular, the anterior cingulate cortex and insular cortex have been found to be related in all reports, which shows that they are key brain regions for the neural basis of the interaction between the mind and the body.

3.1 Brain Changes Associated With Psychiatric Symptoms

A meta-analysis of brain changes common to psychiatric disorders has reported that the volume of the anterior cingulate cortex and insular cortex is reduced, and that the functional connectivity between the anterior cingulate cortex and insular cortex is strong (Goodkind et al., 2015). Functional connectivity indicates that brain activity, as demonstrated by blood oxygen level-dependent signal (BOLD signal), between distant brain regions is correlated. For example, even if brain regions A and B are located far apart, their brain activity may be synchronized, and the degree of correlation can be quantified as the degree of functional connectivity. When the brain activities of distant regions (A and B in Figure 4) are correlated, it is said that there is functional connectivity, which is distinguished from anatomical connectivity (connection of nerve fibers). In other words, when brain activity in separate areas A and B is correlated, these areas are considered to be functionally connected, regardless of whether they are directly connected or connected via another brain area.

Figure 4. Example of Functional Connectivity.

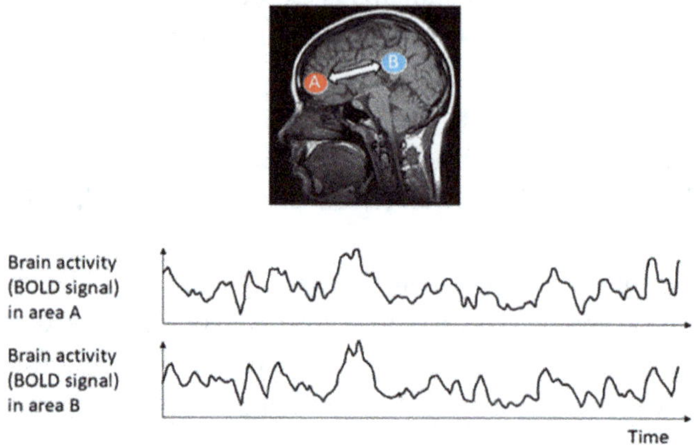

When brain activity in distant regions (A and B in the figure) correlates, it is said to have functional connectivity, which is distinct from anatomical connectivity (connection of nerve fibers).

3.2. Changes in the Brain Related to the Autonomic Nervous System

Note. This section draws on Yoshihara and Sudo (2016).

Activation of the sympathetic nervous system is essential for dealing with stress, such as fearful stimuli. When the sympathetic nervous system is activated, blood pressure and heart rate increase, increasing blood flow to skeletal muscles, while peripheral blood vessels contract, causing a decrease in peripheral body temperature and an increase in core body temperature, allowing people to move more agilely in stressful situations (Kistler et al., 1998; Kreibig et al., 2007; Krumhansl, 1997; Rimm-Kaufman & Kagan, 1996). When a frightening situation is encountered, the amygdala is the first brain structure to be activated, triggering these stress responses (Phan et al., 2002; Phan et al., 2004). The general mechanism of sympathetic nervous responses to fearful stimuli is thought to be that the amygdala, which is involved in fearful emotions, transmits information to the hypothalamus and brainstem—the centers of autonomic nervous function—causing a sympathetic response (Nolte, 2009; Rodrigues et al., 2009). Animal experiments have confirmed that electrical stimulation of the amygdala can cause a sympathetic response (Nolte, 2009). Furthermore, sympathetic nervous activity can be induced not only by electrical stimulation of the amygdala, but also by electrical stimulation of the anterior cingulate cortex and insular cortex (Pool & Ransohoff, 1949; Yasui et al., 1991).

Brain imaging research to elucidate these brain mechanisms began with functional brain mapping research to investigate the function of certain brain regions and to isolate and extract brain regions specialized for a given function. However, brain functions are not limited to a single brain region but are performed by several regions forming a network. Therefore, in order to clarify how information is exchanged between distant brain regions connected by nerve fiber connections, it has become important to investigate the degree of correlation (functional connectivity) in brain activity patterns between distant brain regions. Elucidating sympathetic nervous activity induced by fear stimuli by analyzing this functional connectivity is useful for understanding the brain network system in which emotional stress affects the body via the sympathetic nervous system.

Previous human brain imaging studies have shown that activity in the anterior cingulate cortex and anterior insular cortex is related to sympathetic nervous activity during cognitive task performance (Critchley et al., 2000; Critchley et al., 2003). Because the anterior cingulate cortex and anterior insular cortex are activated by fearful stimuli, these brain regions are likely to be the connection areas that link fear emotion and sympathetic nervous activity. It is therefore suggested that information about fearful stimuli is transmitted from the amygdala to the autonomic nervous center via the anterior cingulate cortex and anterior insular cortex. In particular, the anterior cingulate cortex has been reported to be involved in the recognition and control of emotions (Devinsky et al., 1995), so it is thought that the functional connectivity between the amygdala and the anterior cingulate cortex plays an important role in the relationship between fear and the sympathetic nervous system. However, the neural basis for the sympathetic nervous activity response to fearful stimuli had not been fully elucidated.

Therefore, Yoshihara and colleagues used functional magnetic resonance imaging (MRI) to investigate brain activity and brain networks related to fear-induced sympathetic nervous activity in 32 healthy subjects while they watched a horror movie and a control movie for approximately 10 minutes each. During MRI imaging, changes in fingertip temperature (peripheral body temperature) were measured as an index of sympathetic nervous response. After MRI imaging, the subjects watched the movies again and rated the degree of fear from 1 (not at all) to 9 (maximum) every 3 seconds.

As a result, a significant negative correlation was found between the degree of fear and the rate of change in fingertip temperature, and the anterior cingulate cortex and insular cortex were identified as brain regions related to sympathetic nervous activity, as indexed by the rate of change in fingertip temperature (Figure 5). In addition, the amygdala was activated in proportion to the degree of fear, and an analysis of functional connectivity between brain regions showed that the functional connectivity between the amygdala and anterior cingulate cortex, and between the amygdala and insular cortex, was stronger when participants watched a horror movie compared to when they watched a control movie. Furthermore, the greater the degree of fear, the stronger the functional connectivity between the left amygdala and anterior cingulate cortex. These results suggest that the greater the degree of fear, the stronger the functional connectivity from the left amygdala to the anterior cingulate cortex, which regulates the sympathetic nervous system.

Figure 5. Brain Areas Related to the Autonomic Nervous System.

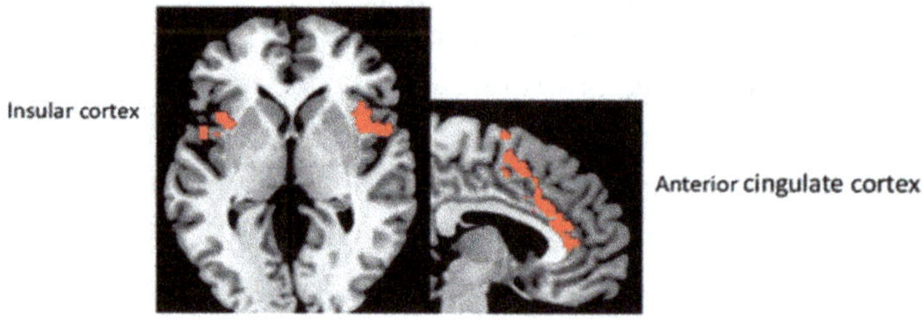

Brain regions correlated with sympathetic nerve activity (rate of change in peripheral body temperature).

3.3 Pain-Related Changes in the Brain

Pain is classified into two types: pain as a sensation (sensory aspect) and pain as an emotion (emotional aspect). A review of brain functions related to pain has reported that the primary and secondary somatosensory cortex and the posterior insular cortex are related to the sensory aspect of pain, and the anterior cingulate cortex and anterior insular cortex are related to the emotional aspect of pain (Eisenberger, 2012).

3.4 Brain Changes Associated With Social Distress

The anterior cingulate cortex and insular cortex are involved in social pain, which is the distress caused by being isolated from society or being unable to engage in social activities. A correlation has been found between social distress and activity in the anterior cingulate cortex (Eisenberger et al., 2004).

3.5 Psychosomatic Correlation of Bronchial Asthma

Recently, the psychological effects of human bronchial asthma have also been studied using brain imaging. Rosenkranz et al. measured the forced expiratory volume in one second and brain activity using functional MRI 1 and 4 hours after inhalation of saline, methacholine, or an antigen in asthmatic patients, and measured the number of eosinophils in sputum 24 hours after inhalation. The image stimulus task used during MRI imaging consisted of 10 randomly presented words from three categories: asthma-related words (20 such as "asthma"), negative words (20 such as "loneliness"), and neutral words (20 such as "curtain"), created in one of four colors: blue, yellow, green, and red, each presented for 2 seconds with an interval of 8–12 seconds. Subjects were instructed to press a button of the same color as the word. As a result, it has been reported that changes in brain activity in the anterior cingulate cortex and insular cortex due to stimulation with "asthma-related words" after exposure to allergens in asthma patients were related to changes in the percentage of eosinophils in sputum and forced expiratory volume in one second.

Brain imaging studies in humans have reported that autonomic nervous activity is related to higher centers such as the anterior cingulate cortex and insular cortex (Critchley et al., 2000; Critchley et al., 2003; Critchley et al., 2005), and it has also been suggested that activity of the anterior cingulate cortex is related to inflammation and behavior (Capuron et al., 2005). Anatomically, it has been reported that neurons in the anterior cingulate cortex project to the hypothalamus and brainstem, which are centers of homeostasis and autonomic nervous function (An et al., 1998; Öngür et al., 1998). It has also been suggested that the insular cortex plays an important role in monitoring the internal state of the body and maintaining homeostasis (Craig, 2002; Critchley et al., 2004). These reports suggest that activity in the anterior cingulate cortex and insular cortex may be related to changes in the autonomic nervous system and increased airway inflammation and hyperresponsiveness due to the interaction between allergens and asthma-related stress stimuli. Thus, brain imaging research is likely to be a useful tool for elucidating the pathology of the mind–body correlation in bronchial asthma.

4. PROCEDURES FOR EVALUATION AND TREATMENT OF PSYCHOSOMATIC DISORDERS

Excessive stress leads to mental and physical disorders, and causes stress-related illnesses such as psychosomatic disorders. Since various stresses affect physical symptoms via the endocrine, immune, and nervous systems, it is highly likely that symptoms of stress-related illnesses worsen through the accumulation and interaction of these stresses. Therefore, it is important to evaluate the pathological condition of both the mind and body in stress-related illnesses such as psychosomatic disorders and provide treatment according to the condition.

4.1 Classification of Psychosomatic Disorders

Psychological factors affect physical illnesses by altering not only the central nervous system, but also the autonomic nervous system, immune system, and endocrine system. Conversely, biological changes caused by physical illness also affect psychological states, so there is a two-way interaction between the mind and the body. When diagnosing psychosomatic disorders in Japan, the focus is on the unidirectional effect of the psychological state on the body. If this is defined as psychosomatic disorder in the narrow sense, psychosomatic disorders in the broad sense can be classified into three categories in the Japanese medical context, though this classification is not universally accepted internationally (Yoshihara et al., 2008). These three categories are not unrelated to each other but are interrelated.

Category 1: *A group in which stress causes the onset, recurrence, worsening, or persistence of a physical illness (psychosomatic disorder in the narrow sense).* This is the case when psychosocial stress is one of the factors that worsens or develops a physical illness. Changes in life events (birth, marriage, divorce, moving, employment, job change, continuing education, illness or death of a close relative, etc.) and stress in daily life (problems with interpersonal relationships at home, work, or school; burdens of study or work; etc.) precede the onset or recurrence of the disease. There is also a close relationship between psychological states (anxiety, tension, anger, depression, etc.) and the exacerbation or remission of symptoms.

Category 2: *Those experiencing psychological distress or social dysfunction due to physical illness—a category that represents a causal direction opposite to the narrow definition of psychosomatic disorders, yet is included within the broad sense.* Among physical illnesses, chronic illnesses such as bronchial asthma, atopic dermatitis, rheumatoid arthritis, and ulcerative colitis can be difficult to predict for improvement, and therefore involve a large physical, mental, and economic burden in treatment. These conditions can cause significant psychological distress and impaired social and occupational functioning in patients, making them candidates for psychosomatic treatment. Symptoms include sleep disorders, avoidance or social withdrawal from social situations, impaired academic and work performance, depressed mood, and anxiety.

Category 3: *Psychosocial factors that impede the treatment and management of physical illnesses.* In cases of bronchial asthma, atopic dermatitis, and autoimmune diseases, there is irrational anxiety and fear about steroid therapy and other drugs and procedures, a sense of powerlessness in controlling symptoms, and strong distrust in medical care and medical professionals. In such cases, psychosocial factors can cause poor adherence to physicians' prescriptions and instructions, preventing appropriate treatment and management of physical illnesses and significantly affecting treatment and progression.

4.2 Pathological Assessment of Psychosomatic Disorders

4.2.1 Pre-Onset Factor

A pre-onset factor is a factor that does not immediately cause a disease but creates conditions that make it easy for a disease to occur when various triggering factors are added. Psychological pre-onset factors include the conscious or unconscious suppression of negative emotions (repression), the difficulty in identifying or expressing emotions (alexithymia), and the continued effort to adapt more than necessary to meet the expectations of others (over-adaptation).

4.2.2 Triggering Factor

A triggering factor is an acquired factor that, when added to the pre-onset state, makes the disease manifest. Psychological triggering factors include strong emotions such as anxiety, anger, and sadness, which are thought to cause acute reactions in the body's nervous, immune, and endocrine systems. Keeping in mind that clinical symptoms will not become apparent even if triggering factors are present when the pre-onset state is eliminated, it is important in treatment not to focus excessively on triggering factors but instead to work to eliminate pre-onset factors.

4.2.3 Persistent and Aggravating Factors

Persistent or aggravating factors are acquired factors that act to sustain or aggravate a disease once it has been caused. In particular, there are many cases where problems at home, work, or school serve in this role.

4.3 Procedures for Treating Psychosomatic Disorders

Treatment that takes into account psychosocial factors has been systematized by Ago and summarized in an easy-to-understand five-stage treatment format (Ago, 2009).

Stage 1: *Establishing a therapeutic relationship and motivation for treatment.* Because patients may be resistant to psychological issues, physical examinations and treatments are performed to alleviate or eliminate physical symptoms as quickly as possible, building a trusting relationship between the patient and the doctor. At the same time, a detailed medical history is taken and the onset and progression of symptoms are examined from both the mental and physical perspectives, which can help patients realize the importance of a mind–body perspective and motivate them to undergo psychosomatic treatment. For patients who do not comply with treatment, it is important to listen carefully to the patient's concerns and reasons for non-adherence without criticizing them, and to explain things carefully again after understanding the patient's feelings.

Stage 2: *Experience of relaxation and relief of symptoms.* If the patient's environment is stressful, hospitalization may be necessary if circumstances permit, placing them in a state where they can relax both physically and mentally. If the patient is an outpatient, the environment is adjusted as much as possible. They may also be trained in relaxation techniques such as autogenic training (described below). Furthermore, through interviews, they are encouraged to express the frustration and negative emotions they have been suppressing, and empathic understanding is shown to help release internal tension. If there is severe sleep disorder, anxiety, depression, or physical complaints, drug therapy with sleeping pills, anti-anxiety drugs, or antidepressants is administered. As a result, the patient's motivation for treatment is often increased by experiencing a reduction or disappearance of physical symptoms and a reduced likelihood of recurrence.

Stage 3: *Understanding the mind–body correlation and reexamining adaptive patterns.* Focus is placed on the external factors that tend to cause symptoms and the patient's own patterns of thinking and behavior. By doing so, the patient can objectively view these patterns and realize that previous thoughts and behaviors have not necessarily been appropriate. From this stage, it is effective to use cognitive behavioral therapy (described below) or transactional analysis (described below).

Stage 4: *Acquiring better adaptive patterns.* Medical professionals—such as doctors and psychologists—support the patients in modifying the patterns of thinking and behavior that were related to the appearance or worsening of symptoms into more appropriate ones, or in acquiring new, more appropriate adaptive behaviors. When the patient is able to successfully acquire adaptive behaviors, they will often be able to see things objectively and from multiple perspectives, change from self-blaming or blaming thoughts to self-acceptance or acceptance of others, and become able to assert themselves appropriately.

Stage 5: *Gradual withdrawal of the therapeutic relationship.* Treatment can be terminated once it has been confirmed that more appropriate patterns of thinking and behavior have been acquired and that the gradual reduction or cessation of medication does not result in a recurrence or worsening of symptoms.

5. PSYCHOLOGICAL APPROACH (PRACTICAL METHODS THAT AFFECT THE MIND) - HEALING THE MIND AND REGAINING HEALTH

In Japan, psychosomatic therapy is defined as "a treatment method for psychosomatic patients that, based on a set treatment plan, clarifies the relationship between physical injuries and illnesses and psychological and social factors, and exerts a psychological influence on the patient, thereby improving symptoms or recovering from the injury or illness." This psychosomatic therapy includes autogenic training, counseling, behavioral therapy, hypnotherapy, biofeedback therapy, transactional analysis, Gestalt therapy, bioenergetic therapy, Morita therapy, fasting therapy, general psychotherapy, and simplified psychoanalytic therapy. The following sections briefly explain the main psychosomatic therapies: autogenic training, cognitive behavioral therapy, transactional analysis, and other psychotherapies.

5.1 Autonomic Training Method

Autogenic training is one of the relaxation techniques used in Japanese psychosomatic medicine. In a relaxed state, the hands and feet feel heavy and warm. This method leads the mind and body to a relaxed state by repeating phrases such as "both my hands and feet feel heavy" and "both my hands and feet are warm." Examples of phrases include the background formula "I feel calm," the first formula "both my hands and feet feel heavy," and the second formula "both my hands and feet are warm." Autogenic training is said to have effects such as reducing tension and anxiety, recovering from fatigue, improving concentration, reducing impulsive behavior, and easing physical pain and mental distress.

5.2 Cognitive Behavioral Therapy

Behavioral therapy is a behavioral modification technique based on learning theory, and includes treatments such as exposure therapy and systematic desensitization. Recently, it has been integrated with cognitive therapy and is often called cognitive behavioral therapy. Cognitive therapy is a therapeutic technique that helps patients realize that there are several adaptive and realistic thoughts (adaptive thoughts) that emerge from objectively viewing a situation or viewing it from multiple perspectives when negative emotions arise due to automatic thoughts in a certain situation (*What is Cognitive Therapy?*, 2025). This adaptive thinking often reduces negative emotions. Treatment may also be performed using mindfulness—intentionally focusing attention on the experience of the present moment, without evaluation, and simply observing in a state of detachment (*Japan Mindfulness Association*, 2025).

5.3 Transactional Analysis

Note. This section draws on What is Transactional Analysis? (2025).

Transactional analysis is a psychotherapy that has a dynamic perspective based on psychoanalysis, focuses on observable behavior, and analyzes "interactions between people." There are four basic theories of transactional analysis: structural analysis, interaction pattern analysis, game analysis, and script analysis. In interactions between people, there are stimuli (strokes) such as conversation and contact; positive words and actions such as encouragement and praise are called positive strokes, and negative words and actions are called negative strokes.

In structural analysis, ego states (ways of being) are classified into parent ego states (P), adult ego states (A), and child ego states (C), and P is further divided into critical parents (CP) and protective parents (NP), and C is divided into free children (FC) and adaptive children (AC). The egogram is a questionnaire that measures the amount of mental energy in these ego states; by informing patients of the results, patients can objectively view their ego states, become aware of them, and may be motivated to change their behavior. Exchange pattern analysis (analyzing the exchange patterns between each ego state of oneself and the other person) can serve as an opportunity to improve inappropriate behavior patterns in patients' communication. Furthermore, inappropriate communication that has become habitual, and words and actions that make people feel bad (negative strokes), are called "games." Game analysis allows people to become aware of these games and stop them to learn appropriate communication. Many of these negative stroke interactions are based on the life scripts people write as children, so script analysis helps them to let go of these negative scripts and build closer relationships with positive stroke interactions.

Forgiving oneself and others ("I'm OK, You are OK") is also said to lead to stress reduction. People with high AC (over-adaptation) often find it difficult to refuse when asked or invited by others, so assertiveness training can be effective. Assertiveness training is "understanding and respecting the other person's feelings and opinions before conveying your own."

5.4 Other Psychological Therapies

In addition to the above, Japanese Naikan therapy may also be used as a form of psychotherapy. Naikan therapy is said to promote inner growth by introspecting along three introspection items (things one has received help from, things one has repaid, and things one has been a nuisance about), realizing one's own "self-centered way of life" and "the fact that one has lived a life of being loved," and reaffirming one's sense of security and basic trust in others (Yoshihara, 2009). In addition, if the relationship with family is thought to be related to the pathology, a family interview may be conducted

6. NEURAL BASIS OF PSYCHOLOGICAL APPROACHES (PRACTICES THAT AFFECT THE MIND) – NEUROPLASTICITY THROUGH PSYCHOTHERAPY

Psychological approaches are used to improve the physical and mental symptoms of patients with psychosomatic disorders. However, little is known about what happens in the patient's brain when a psychological approach improves physical and mental symptoms. The following sections introduce active listening—the basis of psychological approaches—and changes in the brain caused by mindfulness.

6.1 Changes in the Brain Caused by Active Listening

Note. This section draws on Kawamichi et al. (2015).

Active listening is defined as empathic understanding, unconditional positive regard, and behavior consistent with it (Rogers, 1959). Being listened to has also been shown to have a positive effect on future behavior (Rogers, 1959). Active listening is a fundamental technique in psychotherapy, and it is known that active listening can bring about personality changes (Duan & Hill, 1996; Gladstein, 1977) and improve impressions of the experiences discussed (Rogers, 1957). By being listened to, a person feels that the other party is interested in them (Rogers, 1959), and such positive social interactions are thought to be rewarding (Baumeister & Leary, 1995). Therefore, Kawamichi et al. (2015) used functional MRI to investigate changes in brain activity and impressions of the contents of the conversation and the other person when subjects were listened to and not listened to.

Twenty-two right-handed healthy subjects were asked to talk about their experiences, which involved positive or negative emotions, for at least 20 seconds in front of a video camera on the first day. Before the experiment began, videos were created in which 10 evaluators (actors) acted out six different attitudes, one in which they listened attentively and the other in which they did not listen attentively. The subjects were told that the evaluators would watch a video of them speaking, and when they came back later, they were shown a video of the evaluators listening attentively or not listening attentively in an MRI machine, while hearing their own voice from the previous recording. After that, the subjects were asked to indicate their impression of the story they had told using a visual analog scale (VAS), with the left end being negative and the right end being positive.

As a result, when someone listened to them attentively, activity in the ventral striatum (reward system) and insular cortex increased compared to when they were not listened to. In addition, when someone listened to them attentively, their impression of the experience they shared changed to a more positive one. Furthermore, when someone listened to them attentively, their impression of the other person improved compared to when they were not listened to, and they felt a stronger desire to collaborate.

6.2 Changes in the Brain Caused by Mindfulness

A meta-analysis of brain imaging studies before and after mindfulness-based stress management and cognitive therapy reported increased brain activity and brain volume in the anterior cingulate cortex and insular cortex after treatment (Gotink et al., 2016; Manuello et al., 2016).

6.3 Brain Changes Common to Psychological Approaches

It is thought that psychosomatic therapies such as cognitive therapy using active listening and mentalization, and mindfulness, act on the anterior cingulate cortex and insular cortex—brain areas related to mental and physical symptoms—and may improve the mental and physical symptoms of psychosomatic patients. In other words, it is speculated that psychosomatic therapies induce structural and functional changes in the patient's brain (anterior cingulate cortex and insular cortex), and that mental and physical symptoms improve through these changes in the brain.

7. SOMATIC APPROACHES (PRACTICES THAT WORK ON THE BODY) - AWAKENING HEALTH THROUGH WORKING WITH THE BODY

Commonly used psychotherapy is a psychological approach that affects the body from the mind. On the other hand, yoga and qigong are physical approaches that affect the mind from the body, and since they do not directly intervene in psychological matters, they can often be relatively easily introduced to patients who believe that their physical symptoms are not related to psychological factors. However, yoga and qigong require patients to actively continue practicing, including at home, so it is necessary to motivate them for treatment in advance. By continuing to practice yoga or qigong, patients often become able to control their physical and mental symptoms themselves.

The following sections present evidence on the effects of yoga and qigong on the mind and body, as well as their therapeutic effects and adverse events, and introduce the yoga practiced at the Department of Psychosomatic Medicine at Kyushu University Hospital.

7.1 History of Yoga and Qigong

7.1.1 History of Yoga

Note. This section draws on Overview of Yoga (2025).

The origins of yoga are unknown, but it is believed to have arisen in ancient India around 300 BC as a religious training method. In the 11th century, Hatha Yoga developed and physical movements were introduced. In the first half of the 20th century, several Indian yogis introduced Hatha Yoga to the West, and it also began to be practiced in Japan. Much of the yoga practiced today is aimed at improving physical and mental health, with no religious elements in place.

7.1.2 The History of Qigong

Note. This section draws on Ma and Akira (1990).

The origins of qigong are similarly unclear, but there are records from around 200 BC indicating that it originated from the movements of an ancient dance. The *Huangdi Neijing* also contains a description of Doin (a dynamic or static training method involving moving the limbs, training the breath, and self-massage), which is thought to be similar to modern qigong. There are two types of qigong: internal qigong, which involves controlling the "qi" (energy that circulates through the body and has some kind of function), and external qigong, which aims to use "qi" taken in from the outside to affect the outside world. Internal qigong is used in medical treatment and is recognized as a health regimen.

7.2 Components of Yoga and Qigong

7.2.1 Components of Yoga

Yoga consists of three main components: postures (asanas), breathing techniques (pranayama), and meditation (Table 2). Yoga has numerous postures (asanas), and simple postures are equivalent to gentle stretching. Breathing techniques (pranayama) are generally considered to involve slow, deep abdominal breathing. Meditation used in yoga is similar to mindfulness, which is defined as awareness that arises by paying attention to the present without judgment or evaluation.

Table 2. Components of yoga and qigong

Components of Yoga	Components of Qigong
Pose (Asana)	Adjustment of posture and certain movements
Breathing exercises (Pranayama)	Breath control (breathing regulation)
Meditation	Attunement (not being distracted by distracting thoughts)

Note. Components adapted from Ma and Akira (1990) for qigong and from *Overview of Yoga* (2025) for yoga.

7.2.2 Components of Qigong

Note. This section draws on Ma and Akira (1990).

Qigong is made up of three elements: adjusting the body by adjusting posture and certain movements, adjusting the breath, and adjusting the mind by not being distracted by distracting thoughts (Table 2). Internal Qigong can be divided into static Qigong, which does not involve physical movement, and dynamic Qigong, which involves physical movement. In static Qigong, the body is adjusted by sitting, lying down, or standing, while in dynamic Qigong, movements include bending and straightening the limbs, rotating, and bending forward and backward. Breath adjustment includes breathing techniques such as natural breathing and abdominal breathing. In static Qigong, breathing is done according to the situation, while in dynamic Qigong, breathing is synchronized with movement. In both types, the mind is adjusted by focusing attention and not being distracted by distracting thoughts

7.3 Effects of Yoga and Qigong

Several effects of yoga and qigong have been reported regarding improvements in physiological indicators such as the nervous, immune, and endocrine systems. In addition, there is not much high-quality evidence on the therapeutic effects of yoga and qigong for specific diseases. Yoga has been shown to improve moods such as anxiety and depression, and to reduce stress. Yoga and qigong have also been shown to improve pain, fatigue, insomnia, and quality of life (QOL). They are also useful as a means of disease prevention and self-control.

7.3.1 Effects of Yoga on the Nervous System

A meta-analysis of studies examining whether differences in brain morphology can be seen in people who practice meditation—one of the components of yoga—showed that the volume of the anterior cingulate cortex, middle cingulate cortex, orbitofrontal cortex, and insular cortex was larger (Fox et al., 2014). The anterior cingulate cortex and insular cortex are important brain regions related to psychosomatic symptoms and psychosomatic medicine therapy. It has also been shown that yoga increases parasympathetic nervous activity in patients with chronic fatigue (Oka et al., 2018).

7.3.2 Effects of Yoga and Qigong on the Immune System

Yoga and qigong have been reported to reduce inflammatory markers (Morgan et al., 2014). They have also been shown to downregulate gene expression involved in chronic stress-induced inflammatory responses (Buric et al., 2017).

7.3.3 Effects of Yoga on the Endocrine System

It has been reported that practicing yoga reduces blood and salivary cortisol levels in patients with chronic fatigue and breast cancer (Banasik et al., 2011; Oka et al., 2018).

7.3.4 Effects of Qigong on the Autonomic Nervous System and Immune System

Objective studies using topical Qigong have reported increased parasympathetic activity (suggesting relaxation) and enhanced natural killer (NK) cell activity (suggesting immune modulation). Anecdotal reports, such as the disappearance of viral warts after Qigong practice, further suggest possible physiological effects.

7.3.5 Improvement of Mood (Anxiety, Depression, Anger), Fatigue and Physical Symptoms

Several meta-analyses and recent randomized controlled trials have suggested that yoga may be effective as a monotherapy or add-on therapy for patients with unipolar major depression (*Overview of Yoga*, 2025). In a study of healthy subjects, 12 weeks of yoga improved not only anxiety, but also depression, anger, fatigue, and physical symptoms (Yoshihara et al., 2014). It was also shown that people who had been practicing yoga for more than two years had lower levels of anxiety, anger, and fatigue than those who had not practiced yoga (Yoshihara et al., 2011).

7.3.6 Stress Reduction and Improvement Of QOL

A study on people who were stressed showed that doing yoga for 10 weeks reduced stress (Smith et al., 2007). Yoga has also been shown to improve QOL, similar to mindfulness-based cognitive therapy and cognitive behavioral therapy (Grensman et al., 2018).

7.3.7 Pain Relief Effect

A 2012 meta-analysis showed that yoga is effective for pain (Büssing et al., 2012). In a randomized controlled trial of patients with fibromyalgia, eight weeks of yoga improved pain, fatigue, mood, and pain catastrophizing (Carson et al., 2010). At a three-month follow-up, many of the improvements from yoga were sustained, with those who practiced yoga more experiencing greater improvement (Carson et al., 2012). In addition, a systematic review of the effects of qigong on patients with fibromyalgia found improvements in pain, quality of life, sleep quality, and fatigue (Lauche et al., 2013).

7.3.8 Improvement of Hypertension

A meta-analysis of the effects of yoga on hypertensive patients reported that it lowered systolic blood pressure by 5 mmHg and diastolic blood pressure by 4 mmHg (Park et al., 2017). The blood pressure lowering effect was greater in patients under 60 years of age.

7.3.9 Other Improvement Effects

Numerous reviews have shown that qigong is effective in improving anxiety, depression, sleep quality, fatigue, and quality of life in a variety of populations, including people with fibromyalgia, cancer, and chronic fatigue syndrome (CFS), students, and healthy adults.

7.4 Adverse Events

7.4.1 Adverse Events From Yoga in the United States

Note. This section draws on Swain and McGwin (2016).

A U.S. survey found that 0.6% of people who practiced yoga reported adverse events that led to discontinuation of practice, 0.2% required medical attention, and 0.01% visited an emergency department. The frequency of adverse events due to yoga was not different from that of other similar levels of exercise. However, since adverse events have been reported more frequently in the elderly and those with illnesses or injuries, caution is advised when introducing yoga to the elderly and patients.

7.4.2 Adverse Events Associated With Yoga in Japan

Note. This section draws on Guide to the Use of Yoga for Stress-Related Illnesses for Medical Professionals (2025).

In a Japanese survey, 28% of participants reported adverse events during a single yoga class. The most common symptoms were musculoskeletal (muscle pain, joint pain, etc.), nervous (dizziness, numbness, faintness, heavy head), and respiratory (cough, nasal congestion, runny nose) symptoms. Sixty-four percent of participants who reported adverse events had minor symptoms, but 2% of participants (0.6% of the total) discontinued practice due to pain, darkness in front of their eyes, cough, dizziness, or feeling unwell.

7.5 Treatment Practice

Since the 1970s, the Department of Psychosomatic Medicine at Kyushu University has incorporated yoga, qigong, and tai chi into its treatment. Basically, a yoga or qigong instructor is in charge of treatment, separate from the attending physician. Currently, yoga is offered to inpatients or outpatients of the Department of Psychosomatic Medicine twice a month, one-on-one for 20–30 minutes by an instructor with over 30 years of yoga experience, without background music, in a soundproof room in the outpatient building.

7.5.1 Adaptation

Yoga treatment has relatively few adverse events, so it can be used for a variety of illnesses, except when rest and relaxation are necessary. Many of the patients who have been introduced to yoga in our department are those with chronic fatigue, chronic pain, depression, anxiety, and insomnia, for which yoga has been shown to have a certain degree of therapeutic effect. However, caution is required when meditating, as even healthy people may experience auditory and visual hallucinations.

As a rule, it is more effective to start yoga after symptoms have subsided to a certain extent. Since yoga may temporarily worsen symptoms such as pain and anxiety, it is advisable to inform the patient of this possibility in advance. The content of yoga needs to be individually adjusted to suit the symptoms and characteristics of each patient. For example, for patients who are very tired, yoga can be changed to one that can be done while sitting or lying down, or isometric yoga (in which poses are performed while maintaining the same posture and putting stress on certain muscles), so as not to worsen fatigue. In addition, for patients with pain, yoga postures can sometimes worsen pain, so yoga should be performed in a posture that does not increase pain.

Yoga and qigong have relatively few adverse events, but difficult poses and postures should be avoided. Even simple poses and postures can cause adverse events, so they should be performed under the supervision of a skilled instructor.

7.5.2 Sharing Information on Implementation and Implementation Status

Before introducing yoga, the doctor must establish a good patient–physician relationship. Once the doctor decides to introduce yoga, he or she creates a yoga application form in the electronic medical record that includes the patient's information (ID, name, age, diagnosis, main symptoms and problems) and specific treatment goals, requests, and precautions, and gives the printed form to the yoga instructor. The yoga instructor begins yoga lessons based on this information. The patient is instructed to record their home practice on a yoga record sheet, on which they are instructed to write (freely) the date and time, the time and number of times yoga was performed, the content of yoga, the location and posture of yoga, the effects (choose from three options: +, ±, −), physical reactions during practice, psychological reactions, and any physical or psychological changes or sensations that occurred during practice, including reactions unrelated to yoga.

The yoga instructor reads and comments on the contents of the yoga record sheet. The yoga record sheet is also reviewed by the patient's doctor to check the effects of yoga, adverse events, and treatment status.

7.6 Summary of Physical Approaches (Yoga and Qigong)

Both yoga and qigong are known to have a relaxing effect on the mind and body. The three elements that yoga and qigong have in common—taking a fixed posture, regulating breathing, and not being distracted by distracting thoughts—may calm the state of the brain by feeling one's own body, focusing on breathing, balancing the autonomic nervous system, and reducing rumination.

In treatment, patients can relax and easily reflect on themselves in a state conducive to self-reflection, which often leads to realizations and insights. For example, asking about the patient's psychosocial background while they are practicing yoga or qigong can provide an opportunity to realize that their childhood relationship with their parents is affecting their current relationships. In this way, yoga and qigong can be a trigger or clue for treatment, and can help progress in cases where treatment has reached a deadlock with conventional psychotherapy.

For psychosomatic patients with physical symptoms, therapies that approach the body, such as yoga and qigong, may act on the insular cortex in the brain by focusing attention on bodily sensations and movements, and may also affect emotions. Further research is needed to clarify the detailed mechanisms by which yoga and qigong improve mental and physical symptoms.

8. CONCLUSION

This chapter has examined the concept of mind–body interaction, various techniques for working with the mind and body, and their neural basis. The relationship between the mind and body, which can be viewed from different perspectives such as mind–body correlation, mind–body oneness, and psychosomatic disorders, is gradually becoming clearer through modern neuroscience research in terms of its biological mechanisms. The effects of approaches to the mind and body on the brain, changes in the autonomic and endocrine systems, and the processes by which they interrelate provide scientific support for the ancient intuitive understanding of the unity of mind and body. In particular, the concept of neuroplasticity suggests that mind–body techniques can bring about lasting healing through structural and functional changes in the brain, rather than merely a temporary effect.

Future research is expected to optimize mind–body approaches that take into account individual differences and cultural backgrounds, develop integrated approaches that combine multiple techniques, and create new intervention methods based on neuroscientific knowledge. Advances in digital technology are also making it possible to monitor brain activity in real time and provide individualized intervention programs. The relationship between the mind and the body is important not only for the treatment of disease, but also for health promotion and preventive medicine. It is hoped that the findings outlined in this chapter will contribute to the development and practice of mind–body medicine.

REFERENCES

Ago, Y. (2009). Treatment of psychosomatic disorders—overview. [in Japanese] In Kubo, C. (Ed.), *Standard textbook of psychosomatic medicine* (3rd ed., pp. 238–245). Igaku-Shoin.

Amore, M., Antonella, C., Bettini, E., Boracchia, L., Innamorati, M., Montali, A., Parisoli, C., Pisi, R., Ramponi, S., & Chetta, A. (2013). Disease control in patients with asthma is associated with alexithymia but not with depression or anxiety. *Behavioral Medicine (Washington, D.C.), 39*(4), 138–145. https://www.tandfonline.com/doi/10.1080/08964289.2013.818931 PMID: 24236811

An, X., Bandler, R., Öngür, D., & Price, J. L. (1998). Prefrontal cortical projections to longitudinal columns in the midbrain periaqueductal gray in macaque monkeys. *The Journal of Comparative Neurology, 401*(4), 455–479. https://onlinelibrary.wiley.com/doi/10.1002/(SICI)1096-9861(19981130)401:4%3C455:AID-CNE3%3E3.0.CO;2-6 PMID: 9826273

Banasik, J., Williams, H., Haberman, M., Blank, S. E., & Bendel, R. (2011). Effect of Iyengar yoga practice on fatigue and diurnal salivary cortisol concentration in breast cancer survivors. *Journal of the American Academy of Nurse Practitioners, 23*(3), 135–142. DOI: 10.1111/j.1745-7599.2010.00573.x PMID: 21355946

Baumeister, R. F., & Leary, M. R. (1995). The need to belong: Desire for interpersonal attachments as a fundamental human motivation. *Psychological Bulletin, 117*(3), 497–529. DOI: 10.1037/0033-2909.117.3.497 PMID: 7777651

Buric, I., Farias, M., Jong, J., Mee, C., & Brazil, I. A. (2017). What is the molecular signature of mind–body interventions? A systematic review of gene expression changes induced by meditation and related practices. *Frontiers in Immunology, 8*, 670. Advance online publication. DOI: 10.3389/fimmu.2017.00670 PMID: 28670311

Büssing, A., Ostermann, T., Lüdtke, R., & Michalsen, A. (2012). Effects of yoga interventions on pain and pain-associated disability: A meta-analysis. *The Journal of Pain, 13*(1), 1–9. DOI: 10.1016/j.jpain.2011.10.001 PMID: 22178433

Capuron, L., Pagnoni, G., Demetrashvili, M., Woolwine, B. J., Nemeroff, C. B., Berns, G. S., & Miller, A. H. (2005). Anterior cingulate activation and error processing during interferon-alpha treatment. *Biological Psychiatry, 58*(3), 190–196. DOI: 10.1016/j.biopsych.2005.03.033 PMID: 16084839

Carson, J. W., Carson, K. M., Jones, K. D., Bennett, R. M., Wright, C. L., & Mist, S. D. (2010). A pilot randomized controlled trial of the Yoga of Awareness program in the management of fibromyalgia. *Pain, 151*(2), 530–539. DOI: 10.1016/j.pain.2010.08.020 PMID: 20946990

Carson, J. W., Carson, K. M., Jones, K. D., Mist, S. D., & Bennett, R. M. (2012). Follow-up of yoga of awareness for fibromyalgia: Results at 3 months and replication in the wait-list group. *The Clinical Journal of Pain, 28*(9), 804–813. DOI: 10.1097/AJP.0b013e31824549b5 PMID: 22751025

Chen, E., Fisher, E. B., Bacharier, L. B., & Strunk, R. C. (2003). Socioeconomic status, stress, and immune markers in adolescents with asthma. *Psychosomatic Medicine, 65*(6), 984–992. https://journals.lww.com/bsam/abstract/2003/11000/socioeconomic_status,_stress,_and_immune_markers.9.aspx PMID: 14645776

Chida, Y., Sudo, N., Sonoda, J., Hiramoto, T., & Kubo, C. (2007). Early-life psychological stress exacerbates adult mouse asthma via the hypothalamus-pituitary-adrenal axis. *American Journal of Respiratory and Critical Care Medicine, 175*(4), 316–322. DOI: 10.1164/rccm.200607-898OC PMID: 17110645

Chijiwa, T., Oka, T., Tominaga, M., Matsumura, S., Tsuzuki, S., Iida, H., & Fuchigami, T. (2015). Prior chronic stress induces persistent polyI:C-induced allodynia and depressive-like behavior in rats: Possible involvement of glucocorticoids and microglia. *Physiology & Behavior, 147*, 264–273. https://www.sciencedirect.com/science/article/abs/pii/S0031938415002577?via%3Dihub PMID: 25936823

Clauw, D. J. (2014). Fibromyalgia: A clinical review. *Journal of the American Medical Association, 311*(15), 1547–1555. DOI: 10.1001/jama.2014.3266 PMID: 24737367

Craig, A. D. (2002). How do you feel? Interoception: The sense of the physiological condition of the body. *Nature Reviews. Neuroscience, 3*(8), 655–666. DOI: 10.1038/nrn894 PMID: 12154366

Critchley, H. D., Corfield, D. R., Chandler, M. P., Mathias, C. J., & Dolan, R. J. (2000). Cerebral correlates of autonomic cardiovascular arousal: A functional neuroimaging investigation in humans. *The Journal of Physiology, 523*(Pt 1), 259–270. DOI: 10.1111/j.1469-7793.2000.t01-1-00259.x PMID: 10673560

Critchley, H. D., Mathias, C. J., Josephs, O., O'Doherty, J., Zanini, S., Dewar, B. K., Cipolotti, L., Shallice, T., & Dolan, R. J. (2003). Human cingulate cortex and autonomic control: Converging neuroimaging and clinical evidence. *Brain, 126*(Pt. 10), 2139–2152. DOI: 10.1093/brain/awg216 PMID: 12821513

Critchley, H. D., Tang, J., Smyth, S., Mathias, C. J., & Dolan, R. J. (2005). Anterior cingulate activity during error and autonomic response. *NeuroImage, 27*(4), 885–895. DOI: 10.1016/j.neuroimage.2005.05.047 PMID: 15996878

Critchley, H. D., Wiens, S., Rotshtein, P., Öhman, A., & Dolan, R. J. (2004). Neural systems supporting interoceptive awareness. *Nature Neuroscience, 7*(2), 189–195. DOI: 10.1038/nn1176 PMID: 14730305

Devinsky, O., Morrell, M. J., & Vogt, B. A. (1995). Contributions of anterior cingulate cortex to behaviour. *Brain, 118*(Pt 1), 279–306. DOI: 10.1093/brain/118.1.279 PMID: 7895011

Duan, C., & Hill, C. E. (1996). The current state of empathy research. *Journal of Counseling Psychology, 43*(3), 261–274. DOI: 10.1037/0022-0167.43.3.261

Eisenberger, N. I. (2012). The pain of social disconnection: Examining the shared neural underpinnings of physical and social pain. *Nature Reviews. Neuroscience, 13*(6), 421–434. DOI: 10.1038/nrn3231 PMID: 22551663

Eisenberger, N. I., Lieberman, M. D., & Williams, K. D. (2004). Why rejection hurts: A common neural alarm system for physical and social pain. *Trends in Cognitive Sciences, 8*(7), 294–300. DOI: 10.1016/j.tics.2004.05.010 PMID: 15242688

Fox, K. C. R., Nijeboer, S., Dixon, M. L., Floman, J. L., Ellamil, M., Rumak, S. P., Sedlmeier, P., & Christoff, K. (2014). Is meditation associated with altered brain structure? A systematic review and meta-analysis of morphometric neuroimaging in meditation practitioners. *Neuroscience and Biobehavioral Reviews, 43*, 48–73. DOI: 10.1016/j.neubiorev.2014.03.016 PMID: 24705269

Gladstein, G. A. (1977). Empathy and counseling outcome: An empirical and conceptual review. *The Counseling Psychologist, 6*(4), 70–79. 10.1177/001100007700600427

Goodkind, M., Eickhoff, S. B., Oathes, D. J., Jiang, Y., Chang, A., Jones-Hagata, L. B., Ortega, B. N., Zaiko, Y. V., Roach, E. L., Korgaonkar, M. S., Grieve, S. M., Galatzer-Levy, I., Fox, P. T., & Etkin, A. (2015). Identification of a common neurobiological substrate for mental illness. *JAMA Psychiatry, 72*(4), 305–315. DOI: 10.1001/jamapsychiatry.2014.2206 PMID: 25651064

Gotink, R. A., Meijboom, R., Vernooij, M. W., Smits, M., & Hunink, M. G. M. (2016). 8-week mindfulness based stress reduction induces brain changes similar to traditional long-term meditation practice—A systematic review. *Brain and Cognition, 108*, 32–41. DOI: 10.1016/j.bandc.2016.07.001 PMID: 27429096

Grensman, A., Acharya, B. D., Wändell, P., Nilsson, G. H., Falkenberg, T., Sundin, Ö., & Werner, S. (2018). Effect of traditional yoga, mindfulness-based cognitive therapy, and cognitive behavioral therapy, on health related quality of life: A randomized controlled trial on patients on sick leave because of burnout. *BMC Complementary and Alternative Medicine*, *18*(1), 80. Advance online publication. DOI: 10.1186/s12906-018-2141-9 PMID: 29510704

Guide to the use of yoga for stress-related illnesses for medical professionals [in Japanese]. (2025). Evidence-based Japanese Integrative Medicine Information Site. https://www.ejim.mhlw.go.jp/doc/pdf/y01.pdf

Han, Y. Y., Yan, Q., Forno, E., Cortez, M., & Celedón, J. C. (2022). Child maltreatment, anxiety and depression, and asthma among British adults in the UK Biobank. *The European Respiratory Journal*, *60*(4), 2103160. Advance online publication. DOI: 10.1183/13993003.03160-2021 PMID: 35301250

Japan Mindfulness Association [in Japanese]. (2025). https://mindfulness.smoosy.atlas.jp/ja

Jones, M. P., & Creed, E. (2013). A multidimensional model of psychobiological interactions in functional dyspepsia: A structural equation modelling approach. *Gut*, *62*(11), 1573–1580. DOI: 10.1136/gutjnl-2012-302741 PMID: 22917658

Katon, W. J., Richardson, L., Lozano, P., & McCauley, E. (2004). The relationship of asthma and anxiety disorders. *Psychosomatic Medicine*, *66*(3), 349–355. DOI: 10.1097/01.psy.0000126202.89941.2c PMID: 15184694

Kawamichi, H., Yoshihara, K., Sasaki, A. T., Sugawara, S. K., Tanabe, H. C., Shinohara, R., Sugisawa, Y., Tokutake, K., Mochizuki, Y., Anme, T., & Sadato, N. (2015). Perceiving active listening activates the reward system and improves the impression of relevant experiences. *Social Neuroscience*, *10*(1), 16–26. DOI: 10.1080/17470919.2014.954732 PMID: 25188354

Kick, L., Stegmann, S., Diedrich, A., & Galatzer-Levy, I. (2024). Alexithymia as a mediator between adverse childhood events and the development of psychopathology: A meta-analysis. *Frontiers in Psychiatry*, *15*, 1412229. https://www.frontiersin.org/journals/psychiatry/articles/10.3389/fpsyt.2024.1412229 PMID: 39011338

Kistler, A., Mariauzouls, C., & von Berlepsch, K. (1998). Fingertip temperature as an indicator for sympathetic responses. *International Journal of Psychophysiology*, *29*(1), 35–41. DOI: 10.1016/S0167-8760(97)00087-1 PMID: 9641246

Kreibig, S. D., Wilhelm, F. H., Roth, W. T., & Gross, J. J. (2007). Cardiovascular, electrodermal, and respiratory response patterns to fear- and sadness-inducing films. *Psychophysiology, 44*(5), 787–806. DOI: 10.1111/j.1469-8986.2007.00550.x PMID: 17598878

Krumhansl, C. L. (1997). An exploratory study of musical emotions and psychophysiology. *Canadian Journal of Experimental Psychology, 51*(4), 336–353. DOI: 10.1037/1196-1961.51.4.336 PMID: 9606949

Lauche, R., Cramer, H., Häuser, W., Dobos, G., & Langhorst, J. (2013). A systematic review and meta-analysis of qigong for the fibromyalgia syndrome. *Evidence-Based Complementary and Alternative Medicine : eCAM, 2013*, 635182. Advance online publication. DOI: 10.1155/2013/635182 PMID: 24288564

Ma, J., & Akira, K. (1990). *Chinese qigong studies.* Toyo Gakujutsu Shuppansha.

Manuello, J., Vercelli, U., Nani, A., Costa, T., & Cauda, F. (2016). Mindfulness meditation and consciousness: An integrative neuroscientific perspective. *Consciousness and Cognition, 40*, 67–78. DOI: 10.1016/j.concog.2015.12.005 PMID: 26752605

Morgan, N., Irwin, M. R., Chung, M., & Wang, C. (2014). The effects of mind–body therapies on the immune system: Meta-analysis. *PLoS One, 9*(7), e100903. Advance online publication. DOI: 10.1371/journal.pone.0100903 PMID: 24988414

Nagano, J., Kakuta, C., Motomura, C., Odajima, H., Sudo, N., Nishima, S., & Kubo, C. (2010). The parenting attitudes and the stress of mothers predict the asthmatic severity of their children: A prospective study. *BioPsychoSocial Medicine, 4*, 12. Advance online publication. DOI: 10.1186/1751-0759-4-12 PMID: 20929533

Niti, M., Ng, T. P., Mahendran, R., & Kua, E. H. (2007). Depressive disorder in older adults: The role of sub-threshold depression and neuroticism. *International Journal of Geriatric Psychiatry, 22*, 1040–1047. DOI: 10.1002/gps.1790

Nolte, J. (2009). *The human brain: An introduction to its functional anatomy* (6th ed.). Mosby/Elsevier.

Oka, T., Tanahashi, T., Chijiwa, T., Lkhagvasuren, B., Sudo, N., & Oka, K. (2018). Changes in fatigue, autonomic functions, and blood biomarkers due to sitting isometric yoga in patients with chronic fatigue syndrome. *BioPsychoSocial Medicine, 12*, 3. Advance online publication. DOI: 10.1186/s13030-018-0123-0 PMID: 29643935

Öngür, D., An, X., & Price, J. L. (1998). Prefrontal cortical projections to the hypothalamus in macaque monkeys. *The Journal of Comparative Neurology, 401*, 480–505. PMID: 9826274

Overview of yoga. (2025). UpToDate. https://www.uptodate.com/contents/overview-of-yoga

Park, S. H., Han, K. S., & Kang, C. B. (2017). Blood pressure response to meditation and yoga: A systematic review and meta-analysis. *Journal of Alternative and Complementary Medicine (New York, N.Y.)*, *23*(9), 685–695. DOI: 10.1089/acm.2016.0217 PMID: 28384004

Psychological factors affecting other medical conditions: Clinical features, assessment, and diagnosis. (2025). UpToDate. https://www.uptodate.com/contents/psychological-factors-affecting-other-medical-conditions-clinical-features-assessment-and-diagnosis

Phan, K. L., Wager, T., Taylor, S. F., & Liberzon, I. (2002). Functional neuroanatomy of emotion: A meta-analysis of emotion activation studies in PET and fMRI. *NeuroImage*, *16*(2), 331–348. DOI: 10.1006/nimg.2002.1087 PMID: 12030820

Phan, K. L., Wager, T. D., Taylor, S. F., & Liberzon, I. (2004). Functional neuroimaging studies of human emotions. *CNS Spectrums*, *9*(4), 258–266. DOI: 10.1017/s1092852900009196 PMID: 15048050

Pool, J. L., & Ransohoff, J. (1949). Autonomic effects on stimulating rostral portion of cingulate gyri in man. *Journal of Neurophysiology*, *12*(6), 385–392. DOI: 10.1152/jn.1949.12.6.385 PMID: 15408005

Prins, J. B., van der Meer, J. W. M., & Bleijenberg, G. (2006). Chronic fatigue syndrome. *Lancet*, *367*(9507), 346–355. DOI: 10.1016/S0140-6736(06)68073-2 PMID: 16443043

Rimm-Kaufman, S. E., & Kagan, J. (1996). The psychological significance of changes in skin temperature. *Motivation and Emotion*, *20*, 63–78. 10.1007/BF02251007

Rodrigues, S. M., LeDoux, J. E., & Sapolsky, R. M. (2009). The influence of stress hormones on fear circuitry. *Annual Review of Neuroscience*, *32*, 289–313. DOI: 10.1146/annurev.neuro.051508.135620 PMID: 19400714

Rogers, C. (1959). A theory of therapy, personality and interpersonal relationships as developed in the client-centered framework. In Koch, S. (Ed.), *Psychology: A study of a science* (Vol. 3). McGraw-Hill.

Rogers, C. R. (1957). The necessary and sufficient conditions of therapeutic personality change. *Journal of Consulting Psychology*, *21*(2), 95–103. DOI: 10.1037/h0045357 PMID: 13416422

Saygideger, Y., Özdemir, H., Ekinci, R. M. K., & Yücel, G. Y. (2022). Adulthood asthma as a consequence of childhood adversity: A systematic review of epigenetically affected genes. *Journal of Developmental Origins of Health and Disease, 13*(6), 674–682. DOI: 10.1017/S2040174422000058 PMID: 35256035

Scott, K. M., Von Korff, M., Alonso, J., Angermeyer, M. C., Bromet, E., Fayyad, J., de Girolamo, G., Demyttenaere, K., Gasquet, I., Gureje, O., Haro, J. M., He, Y., Kessler, R. C., Levinson, D., Medina Mora, M. E., Oakley Browne, M., Posada-Villa, J., Watanabe, M., Williams, D., & Karam, A. N. (2007). Mental disorders among adults with asthma: Results from the World Mental Health Survey. *General Hospital Psychiatry*, *29*(2), 123–133. DOI: 10.1016/j.genhosppsych.2006.12.006 PMID: 17336661

Sifneos, P. E. (1973). The prevalence of "alexithymic" characteristics in psychosomatic patients. *Psychotherapy and Psychosomatics*, *22*(2), 255–262. DOI: 10.1159/000286529 PMID: 4770536

Silvestro, O., Raffaele, L., & Vicario, C. M. (2023). Alexithymia and asthma: A systematic review. *Frontiers in Psychology*, *14*, 1221648. Advance online publication. DOI: 10.3389/fpsyg.2023.1221648 PMID: 37609491

Smith, C., Hancock, H., Blake-Mortimer, J., & Eckert, K. (2007). A randomised comparative trial of yoga and relaxation to reduce stress and anxiety. *Complementary Therapies in Medicine*, *15*(2), 77–83. DOI: 10.1016/j.ctim.2006.05.001 PMID: 17544857

Sorrells, S. F., Caso, J. R., Munhoz, C. D., & Sapolsky, R. M. (2009). The stressed CNS: When glucocorticoids aggravate inflammation. *Neuron*, *64*(1), 33–39. DOI: 10.1016/j.neuron.2009.09.032 PMID: 19840546

Swain, T. A., & McGwin, G. (2016). Yoga-related injuries in the United States from 2001 to 2014. *Orthopaedic Journal of Sports Medicine*, *4*(11), 2325967116671703. Advance online publication. DOI: 10.1177/2325967116671703 PMID: 27896293

VanderWeele, T. J. (2017). On the promotion of human flourishing. *Proceedings of the National Academy of Sciences of the United States of America*, *114*(31), 8148–8156. DOI: 10.1073/pnas.1702996114 PMID: 28705870

What is cognitive therapy? [in Japanese]. (2025). Japan Cognitive Therapy Association. https://jact.jp/introduction/

What is transactional analysis? [in Japanese]. (2025). Japan Transactional Analysis Association. http://www.js-ta.jp/analysis.html

Yasui, Y., Breder, C. D., Saper, C. B., & Cechetto, D. F. (1991). Autonomic responses and efferent pathways from the insular cortex in the rat. *The Journal of Comparative Neurology, 303*(3), 355–374. DOI: 10.1002/cne.903030303 PMID: 2007654

Ye, G., Baldwin, D. S., & Hou, R. (2021). Anxiety in asthma: A systematic review and meta-analysis. *Psychological Medicine, 51*(1), 11–20. DOI: 10.1017/S0033291720003037 PMID: 33431086

Yoshihara, K. (2015). Psychosomatic treatment for allergic diseases. *BioPsychoSocial Medicine, 9*, 8. Advance online publication. DOI: 10.1186/s13030-015-0036-8 PMID: 25844089

Yoshihara, K., Hiramoto, T., Oka, T., Kubo, C., & Sudo, N. (2014). Effect of 12 weeks of yoga training on the somatization, psychological symptoms, and stress-related biomarkers of healthy women. *BioPsychoSocial Medicine, 8*(1), 1. Advance online publication. DOI: 10.1186/1751-0759-8-1 PMID: 24383884

Yoshihara, K., Hiramoto, T., Oka, T., & Sudo, N. (2011). Profile of mood states and stress-related biochemical indices in long-term yoga practitioners. *BioPsychoSocial Medicine, 5*(1), 6. Advance online publication. DOI: 10.1186/1751-0759-5-6 PMID: 21635790

Yoshihara, K., & Kubo, C. (2008). Stress, fatigue, and psychosomatic illnesses [in Japanese]. *Psychiatry, 50*, 597–602.

Yoshihara, K., & Sudo, N. (2016). Mental health related diseases and treatment: Psychosomatic diseases [in Japanese]. *Clinical Research, 3*, 600–604.

Yoshihara, K. (2009). Naikan therapy [in Japanese]. In K. C. (Ed.), *Standard textbook of psychosomatic medicine* (3rd ed., pp. 339–343). Igaku-Shoin.

Chapter 3
Travelling Body, Travelling Mind:
Alexandra David-Neel's Spiritual Walk Through Asia

Oriane Chevalier
http://orcid.org/0009-0005-5403-2096
Université Clermont Auvergne, France

ABSTRACT

After fourteen years of wandering across Asia, Alexandra David-Neel became the first Western woman to enter the forbidden city of Lhasa in 1924. To get there, the explorer passed herself off as an old Tibetan beggar, a metamorphosis that was not only physical but also spiritual, marking her identity and enabling her to transcend cultural boundaries. The body certainly affects the mind by transforming its identity, but the mind also affects the body. The Buddhist explorer's walk was close to a physical feat, as her body was constantly tested by hunger and cold. The mind can also plunge the body into a state of half-dream, leading the explorer to have hallucination and mystical apparition. Therefore, the experience of the environment takes on a magical dimension that can be apprehended through the motif of walking, whose writing is marked by hesitation and exaggeration. This paper will consider Alexandra David-Neel's walk as an artistic and spiritual performance through an itinerary influenced by divine apparitions and natural events interpreted as prodigies.

INTRODUCTION

In his *Essays*, Montaigne writes about walking: "My thoughts sleep if I sit still: my mind does not go by itself, as when my legs move it"[1] (1965, p. 72). This state-

DOI: 10.4018/979-8-3373-3521-6.ch003

ment could also have been Alexandra David-Néel's, who travelled all her life in a constant movement that is part of her works. Alexandra David-Néel (1868–1969) was a French explorer, writer, and Orientalist whose work had a major impact on the popularization of Buddhism and Asian cultures in the West. She undertook several journeys in Asia, where she studied Buddhism, learned Tibetan language, befriended lamas, and met the Dalai Lama. This study will focus on her most famous journey, which lasted fourteen years, from 1911 to 1925. During this journey, she stayed in Sikkim to study under the gomchen of Lachen, then travelled to Japan, Korea, and China before returning to a land that exerted an irresistible pull on her, Tibet, to which she dedicated two of her major literary successes, *My Journey to Lhasa* (1927) and *Magic and Mystery in Tibet* (1929).

This work will draw on these two works, as well as her correspondence, to trace her spiritual journey, which, after fourteen years of wandering across Asia, made her the first Western woman to enter the forbidden city of Lhasa in 1924. To get there, she passed herself off as an old Tibetan beggar, a metamorphosis that was not only physical but also spiritual, marking her identity and enabling her to transcend cultural boundaries. Besides, her walk was close to a physical feat, as her body was constantly tested by hunger and cold: she walked more than 2,000 kilometres from Yunnan to Lhasa, including summits at altitudes of more than 5,200 metres in the middle of winter. In David-Néel's writings, well-being is achieved through the movement of both body and mind: this movement is not only a source of well-being, but it is also vital. During her journey, the writer's well-being was developed through strategies to heal the body through the mind, so that she could keep walking. Thus, she acquired the *tummo* technique, to warm her body with her mind and survive the very low temperatures of the Himalayan peaks.

Even though the body affects the mind, the mind also affects the body by plunging it into a "state of half-dream[2]" (David-Néel, 1983, p. 41) which leads the explorer to hallucinate and see mystical apparitions. Therefore, the experience of the environment takes on a mystical dimension that can be apprehended through the motif of walking, whose writing is marked by hesitation and exaggeration while "showing the link between life and art[3]" (Locatelli, 2021, p. 18). This chapter aims at considering Alexandra David-Néel's walk as an artistic and spiritual performance, enabling a "re-enchantment of the world" (Fischer-Lichte, 2008) through an itinerary influenced by divine apparitions and natural events interpreted as prodigies. Well-being is therefore understood from a holistic perspective, since the interactions between body and spirit extend to the geographical and spiritual environment. These interactions seem also to extend beyond the physical environment since Alexandra David-Néel's beliefs blur the line between mystical apparition, present to the mind, and hallucination, due to the trials endured by the body. Thus, this chapter aims to explore body-mind interactions in David-Néel's travel writings, combining anthropology, religious studies, gender studies, and postcolonial studies, in order to demonstrate that walking is not just a physical gesture but a transformative practice, a metaphor for spiritual growth.

TRANSMISSION OF BODY-MIND INTERACTIONS FROM EAST TO WEST

Testifying Buddhist and Mystic Practices

Although posterity retains the image of Alexandra David-Néel as an intrepid explorer who braved danger, her real path is that of "a philosophical and mystical quest, made up of the doubts of one who is progressing along the Buddhist path, which is her own[4]" (David-Néel, 2004, p. 16). It was through this bridge-builder between East and West that the Western public discovered Buddhist and mystical practices, in which body and mind interact. Alexandra David-Néel underlines this reciprocity in that the mind can indeed "regulate breathing", but breathing can also be regulated "by making the mind calm[5]" (2004, p. 264).

She describes a number of practices in which body and mind interact, starting with those of the *lung-gom-pa* (རླུང་སྒོམ་པ), that is to say "an athlete capable of running, with extraordinary speed, considerable distances, without sustenance or rest", over "several hundred kilometres[6]" (2004, p. 214-215). This type of runner is in fact the result of "half-psychic, half-physical training designed to give the practitioner supra-normal lightness and celerity."[7] Alexandra David-Néel not only describes this psychic sport, she also witnesses it first-hand, describing her first encounter with a *lung-gom-pa*:

> *I could clearly see his impassive face and his wide-open eyes high up, which seemed to be gazing steadily at a point somewhere high above the empty space. The lama was not running. He seemed to lift himself off the ground with each step, and to advance by bounds, as if he had had the elasticity of a ball [...] the astonishing regularity of his successive elastic steps, as measured as the oscillations of a pendulum.[8] (2004, p. 217)*

The adverb "clearly" underlines the reliability of this eyewitness account, while the two comparisons help Western audiences to imagine superhuman activity. David-Néel also manages to estimate the *lung-gom-pa*'s speed by explaining that he had walked at a brisk pace "all night and the next day, without stopping[9]" (2004, p. 218). She also explains the training these men undergo, which consists of remaining motionless in total darkness for three years, three months, three weeks and three days (2004, p. 221). The explorer nevertheless points out that the *lung-gom-pa* apprentices are less interested in "physical development[10]" (2004, p. 222) than in an incantatory formula that "gives rhythm to the play of breathing while walking, the steps being taken in time with the syllables of the formula[11]" (2004, p. 226). *Logos* and words condition the body's rhythm, having a real effect on the runner's speed and steadiness.

Alexandra David-Néel also witnesses the split between the spirit and the body, when it becomes a corpse. To illustrate this journey of the spirit into the afterlife, she translates a passage from the *Guide to the Spirit of the Dead in the Afterlife* (*Bardo Thödol*, བར་དོ་ཐོས་གྲོལ), which explains that the body is first dismembered, thrown into a sacred river and then burned before being buried, each of these steps aiming to nourish the animal, vegetable and divine worlds (David-Néel, 2004, 59). Finally, this Buddhist ritual aims to extract the spirit of the dead from their body to project it in the other world: David-Néel herself practices this ritual several times in her travelogues, the direct testimony complementing the information transmitted by book translation.

Alexandra David-Néel completes these accounts of Buddhism with other Tibetan rituals. This is the case of the "ro-lang" (རོ་ལང) rite, which can be translated as "the rising corpse". According to the explorer, this rite was practised by sorcerers, even before Buddhism was introduced into Tibet. This is her account:

> *The officiant of the rite is locked up, alone with a corpse, in a dark room. He has to revive the corpse by lying on top of it, putting his mouth on it [...] After a few moments, the corpse begins to move. He gets up and wants to escape. [...] In the end, the corpse's tongue points outwards. This is the critical moment. The sorcerer has to grab it with his teeth and pull it out. Immediately the corpse falls back inert and its tongue [...] becomes a powerful magical weapon.*[12] *(David-Néel, 2004, p. 181)*

David-Néel's writing tends to interweave Buddhist rites with other mystical beliefs rooted in Tibetan folklore, adding to Western knowledge of Tibet while offering a decentred gaze.

Becoming a Woman Orientalist at the Dawn of the 20th Century: A Partially Decentered Gaze

While Edward Said tends to focus on men writing about the Orient, showing reluctance to take into account the Orientalist writings of women, Reina Lewis points out that "women did play a part in the textual production that constituted Orientalism" (1995, p. 18). David-Néel's writings are thus representative of this Gendered Orientalism, which contributes to the diversity of representations since it is at once "heterogeneous," "polyglot," and "polysemic" in the images it conjures up (1995, p. 184). Furthermore, although Women Orientalists often retain a dominant position due to their Western identity, their writings often reveal a shift in perspective in that they also write from a position of subordination as women: this dual position therefore complexifies the reading of Gendered Orientalism. In the case of Alexandra David-Néel, another parameter must be taken into account: she is generally accompanied on her travels by her adopted son, Aphur Yongden: they therefore form a couple of both insiders-foreigners, Yongden not being from Tibet proper but from a distant part of the Tibetophone world (Sikkim). Although Yongden may have been instrumentalised for David-Néel's "success story," the writer shows herself to be attentive to her adopted son's beliefs, with the two companions mutually influencing each other's perspectives on Buddhism.

Alexandra David-Néel played a major role in the circulation of Buddhist thought in France[13], and more widely around the world[14], bringing Buddhism out of the "closed circle of scholars[15]" (Delaunay, 2015, p. 136). Her travelogues contributed to renew Western Orientalism and to deconstruct many prejudices, such as in *Magic and Mystery in Tibet*:

> *Lay people generally imagine that Buddhists believe in the reincarnation of the soul, or even in metempsychosis. This is a mistake. What Buddhism teaches is that the energy produced by a being's mental and physical activity causes new mental and physical phenomena to appear after that being has been dissolved by death.[16] (2004, p. 53)*

David-Néel thus redefines the interactions between body and mind in a holistic approach, offering a decentered gaze on Buddhism. This deconstruction does not, however, prevent a rapprochement between certain mystical practices and Western references. The writer regularly resorts to comparisons, not without humor, between her experience of telepathy and the role played by "wireless telegraphy[17]" (2004, p. 241) in the West. She adds, about *lung-gom-pa*, that they experience "that pleasant excitement well known to speeding drivers[18]" (p. 228): from then on, the comparison functions as a method of bringing East and West closer together.

Alexandra David-Néel also strives to distance herself from the hermetic and esoteric representations of Buddhism: on the contrary, she sheds light on these practices through an approach that can be described as both cartesian and empirical. Indeed, she writes: "The study of psychic phenomena must, it seems to me, be inspired by the same spirit as any scientific research[19]" (2004, p. 306). This is how she explains the practice of telepathy in two steps: first by "certain physical influences due to high altitude[20]" (2004, p. 246) and then by an empirical approach. Indeed, she writes: "As far as I am concerned, I am certain that I have received telepathic messages from lamas with whom I have been in contact[21]" (2004, p. 246). A similar approach can be observed regarding the writer's hallucinations, which she explains successively because of fever, neurasthenia and cerebral overwork, and then as the effect of occult forces[22] (2004, p. 73).

In addition to this dual approach, there is a decentered gaze, with Western beliefs in telepathy being judged by Tibetans. For example, when the explorer explains to a lama that foreigners "believe in the possibility of communicating in this way with the spirits of the dead and even with certain Tibetan mystical masters", he exclaims: "And these are the people who conquered India[23]!" (2024, p. 245-246). Alexandra David-Néel's anti-colonialism is a recurrent theme in her travel writings, and it reflects the anti-Western xenophobia of the Tibetan people. She underlines [the Dalai Lama's] "conviction of the mental inferiority of Whites [...], shar[ing] the opinion common to all Asians, from Ceylon to the northern confines of Mongolia[24]" (2024, p. 35). This anti-colonial stance is also reflected in the relationship between colonial presence, on the one hand, and the natural and spiritual world, on the other, threatened by the Anthropocene era[25] (2004, p. 40).

Alexandra David-Néel's decentered gaze is based on the principle of *tabula rasa*, which enables the Orientalist to embrace another doxa, beyond the dichotomy between possible and impossible that is characteristic of Western thought[26]. Thus, the place of the spirit, assigned to the head in Western doxa, becomes illusory in the eyes of a Tibetan lama whom David-Néel meets: "As you can see, the mind can be felt in different places. Since these people experience the sensation of 'thinking in their head' and I experience it 'in my heart', we can assume that it is just as possible to have the impression of thinking 'in our foot[27]'" (2004, p. 276). Alexandra David-Néel's decentered gaze offers a new version of Buddhism for the West, one that also reveals the writer's political convictions.

Anarchist and Feminist Buddhism

Another particularity of the Buddhism transmitted by Alexandra David-Néel concerns its dual anarchist and feminist dimensions. According to the writer, there are different Buddhisms, among which she chooses to retain an original Buddhism, devoid of notions of hierarchy and authority. Although she was the first non-Tibetan woman to be received by the Dalai Lama, she nevertheless wrote in a letter to her husband: "I do not like *popes*, I do not like the kind of Buddhist Catholicism over which this one presides[28]" (David-Néel, 1975, p. 190-191). Nor did Alexandra David-Néel hesitate to stress the superiority of the *Bön* sorcerer and *Ngagpa* magician over the lama in dealing with the demons, abolishing any hierarchy between pre-Buddhist practices, original Buddhism and clerical Buddhism[29] (2004, p. 43). Moreover, her forbidden march to Lhasa was less a Buddhist pilgrimage than a provocative transgression against the ban. In *Voyage d'une parisienne à Lhassa*, she writes that she "endeavoured to reach the capital of Thibet more to meet the challenge of travelers than out of a strong desire to visit it[30]" (1983, p. 319). Throughout her peregrinations in Asia, she and her adopted son Yongden never cease to "shake the superstitious beliefs deeply rooted in the minds of her listeners" by instilling in them "the true Buddhist doctrine[31]" (1983, p. 76): in this way, the two companions transmit a Buddhist conception that is their own.

Another distinctive feature of Alexandra David-Néel's writings concerns the feminine practice of Buddhism, which she constantly expounds. She reminds us that women play an important role not only in communication between the human and spiritual worlds, as witnessed by the *pamos* who lend their bodies to the deceased so that they can express themselves[32] (2004, p. 64), but also in the interactions between body and mind. For example, she recounts her encounter with a *Delog* woman, meaning "returned from the beyond," to whom it was "enough to want to transport herself to a place to be immediately returned[33]" (2004, p. 58). The orientalist also reveals that female deities, called "*Dâkinis*" (or *khandroma* མཁའ་འགྲོ་མ in Tibetan), dispense the secret doctrines of Lamaist mysticism (2004, p. 191). Moreover, the spiritual life of women is not incompatible with married and family life, since, as David-Néel explains, "[t]he women who embody the *kandhomas* (fairies) can indifferently be nuns or married women[34]" (2004, p. 129). In addition to these "fairies," Alexandra David-Néel mentions various female demons, such as the possessed poisoners who keep poison under their breasts[35] (2004, p. 173), in a small invisible sachet, as well as the eaters of "vital breaths" (2004, p. 172).

David-Néel also reshapes representations of female religious communities in Tibet. She explains how she admires "the quiet bravery of these women", who, without ignoring brigands and ferocious beasts, decide to "form communities of less than a dozen members, living in isolated convents [...] blocked by snow for eight months of the year[36]" (2004, p. 88-89). This feminine orientalism, which assigns new qualities to Tibetan women in Western representations, is also intended as a source of inspiration for European and American women who, according to David-Néel, would not dare expose themselves to the same dangers as their Tibetan sisters. The writer also adds that some *tulkous* nuns lead monasteries staffed by men (2004, p. 130), which completes this feminine fresco of Tibet by renewing the traditional representations of masculine and Western Orientalism. However, David-Néel is not simply an observer of Tibet, that she represents from a position that is both dominant and dominated: by converting herself to Buddhism, she also welcomes the interactions between body and spirit that she experiences.

EXPERIENCING BODY-MIND INTERACTIONS

Changing Body, Changing Mind: The Self becoming the Other

While she wears various Lamaist outfits throughout her peregrinations in Asia, it was during her incognito journey to Lhasa that Alexandra David-Néel most embraced the Tibetan identity in what we can describe as an age, class and ethnic passing (Chevalier, 2024). Indeed, she transforms her appearance to pass for an old Tibetan beggar on her pilgrimage to Lhasa. She dyes her hair with a "Chinese ink stick" and adds "yak hair [...] to match her brown tint with their jet-black[37]" (David-Néel, 1983, p. 40), while her face is powdered with "a mixture of powdered ember and cocoa[38]" (p. 40-41). This physical metamorphosis is complemented by a posture and bodily behavior adapted to her condition as a beggar: the body's unconscious must be controlled, even in her sleep. Indeed, Alexandra David-Néel could not "sleep stretched out to the full [which is] a luxury belonging only to people of quality[39]" (David-Néel, 1983, p. 146). Her body also had to get used to a new rhythm of eating and a new calendar. While she had already been given a Tibetan Lamaist first name meaning "Lamp of Wisdom" (*Yéshé Tömé*), this passing as an old beggar woman enables her to transcend all cultural boundaries through "total integration," both "physically and psychically[40]" (Quatremare Martín, 2022, p. 203). However, this "mimétisation" (Ledesma, 2008, p. 220) and this "total integration" is only possible thanks to the presence of Yongden, who distracts attention whenever the writer's incognito is threatened, allowing the duo to continue their journey as "insiders." Thus, her adoptive son played a major role in keeping her identity hidden from the Tibetans who interacted with her or welcome her into their homes, although the body modification enabled her to add to her knowledge as an orientalist. In addition to mastering the Tibetan language, she discovered Tibetan customs that had previously been hidden from her. She writes:

> *Each step took us to other peasants. We spent the night in their homes, [...] studying their habits closely, listening to their conversations, their reflections on events in Thibet.*
>
> *These good people, who considered us to belong to the common people like themselves, spoke and acted quite freely in our presence.[41] (David-Néel, 1983, p. 138)*

During Alexandra David-Néel's travelogue, we observe an evolution in the orientalist's identity and psyche, as she finds herself unconsciously acting like the beggar whose appearance she has taken on. This physical mimicry of the Other eventually infuses her spirit to the point where she feels "a real Tibetan soul rising up inside [her[42]]" (David-Néel, 1983, 232). This evolution in identity is also reflected in her writing, as she gradually uses more and more Tibetan terms in transliteration, restoring the sound of the term within the French language and gradually freeing herself from having to explain its meaning. She also seems to be embracing a new temporality, a new daily rhythm, imposed on her by her borrowed identity: this is why she is forced to impose the "*tsaphog*," which is a stopover that cuts the journey off towards the middle of the day[43] (David-Néel, 1983, p.55). Thus, David-Néel's Tibetan identity set the pace of her walk.

However, this physical transformation chosen by Alexandra David-Néel is not the only physical factor influencing her mind: the 2,000-kilometer journey on foot to Lhasa also pushes the body to its limits, with interactions between body and mind becoming necessary to ensure the explorer's survival.

Interactions Necessary for Survival: A Body Beyond its Limits

Alexandra David-Néel's route from Yunnan to Lhasa presents many geographical and climatic difficulties, even more so in winter, when she must cross peaks at altitudes of over 5,200 meters without any equipment. The writer states: "On several occasions, Lama Yongden and I have completed steps of nineteen to twenty hours, without stopping and without eating or drinking [...] with snow up to our knees[44]" (David-Néel & Aphur, 2004, p. 218). Having to walk in the same conditions as a Tibetan beggar, she ended up with her "toes burnt by the snow and half-frozen," then "covered in blisters and bleeding sores[45]" (David-Néel, 1983, p. 225-226). The writer also explained that she went more than a week without eating, and she even writes to her husband: "Just for the record, today I arrived in Lhasa reduced to a skeleton[46]" (1975, p. 767). The explorer risked her life on several occasions: she came face to face with a panther, hung over a precipice, fell into an icy river, took several falls that left her unconscious, and was even forced to use her pistol against brigands who attacked her. Nevertheless, the greatest danger to her life remains the cold, as she wisely points out: "Spending the winter in a cave, often at an altitude of 4,000 to 5,000 meters, dressed in a thin robe or even naked and not freezing to death, is a complicated problem[47]" (2004, p. 229).

From then on, she turned to the *tummo* technique (གཏུམ་མོ), which consists in mobilizing her internal energy to produce heat. To master this technique, she trained for five months with the Gomchen of Lachen[48] (David-Néel, 1983, p. 184), who sent her to bathe in icy rivers at an altitude of almost 4,000 meters in winter, then to spend a night motionless without drying off (David-Néel & Aphur, 2004, p. 231). During her journey to Lhasa, Alexandra David-Néel used this technique to ensure her own survival. One evening, when she was unable to light a fire, she decided to warm herself using the *tummo* technique:

My mind [...] remained entirely focused on the idea of toumo and, mechanically, but without any other thought diverting it, continued in a state of half-dream, the regular progression of the practice I had begun.

Soon I saw flames rising around me; they grew larger and larger, enveloping me, curving their red tongues over my head. [...] I could feel the fire coming out of my head, escaping from each of my fingers.[49] *(David-Néel, 1983, p. 185-186)*

In this life-threatening climate, the body goes beyond its limits by interacting with the mind. Mysticism is therefore not a matter of magic: on the contrary, it is based on rigorous and methodical practice. On this subject, Françoise Bonardel writes: "David-Néel therefore took care to point out that Tibetan mystics are not believers, but practitioners skilled in forms of spiritual training that engage both the body and the mind[50]" (Bonardel, 2023, p. 43). In the end, whether through mimetic disguise or by learning practices that engage both body and mind, David-Néel implements strategies to ensure and preserve her well-being throughout her journey across Tibet. Yet, despite the rigor that she applies in her interactions between body and mind, the body also happens to be the dupe of the mind when the writer is confronted with hallucinations.

A Body Lured by the Mind: Hallucinations and Ghosts

During her Buddhist training, Alexandra David-Néel learned to fully control her body and mind: this is how she came to experience "the possibility of creating and animating a ghost[51]" (David-Néel & Aphur, 2004, p. 301). This ghost corresponds to a *tulpa* (སྤྲུལ་པ།) and, as Mikles and Joseph explain in their article "Tracking the Tulpa," David-Néel chose to give this *tulpa* the form of a jolly Western monk so it would not be confused with Tibetan deities (p. 88). It took her six months to dispel the ghost, which was not just a "visual" apparition, as she "sometimes felt as if brushed by the fabric of a dress and felt the pressure [...] of a hand on my shoulder[52]" (David-Néel & Aphur, 2004, p. 301-302). Thus, other people can see the ghost she has created, as she adds: "The interesting thing about these cases of "materialization" is that others see the form created by thought[53]" (David-Néel & Aphur, 2004, p.302). Although Alexandra David-Néel's mind is in full control of a materialization in this psychic practice, she can also be struck by hallucinations over which she struggles to regain control. This is particularly the case during her journey to Lhasa, when these hallucinations were linked to her fear of being discovered. For instance, she believes to see a Tibetan soldier in a "state of half-dream":

At all costs, I have to give him the impression that I am a real Thibetan, if that is even possible. And the best way I could think of to do this was to pretend to blow my nose with my fingers. The movement caused by this gesture shook the state of half-dream in which I had been seeing and thinking until then. The soldier disappeared.[54] (David-Néel, 1983, p. 41)

While some hallucinations dissipate easily and are presented as the result of a trick of the mind, others remain ambivalent. On her journey, for example, she meets a traveler she does not recognize, but who immediately identifies her and declares: "Don't search your memory [...] I have as many faces as I want, and you have never seen this one[55]" (David-Néel, 1983, p. 297). The ascetic eventually dissolves into thin air, without the writer attributing this apparition to a hallucination, leaving the reader in doubt.

Apparitions can also have a real impact on the body. For instance, one night the explorer finds herself wrestling with the spirit of a lama to prevent it from stealing a "*pourba*," described as an "enchanted dagger[56]" (David-Néel & Aphur, 2004, p. 176-177). Nevertheless, the "Chöd" (གཅོད), translated as "to cut", remains the rite that the writer presents as the most perilous of all, for both mind and body. This ritual practice, which she refers to by the phrase "macabre sport[57]" (David-Néel & Aphur, 2004, p. 163), is a form of self-sacrifice during which "some are stricken with madness or sudden death in the course of its celebration[58]" (David-Néel & Aphur, 2004, p. 148). The practitioner must then offer himself to deities and demons for what David-Néel describes as a "red feast," during which a deity "detaches his limbs, flays him, and opens his belly[59]" (David-Néel & Aphur, 2004, p. 154-155). This rite can also involve practitioners remaining attached to a rock "for three days and three nights or even longer, fasting, fighting sleep, prey to the hunger and fatigue that so easily engender hallucinations[60]" (David-Néel & Aphur, 2004 p. 149). Alexandra David-Néel explored, observed and experimented with various hallucinatory practices. Nevertheless, it was when she abandoned herself to walking, or more precisely to wandering, that she underwent intense psychic experiences. In that case, what role did walking play in the spiritual path taken by the writer?

A "RE-ENCHANTMENT OF THE WORLD" THROUGH A SPIRITUAL WALK: IN SEARCH OF HOLISTIC WELL-BEING

Erika Fischer-Lichte uses the phrase "reenchantment of the world" (Fischer-Lichte, 2008) to describe the transformation brought about by theatrical performance. This theatrical dimension is consciously staged in David-Néel's writing, whose past as a cantatrice seems to influence the writing of certain scenes, "the explorer exulting *in petto* behind her Tibetan mask" (Chevalier, 2024, p. 19). In addition to the playful aspect of a disguised staging, this notion de "reechantment of the world" can also be applied to the performance of walking and wandering, which act powerfully not only on the mind but also on the writing of Alexandra David-Néel. Thus, what kind of "reenchantment of the world" emerges from her pen?

Ascending Body, Ascending Mind: An Epiphanic Stroll

First, it should be noted that walk is associated with a vital need for Alexandra David-Néel, as when she stops her walk "her rheumatism flares up and her neurasthenia overwhelms her[61]" (Delaunay, 2015, p. 134). Walking is also linked to the writer's happiness and thirst for freedom, as she confesses:

I must admit, the perfect freedom of the ardjopa who [...] sleeps each night wherever he pleases, in the open air, greatly appealed to me. [...] [And I] consider the happiest days I have ever lived to be those when, with my wretched bundle on my back, I roamed the hills and valleys of the marvelous 'Land of Snow.[62]*' (David-Néel, 1983, p. 39)*

The *ardjopa* is a pilgrim who travels on foot and wander through Tibet: David-Néel associates happiness with the freedom of a Tibetan wanderer.

Nevertheless, walking seems to go beyond this therapeutic and joyous dimension, linked with holistic well-being, as the writer often employs the metaphor of walk—and more specifically, of ascent—to describe her spiritual journey. She thus depicts the "direct path" of Buddhism as the ascent of a summit, which one strives to "reach [...] by climbing the sheer rocks and cross[ing] the abysses [...] in [which] the presumptuous alpinist breaks his bones[63]" (David-Néel & Aphur, 2004, p. 253-254), which account for a vivid echo of her own journey through the Himalayas[64]. Walk then becomes the motif of the interaction between body and mind. On this subject, Federica Locatelli writes that "[walking is] a discursive space, showing the link between life and art [...], [where] the traveler-thinker becomes the protagonist of his experience, body and mind, enjoying a sensorial fervor and getting lost in natural spectacles, [...] his sentence adapt[ing] to the rhythm of his steps[65]" (Locatelli, 2021, p. 18). Alexandra David-Néel thus freed herself wandering aimlessly through the mountains, as she writes: "The nocturnal journeys across these deserts are an enchantment; I would walk for pleasure the whole night long[66] [...]" (David-Néel & Aphur, 2004, p. 160).

Walking thus transforms into wandering, into pilgrimage, with the freedom granted to the body being correlated with spiritual openness and a readiness for epiphany. On this subject, Philippe Antoine writes: "It is as if aimless wandering facilitates reflection, or more precisely, is in tune with the free progress of an available mind, open to contradiction and doubt, in search of a wisdom it does not yet possess[67]" (Antoine, 2011, p. 11). Thus, Alexandra David-Néel seems to open her mind to hallucinations mostly when she wanders aimlessly through the mountains. She recounts one of these experiences in these terms:

The first time I ventured out alone on one of these strange peregrinations, I stopped near a clear-water lake [...]
The phantasmagorical procession of moonlit clouds rolled along the nearby peaks, descending towards me, surrounding me with nebulous ghosts. One of them stepped forward [...]. Was he calling me? Was he chasing me? I hesitated... Then he came closer, so real, so alive, that I closed my eyes to dispel the hallucination. I felt myself embraced, wrapped in the folds of a soft, cold cloak whose subtle substance seeped into me, chilling me to the core...[68] *(David-Néel & Aphur, 2004, p. 156-157)*

It is during one of her strolls that she encounters a phantasmagorical procession and feels the grip of a ghost. This abstract reflects a style marked by hesitation and exaggeration, which are two characteristics of walk writing, according to Federica Locatelli, with the act of walking itself "dominated by accident and the unexpected[69]" (Locatelli, 2021, p. 17). However, these mystical experiences are above all the fruit of writing, since writing has a powerful influence on the editorial and media strategies implemented by David-Néel: the recent reedition of *Souvenirs d'une Parisienne au Thibet* reveals how the writer enriched and developed her writing over the course of the editions of *Voyage d'une Parisienne à Lhassa*: as Jeanne Mascolo de Filippis and Samuel Thévoz point out in their introduction, this account evolved between its first publication in Beijing in 1925 and its publication in France in 1927. (David-Néel, 2024). However, this chapter does not aim to distinguish between what David-Néel actually experienced and what is a matter of imaginative writing: its primary purpose is to highlight the various mind-body interactions she describes, while keeping in mind the narrative dimension of her writing. Thus, it seems that walking and wandering are not the only factors fostering David-Néel's spiritual and mystical awakening, as she believes that such awakening is only possible for her when she is in Tibet.

Ontological and Magical Connections with Tibet

In her works, Alexandra David-Néel presents Tibet as a place that welcomes her soul, holding a part of herself. She writes in a letter: "I have visions of Himalaya, of lakes mirroring snowy peaks, of waterfalls in the woods. [...] Tibet! Tibet! A part of me remained up there in the high steppes[70] [...]" (David-Néel, 1975, p. 262). Thus, her connection to Tibet can be considered to be of an "ontological nature" (Thévoz, 2016, p. 179). The writer even goes so far as to weave a genealogy linking herself to Tibet, claiming to have "the atavism of an Asian nomad in [her] veins[71]" (David-Néel, 1975, p. 371) or that she was a master lama in one of her past lives. This connection to Tibet is so strong that in 1917, during her stay in Japan, she writes that this country is haunting her: "The truth is, I am homesick for a country that is not mine. The steppes, the solitudes, the eternal snows and the big clear sky up there are haunting me[72]!" (David-Néel, 1975, p. 445).

She also justifies this power of attraction by suggesting that "the Himalayan landscape is endowed with special qualities that resonate with her own vision of the world" (Thévoz, 2016, p. 179-180). Furthermore, she constantly reminds us that Tibet is populated by local spirits and "demons" whose number exceeds that of the human population:

> *Tibet is the land of demons. If we were to rely on legends and popular beliefs, we would be led to believe that the number of demons here far exceeds that of the human population. Taking on a thousand different forms, these malevolent beings inhabit trees, rocks, valleys, lakes and springs, pursuing men and animals to steal their "vital breath" and feed on it.[73] (David-Néel & Aphur, 2004, p. 147)*

Both land of demons and land of marvels, Tibet stands out as the centripetal force of David-Néel's writing, directing each line and each word at its heart. On this subject, Samuel Thévoz explains that even though she is not the inventor of Tibetan magic, "David-Néel deliberately fashioned Tibet as the elective—and elected—location for magical feats" (David-Néel & Aphur, 2024, p. 199). Believing in the possibility of exchanging with spirits inhabiting the natural elements repeatedly creates a horizon of expectation for David-Néel, who summons these spirits to get her out of perilous situations. From then on, the traveler attributes to nature the role of adjuvant, in a form of spiritual communication[74]. Nature has a duty to protect the writer, who on several occasions uses natural elements to conceal herself: "Left alone, I hid our bags under the branches, lay flat among the dead leaves and strewn my clothes with them. Thus camouflaged, someone walking through the woods could have passed very close to me without spotting me[75]" (David-Néel, 1983, p. 38). The writer disappeared under the leaves and snow to ensure the success of her journey: this immersion of body and spirit in the Tibetan landscapes and natural elements was part of the ontological link that David-Néel forged with the Himalayan peaks.

A Walk Guided by Miracles: Interaction Between Mind and Spirits

Furthermore, the path that Alexandra David-Néel takes throughout her wanderings in Tibet seems traced by the gods and facilitated by some sort of miracles. This series of miracles even begins upon her arrival in Sikkim when a "hail storm" breaks out which is interpreted as "the work of demons or magicians" (David-Néel & Aphur, 2004, p. 41). Thus, the experience of the environment takes on a magical dimension, and David-Néel's walk is "protected by a sort of miracle" until Lhasa:

Our entry into Lhasa seems protected by a sort of miracle.

No sooner have we disembarked than the atmosphere, which had been very calm until then, suddenly becomes troubled. Within a matter of minutes, a furious storm rises, lifting clouds of sand to the sky. [...]

A gigantic yellow curtain, made of suspended sand, is spread out before the Potala, blinding its guests, obscuring Lhasa and the paths that lead to it. I interpret it as a symbol promising me complete safety.[76] *[...] (David-Néel, 1983, p. 317)*

We observe many natural events interpreted as miracles; this is also the case with an eclipse, concerning which Yongden, David-Néel's adopted son, states: "This is even better than the curtain of sand stretched before the Potala on the day of our arrival [...] now 'your gods' are obscuring the moon so that we cannot be seen[77]" (David-Néel, 1983, p. 334).

Furthermore, the role that David-Néel assumes during her journey to Lhasa is that of a "*Ngakpa*" widow, in other words, the widow of a sorcerer, practicing black magic herself. She eventually comes to embody this role and, when two rupees are stolen from her by brigands, she begins to "invoke the most feared gods," and this is what happens:

[...] the surrounding nature seemed to be carried away by my passionate declaration and came into harmony with it. The forest darkened, a light breeze stirred distant murmurs in the underbrush, and mysterious, mournful voices appeared to rise from the unseen torrent rolling at the bottom of the valley, ascending towards us and filling the air with threatening phrases in an unknown language. I was calm, and yet I could not help but shiver at the occult atmosphere that I had created myself. I was, moreover, not the only one to feel its effect. The seven brigands appeared to be petrified.[78] *(David-Néel, 1983, p. 285)*

David-Néel's mystical and supernatural powers thus act not only on nature but are also acknowledged by the Tibetan people. What was initially a performance gradually seems to surpass the writer's own understanding, to the point that Yongden repeatedly asserts his certainty about his adoptive mother's powers[79] (David-Néel, 1983, p. 100).

Finally, the interactions between body and mind in David-Néel's works illuminate not only her position as a witness but also as a medium for mystical and Buddhist practices. Walking, and especially wandering, further establish themselves as catalysts for these interactions, leading to a spiritual ascent guided by miracles that David-Néel stages in her travel writings. It is, moreover, in this way that she distinguishes herself from the Western tradition of female mysticism. As Sara Mills highlights in *Discourses of Difference: An Analysis of Women's Travel Writing and Colonialism,* "[i]t is unusual to find a [Western] woman writing authoritatively about a religion other than Christianity, and claiming mystical and supernatural powers for herself" (1993, p. 208). The final words of *Voyage d'une parisienne à Lhassa* work as an assertion of power, as the writer envisions herself alone in her room, exclaiming in Tibetan: *"Lha gyalo!"* which means "The gods have triumphed!" (David-Néel, 1983, p. 368). David-Néel's physical achievement, through walk, is thus associated with a divine victory, underlining the spiritual link between her and Tibet and the spirits that inhabit its summits.

REFERENCES

Antoine, P. (2011). *Quand le voyage devient promenade*. PUPS.

Bonardel, F. (2023). *Entre mystiques et magiciens*. Fage.

Chevalier, O. (2024). Jeanne Barret, Hester Stanhope et Alexandra David-Néel: Les exploratrices au prisme du passing. *TRANS*, *29*. Advance online publication. DOI: 10.4000/trans.9058

David-Néel, A. (1975). *Lettres à son mari. Journal de voyage 11 août 1904-31 décembre 1940*. Plon.

David-Néel, A. (1983). *Voyage d'une Parisienne à Lhassa: A pied et en mendiant, de la Chine à l'Inde à travers le Tibet*. Plon.

David-Néel, A. (2024). *Souvenirs d'une Parisienne au Thibet*. Plon.

David-Néel, A., & Aphur, Y. (2004). *Dieux et démons des solitudes tibétaines*. Plon.

Delaunay, J. (2015). Alexandra David-Néel: Bouddhisme et drapeau noir. *BALLAST: stand up, federate, initiate, 4*(1), 126-142.

Fischer-Lichte, E. (2008). *The Transformative Power of performance. A new aesthetics*. Routledge.

Ledesma Pedraz, M. (2008). Alexandra David-Néel ou l'art de la fugue et du déguisement. *Clio. Histoire, femmes et sociétés, 28*, 213-22. DOI: 10.4000/clio.8712

Lewis, R. (1995). *Gendering Orientalism: Race, femininity and representation*. Routledge.

Locatelli, F. (2021). Quand la marche se fait écriture: Le voyageur-penseur au milieu des sommets (XVIIIe-XIXe siècles). *Seminario di filologia francese, revue italienne d'études françaises, 11*. DOI: 10.4000/rief.8022

Mikles, N., & Joseph, L. (2015). Tracking the Tulpa: Exploring the Tibetan origins of a contemporary paranormal idea. *Nova Religio*, *19*(1), 87–97.

Mills, S. (1993). *Discourses of difference: An Analysis of women's travel writing and colonialism*. Routledge.

Montaigne, M. (de) (1965). *Les Essais. Livre III*. Gallimard.

Quatremare Martín, F. (2022). Identités plurielles au cours des voyages d'Alexandra David-Néel. *HYBRIDA*, *4*, 195–216.

Said, E. (1978). *Orientalism*. Pantheon Books.

Thévoz, S. (2016). On the Threshold of the "land of marvels": Alexandra David-Neel in Sikkim and the making of global Buddhism. *Transcultural studies, 7* (1), 149-186. DOI: 10.17885/heiup.ts.23541

Thévoz, S. (2024), Trainings for sorcery, magic, mystic philosophy—for that which is called "the great accomplishment": Alexandra David-Neel's written and unwritten Tibetan grimoires. In C. Bailey & A. Wenta (Eds.), *Tibetan magic. Past and present* (pp. 193–220). Bloomsbury..

ENDNOTES

1 [All quotations from David-Néel and Francophone works are our translations]: "Mes pensées dorment, si je les assis. Mon esprit ne va, si les jambes ne l'agitent".

2 "[…] l'état de demi-rêve dans lequel j'avais vu et pensé jusque-là".

3 "[…] montrant le lien entre la vie et l'art".

4 "[…] son cheminement véritable est celui d'une recherche philosophique et mystique faite des doutes de celle qui progresse dans la voie bouddhique, qui est la sienne".

5 "Mais le souffle dirige aussi l'activité du corps et influence celle de l'esprit, d'où s'ensuivent deux méthodes: la plus aisée, celle qui assagit l'esprit en réglant la respiration, et l'autre, plus ardue, consistant à régler la respiration en faisant le calme dans l'esprit".

6 "Le loung-gom-pa est un athlète capable de parcourir, avec une rapidité extraordinaire, des distances considérables, sans se sustenter, ni prendre de repos […] [sur] des distances de plusieurs centaines de kilomètres ».

7 "[…] un genre d'entraînement mi-psychique, mi-physique, destiné à faire acquérir à celui qui le pratique une légèreté et une célérité supra-normales".

8 "Je pouvais distinguer nettement sa face impassible et ses yeux largement ouverts haut qui semblaient contempler fixement un point situé quelque part, haut, dans l'espace vide. Le lama ne courait point. Il paraissait s'enlever de terre à chacun de ses pas et avancer par bonds, comme s'il avait été doué de l'élasticité d'une balle".

9 "[...] toute la nuit et le lendemain, sans s'arrêter".

10 "[...] il faut se dire que le moyen visé n'a rien de commun avec le développement physique".

11 "Le novice concentre ses pensées sur la répétition mentale et cadencée de cette formule qui rythme le jeu de la respiration pendant la marche, les pas s'effectuant en mesure, avec les syllabes de la formule".

12 "Le célébrant du rite est enfermé, seul avec un cadavre, dans une chambre obscure. Il doit ranimer le mort en s'étendant sur lui, posant sa bouche sur la sienne [...] Au bout de quelques instants, le cadavre commence à se mouvoir. Il se lève et veut s'échapper. [...] À la fin, la langue du cadavre pointe au-dehors. C'est le moment critique. Avec ses dents, le sorcier doit la saisir et l'arracher. Aussitôt le cadavre retombe inerte et sa langue [...] devient une puissante arme magique".

13 In his preface to *Dieux et démons des solitudes tibétaines*, Frank Tréguier writes: "Through her inner quest and her journeys, which are experienced as pilgrimages, she must absorb in this life a very hermetic thousand-year-old tradition and restore it [...] to the West" ["Au travers de sa quête intérieure de ses voyages qui sont vécus comme autant de pèlerinages, elle doit absorber en cette vie une tradition millénaire très hermétique et la restituer [...] à l'Occident"] (2004, p.17).

14 It was through Alexandra David-Néel that the Beat Generation was introduced to Buddhism in the United States: Ginsberg later admitted himself that the "Blakean imagery in Alexandra David-Néel's *Magic and Mystery in Tibet* magnetized [him] toward Buddhist meditation" (Foster, 1998).

15 "[...] elle développe un exposé limpide du bouddhisme afin de le rendre accessible au plus grand nombre et de l'extirper du cercle fermé des érudits".

16 "Les profanes imaginent, en général, que les bouddhistes croient à la réincarnation de l'âme, voire même à la métempsycose. C'est là une erreur. Ce que le bouddhisme enseigne, c'est que l'énergie produite par l'activité mentale et physique d'un être cause l'apparition de nouveaux phénomènes mentaux et physiques après que cet être a été dissous par la mort".

17 "La télépathie est l'une des branches de la science secrète des Tibétains. Elle semble remplir dans les hautes régions du 'Pays des Neiges' le rôle que la télégraphie sans fil joue depuis peu en Occident".

18 "Une sorte d'anesthésie amortit aussi les sensations causées par les heurts contre les pierres et les autres obstacles que l'on peut rencontrer, et l'on marche pendant des heures, avec une vitesse inaccoutumée, éprouvant cette agréable griserie bien connue des automobilistes qui font de la vitesse".

19 "L'étude des phénomènes psychiques doit, il me semble, s'inspirer du même esprit que n'importe quelle recherche scientifique".

20 "Peut-être certaines influences physiques dues à la haute altitude du territoire doivent-elles être envisagées".

21 "En ce qui me concerne, je suis certaine d'avoir reçu des messages télépathiques émanant de lamas avec qui j'avais été en relations".

22 "I attributed these phenomena to a feverish state, to neurasthenia caused by annoyance added to cerebral overwork. Some might have seen in it the effect of occult forces. Whatever the case, I could not control this painful haunting that bordered on hallucination" ["J'attribuai ces phénomènes à un état fiévreux, à de la neurasthénie causée par la contrariété s'ajoutant à du surmenage cérébral. Certains y eussent peut-être vu l'effet de forces occultes. Quoi qu'il en pût être, je ne parvenais pas à dominer cette hantise pénible qui côtoyait l'hallucination"].

23 "Je me rappelle de la répartie amusante d'un lama de Trachilhumpo à qui je disais que certains *philings* croyaient à la possibilité de communiquer de cette façon avec les esprits des morts et même, aussi, avec certains maîtres mystiques tibétains: "Et ce sont ces gens-là qui ont conquis l'Inde!" s'écria-t-il, confondu par la naïveté de ces Anglais redoutables".

24 "[...] [la] conviction [du Dalaï-lama] quant à l'infériorité mentale des Blancs demeurait inébranlée, et en cela il ne faisait que partager l'opinion commune à tous les Asiatiques, de Ceylan aux confins septentrionaux de la Mongolie".

25 "The mule track we were following went deep into the Himâlaya, the sacred land of Hindu traditions, populated by sages, ascetic thaumaturges and deities. The summer resorts set up by foreigners on its edge have not yet succeeded in significantly altering its appearance. A few kilometres from the big hotels where people dance to the sound of jazz, the primeval forest reclaims its rights. Drowned in the wandering mists, a ghostly army of trees, draped in long, livid green moss, gestures ominously at the footsteps of travellers" ["Le sentier muletier que nous suivions s'enfonçait dans l'Himâlaya, cette terre sacrée des traditions hindoues qu'elles peuplent de sages, d'ascètes thaumaturges et de déités. Les stations estivales établies par les étrangers à sa bordure n'ont pas

encore réussi à en altérer sensiblement l'aspect. À quelques kilomètres des grands hôtels où l'on danse au son d'un jazz, la forêt vierge reprend ses droits. Noyée parmi les brouillards errants, une armée fantomatique d'arbres, drapés en de longues mousses d'un vert livide, y esquisse des gestes inquiétants devant les pas des voyageurs"].

26 "In Tibet, psychic phenomena are regarded as facts, certainly uncommon, but not so extraordinary as to arouse in those who witness them or hear them recounted the imperative desire to examine them critically. In reality, they do not upset in their minds, as they do in those of Westerners, fixed notions about natural laws and what is possible and what is impossible" ["Les phénomènes psychiques sont considérés au Tibet comme des faits, certainement peu communs, mais pas assez extraordinaires pour susciter, chez ceux qui en sont témoins ou les entendent relater, le désir impérieux de les examiner d'une façon critique. En réalité, ils ne bouleversent pas dans leur esprit, comme dans celui des Occidentaux, des notions arrêtées touchant des lois naturelles et ce qui est possible et ce qui est impossible"] (David-Néel, 2004, p. 252).

27 "Vous voyez bien qu'on peut sentir l'esprit en différents endroits. Puisque ces gens éprouvent la sensation de 'penser dans leur tête' et que moi, je l'éprouve 'dans mon cœur', on peut croire qu'il est tout aussi possible d'avoir l'impression de penser 'dans le pied'".

28 Letter dated June 25, 1912: "Je n'aime pas les *papes,* je n'aime pas l'espèce de catholicisme bouddhiste auquel celui-ci préside".

29 "Although the lama is more respected than the Bön sorcerer, a follower of the ancient religion of the aborigines, or the *ngagpa* magician assimilated to the official clergy, the latter are considered to be more skilful than the lama when it comes to dealing with demons that in any way harm the living or the spirit of the dead" ["Bien que le lama soit plus respecté que le sorcier Bön, sectateur de l'ancienne religion des aborigènes, ou que le magicien *ngagpa* assimilé au clergé officiel, ces derniers sont tenus pour plus habiles que lui lorsqu'il s'agit de traiter avec des démons qui, d'une façon quelconque, nuisent à un vivant ou à l'esprit d'un mort"].

30 "Bien que je me fusse efforcée de parvenir jusqu'à la capitale du Thibet plutôt pour relever le défi porté aux voyageurs, que par l'effet d'un vif désir de la visiter [...]."

31 "Yongden [...] s'efforça[it] ainsi d'ébranler quelque peu les croyances superstitieuses profondément enracinées dans l'esprit de ses auditeurs. Lorsqu'on

le consultait à propos de malades, il ajoutait encore de bons conseils touchant la propreté et l'hygiène."

32 "Some dead people, however, do not observe the same discretion. They frequently appear in dreams to their relatives or friends [...] The dead themselves, they believe, must be heard. To this end, a male or female medium (*pao* or *pamo*) is essential to lend his or her body to the spirit of the deceased and speak for him or her" ["Certains morts, pourtant, n'observent pas la même discrétion. Ils apparaissent fréquemment, en rêve, à leurs proches ou à leurs amis [...] Le mort lui-même, pensent-ils, doit être entendu. À cet effet, un médium homme ou femme (*pao* ou *pamo*) est indispensable pour prêter son corps à l'esprit du défunt et parler pour lui"].

33 "Il lui suffisait de vouloir se transporter dans un endroit pour y être immédiatement rendue".

34 "Les femmes qui incarnent des kandhomas (fées) peuvent indifféremment être des religieuses ou des femmes mariées".

35 "Or, more likely, this poison only exists in the imagination. The woman is said to keep it under her breasts, in a small sachet, but no one has ever seen the sachet, even when the woman who is supposed to be carrying it is undressed" ["Ou, plus vraisemblablement, ce poison n'existe que dans l'imagination. La femme le conserve, dit-on, sous ses seins, dans un petit sachet, mais ce sachet, personne ne l'a jamais vu, même quand celle qui est supposée le porter est déshabillée"].

36 "Parmi les nombreux exemples de bizarrerie paradoxale qu'offre le Tibet, la bravoure tranquille de ses femmes m'a toujours étonnée. Peu d'Européennes ou d'Américaines oseraient vivre en plein désert par petits groupes de quatre ou cinq compagnes, ou même complètement seules. Bien peu oseraient, aussi, entreprendre, dans ces mêmes conditions, des voyages qui durent des mois, voire même des années, à travers une contrée de hautes montagnes solitaires où rôdent des brigands et des bêtes féroces. [...] Cependant, malgré ces raisons bien propres à les retenir dans les villages, l'on trouve, en maints endroits, des religieuses formant des communautés de moins d'une douzaine de membres, habitant des couvents isolés, dont certains, situés à une très haute altitude, sont bloqués par les neiges pendant huit mois de l'année" (2004, p. 88-89).

37 "Des crins de yak emportés pour cet usage s'ajoutèrent à ma chevelure et, pour assortir sa teinte brune à leur noir jais, je la frottai avec un bâton d'encre de Chine légèrement humidifié".

38 “[…] je me poudrai avec un mélange de braise pulvérisée et de cacao emprunté à l’unique boîte que nous possédions”.

39 “Dormir étendue de tout son long est considéré comme un luxe appartenant aux seules personnes de qualité”.

40 “[…] l’intégration totale, c’est à dire physique et psychique”.

41 “Chaque étape nous amenait auprès d’autres paysans. Nous passions la nuit chez eux, […] étudiant leurs habitudes de près, écoutant leurs conversations, leurs réflexions à propos des évènements survenant au Thibet.

Ces bonnes gens qui nous tenaient pour appartenant au petit peuple comme eux, parlaient et agissaient tout à fait librement en notre présence”.

42 “[…] une véritable âme thibétaine surgissant en moi”.

43 “It would have been contrary to Thibetan women’s customs to pass through this area without stopping for our meal, as the time for tsaphog had arrived” [“Il aurait été contraire aux habitudes des thibétaines de traverser cet endroit sans nous arrêter pour prendre notre repas, car le temps du *tsaphog* était arrivé”] (1983, p. 55).

44 “Le Lama Yongden et moi avons, plusieurs fois, effectué des étapes de dix-neuf à vingt heures, sans aucun arrêté et sans manger ni boire […] avec de la neige jusqu’aux genoux”.

45 “[…] orteils brûlés par la neige et à moitié gelés […] couverts d’ampoules et de plaies saignantes”.

46 Letter dated February 28, 1924: “Sache seulement, aujourd’hui, que je suis arrivée à Lhassa réduite à l’état de squelette”.

47 “Passer l’hiver dans une caverne située, souvent, entre 4000 et 5000 mètres d’altitude, vêtu d’une robe mince ou même nu et ne pas périr gelé, est un problème compliqué”.

48 “I learnt the kind of training that makes it possible to perform these bizarre feats of strength and, more curious than ever to see the experiment through to the end, I practiced it myself for five winter months, wearing the thin cotton dress worn by novices at an altitude of 3,900 metres” [“[…] j’appris le genre d’entraînement qui permet d’accomplir ces tours de force bizarres et, plus que jamais curieuse de pousser l’expérience jusqu’au bout, je m’y exerçai moi-même pendant cinq mois d’hiver, portant la mince robe de coton des novices à 3 900 mètres d’altitude”].

49 “Mon esprit [...] restait entièrement concentré sur l’idée de *toumo* et, machinalement, mais sans qu’aucune autre pensée l’en fasse dévier, continuait dans l’état de demi-rêve, la marche régulière de la pratique commencée.

Bientôt je vis des flammes s’élever autour de moi; elles grandirent de plus en plus, m’enveloppèrent, courbant leurs langues rouges au-dessus de ma tête. [...] Je sentais le feu sortir de ma tête, s’échapper de chacun de mes doigts”.

50 “Aussi David-Néel prit-elle soin de préciser que les mystiques tibétains ne sont pas des croyants, mais des pratiquants rompus à des formes d’entraînement spirituel engageant le corps autant que l’esprit”.

51 “[...] la possibilité de créer et d’animer un fantôme”.

52 “[...] mais il m’arriva d’être comme frôlée par l’étoffe d’une robe et de sentir la pression d’une main posée sur mon épaule”.

53 “La chose intéressante dans ces cas de ‘matérialisation’ est que d’autres voient la forme créée par la pensée”.

54 “À tout prix je dois lui donner le change, le convaincre, si la chose est encore possible, que je suis une vraie thibétaine. Et la meilleure façon que j’imaginai pour me montrer telle fut de faire le simulacre de me moucher avec mes doigts. Le mouvement causé par ce geste secoua l’état de demi-rêve dans lequel j’avais vu et pensé jusque-là. Le soldat disparut”.

55 “Ne cherchez pas dans votre mémoire, [...] j’ai autant de visages que je le souhaite, et vous n’avez jamais vu celui-ci”.

56 “poignard enchanté”.

57 “sport macabre”.

58 “certains sont frappés de folie ou de mort subite au cours de sa célébration”.

59 “Le célébrant [...] imagine une déité féminine qui personnifie sa propre volonté. Celle-ci s’élance hors de sa tête, par le sommet du crâne, tenant un sabre à la main. D’un coup rapide, elle lui tranche la tête. Puis, tandis que des troupes de goules s’assemblent, dans une attente gourmande, elle détache ses membres, l’écorche, et lui ouvre le ventre” (2004, p. 154-155).

60 “il est enjoint au disciple de rester attaché pendant trois jours et trois nuits ou même davantage, jeûnant, luttant contre le sommeil, en proie à la faim et à la fatigue qui engendrent si facilement des hallucinations”.

61 “À chaque arrêt qui se fait trop long, les rhumatismes se réveillent et sa neurasthénie l’assaille”.

62 “Mais, je le confesse, la liberté parfaite de l’*ardjopa* qui […] dort chaque nuit où bon lui semble, en plein air, m’attirait énormément. Et […] [je] tiens pour les plus heureux jours que j’aie jamais vécus, ceux où, mon misérable baluchon sur le dos, j’errais par monts et par vaux au merveilleux “Pays des Neiges”.”

63 “C’est comme si […] l’on tentait d’atteindre [le sommet] en ligne droite, en escaladant les rocs à pic et travers[ant] les abîmes […] [une ascension dans] laquelle l’alpiniste présomptueux se brise les os. Par cette image, les Tibétains entendent une chute spirituelle effroyable amenant aux pires degrés de la perversité et de l’égarement et réduisant à la condition d’être démoniaque.”

64 However, the Tibetan people do not indulge in walking or wandering. On this subject, David-Néel writes: “In Thibet, no one wanders for pleasure, and people consider it absurd to travel when one is not called to a specific place on business or performing a pious pilgrimage” (1983, 294).

65 “la marche […] [est un] espace discursif, montrant le lien entre la vie et l’art, […] [où] le voyageur-penseur s’érige en protagoniste de son expérience, corps et esprit, jouissant d’une ferveur sensorielle et s’égarant dans les spectacles naturels […], sa phrase s’adapt[ant] au rythme de ses pas.”

66 “Les courses nocturnes à travers ces déserts sont un enchantement; j’aurais marché pour mon plaisir durant la nuit entière.”

67 “Tout se passe donc comme si une déambulation sans but précis facilitait la réflexion ou, plus exactement, s’accordait avec le libre cheminement d’un esprit disponible, accueillant à la contradiction et au doute, en quête d’une sagesse qu’il ne possède pas encore.”

68 “La première fois où je partis, seule, pour une de ces bizarres pérégrinations, je m’arrêtai près d’un lac aux eaux transparentes, serti entre des rives pierreuses. Le paysage environnant, complètement nu, exprimait une morne impassibilité excluant toute impression de crainte comme de sécurité, de joie comme de tristesse. On s’y sentait sombrer dans l’indifférence infinie des choses. […] La fantasmagorique procession des nuages éclairés par la lune se déroulait le long des cimes voisines, descendait vers moi, m’environnant de fantômes nébuleux. L’un d’eux s’avança, suivant une traînée de lumière soudainement projetée sur l’eau obscure, comme un tapis devant ses pas.

Géant diaphane, dont les yeux étaient deux étoiles, il me fit signe de son long bras, sortant d’une ample manche. M’appelait-il ? Me chassait-il ? J’hésitais…

Alors il se rapprocha, si réel, si vivant, que je fermai les yeux pour dissiper l'hallucination. Je me sentis enlacée, enveloppée dans les replis d'un manteau souple et froid dont la substance subtile s'insinuait en moi, me glaçant jusqu'au tréfonds de mon être…".

69 "[…] la marche s'avère dominée par l'accident et l'imprévu".

70 Letter dated March 19, 1913: "J'ai des visions d'Himalaya, de lacs où se mirent les pics neigeux, de cascades dans les forêts […]. Tibet ! Tibet ! Une partie de moi est restée là-haut dans les steppes, dans cette solitude désolée."

71 Letter dated April 10, 1915: "J'ai de l'atavisme de nomade asiatique dans les veines, c'est certain […] Mais, dans la mémoire de mes cellules chante un passé… Je m'en rends bien compte, il est plus que singulier que […] je sois douée de cette mentalité si étrangère à celle de mon milieu. J'ai eu la nostalgie de l'Asie avant d'y avoir jamais été […]."

72 Letter dated March 12, 1917: "À vrai dire, j'ai le mal du pays pour un pays qui n'est pas le mien. Les steppes, les solitudes, les neiges éternelles et le grand ciel clair de là-haut me hantent !"

73 "Le Tibet est le pays des démons. Si l'on devait s'appuyer sur les légendes et les croyances populaires, l'on serait conduit à penser que le nombre de ceux-ci y dépasse de beaucoup celui de la population humaine. Revêtant mille formes différentes, ces êtres malfaisants habitent les arbres, les rochers, les vallées, les lacs, les sources, Ils poursuivent les hommes et les animaux pour leur ravir leur "souffle vital" et s'en repaître."

74 "We spent the next few hours in the torments of agony, our ears on the alert for any noise that might herald the approach of the dreaded figure, looking desperately left and right to see if, as in the old fairy tales, a rock or a tree might open up to shelter us. But alas, no miracle was forthcoming. The local geniuses remained seemingly indifferent to our misery" ["Nous passâmes les heures qui suivirent dans les tourments de l'agonie, l'oreille aux aguets pour surprendre un bruit qui pût nous annoncer l'approche du personnage redouté, regardant désespérément à droite et à gauche si, comme dans les vieux contes, un rocher ou un arbre ne s'ouvriraient pas pour nous abriter. Mais, hélas! aucun miracle ne se produisit. Les génies locaux restaient, en apparence, indifférents à notre misère"] (1983, p. 99).

75 "Restée seule, je dissimulai nos sacs sous les branches, m'étendis à plat parmi les feuilles morts et en jonchai mes vêtements. Ainsi camouflée, quelqu'un

cheminant, par aventure, à travers les bois, aurait pu passer bien près de moi sans m'apercevoir".

76 "[N]otre entrée à Lhassa semble protégée par une sorte de prodige. À peine avons-nous débarqué que l'atmosphère jusque-là très calme, se trouble soudainement. Dans l'espace de quelques minutes une tempête furieuse se lève, soulevant jusqu'au ciel, des nuages de sable. [...] Un gigantesque rideau jaune, fait de sable suspendu, est étendu devant le Potala, aveuglant ses hôtes, leur masquant Lhassa et les voies qui y conduisent. Je l'interprète comme un symbole me promettant une entière sécurité [...]".

77 "Ceci est encore mieux que le rideau de sable tendu devant le Potala le jour de notre arrivée, me dit Yongden en riant, voici que « vos dieux » se mettent à obscurcir la lune pour qu'on ne nous voie pas".

78 "[...] la nature environnante parut entraînée par ma déclaration passionnée et se mit à l'unisson. La forêt s'assombrit, une légère brise fit courir de lointaines rumeurs dans les taillis, des mystérieuses et lugubres voix semblèrent surgir de l'invisible torrent roulant au fond de la vallée et monter vers nous, emplissant l'air de phrases menaçantes dans un langage inconnu.

J'étais de sang-froid, et pourtant je ne pus me défendre d'un frisson causé par l'atmosphère occulte que j'avais moi-même créée. Je ne fus, d'ailleurs, pas seule à en éprouver l'effet. Les sept brigands paraissaient pétrifiés".

79 "Jetsunema,,Yongden said to me a few minutes later, you were not mistaken when you assured me, in the forests of Kha-Karpo, that you would 'send them dreams and show them mirages'. This fat man and his retinue have certainly been bewitched." ["Jétsunema me dit Yongden quelques minutes plus tard, vous ne vous trompez pas lorsque vous m'assuriez, dans les forêts du *Kha-Karpo*, que vous 'leur enverriez des rêves et feriez voir des mirages'. Certainement ce gros homme et les gens de sa suite ont été ensorcelés"].

Chapter 4
Healing War Trauma From a Holistic Perspective:
Mario Rigoni Stern at the Intersection Between Western and Eastern Traditions

Gianluca Cinelli
http://orcid.org/0000-0002-9805-0908
Independent Researcher, Italy

ABSTRACT

In Western culture, war trauma is generally looked at as a syndrome (PTSD) and mostly treated pharmaceutically. However, war affects the human soul in a variety of ways, and holistic approaches have therefore been practised since ancient times in different cultures, aimed at maintaining the well-being of veterans. In Japanese culture, Bushido, Zen, as well as the tea ceremony or the "swordsmanship" and other forms of ethical education have been traditionally practiced as effective ways of keeping the human in harmonic homeostasis with nature, especially under stressful or potentially traumatic circumstances. This chapter considers the case of Italian WW2 veteran Mario Rigoni Stern: to overcome his war trauma, he undertook holistic healing based on storytelling and reconnecting with the sacred dimension of nature. The author will claim that Rigoni Stern's holistic way of healing war trauma can be understood from a transcultural perspective that blends the Western cognitive theories of emotional intelligence and adaptive storytelling with the Eastern traditions of Bushido and Zen.

DOI: 10.4018/979-8-3373-3521-6.ch004

INTRODUCTION

Speaking of war trauma, one has to deal with a large spectrum of implications—such as moral, political, ideological, psychological, etc.—both public (collective) and private (personal). The very notion of trauma can be interpreted diversely in different cultural systems, insofar as "across cultural contexts, there is a difference in the phenomenology of what is experienced as normal and possible and what disrupts this horizon of possibilities" (Wilde, 2020, p. 226), even though all humans share the universal ability to "normalise" uncomfortable, adverse or even shocking experiences (Hillman, 2004, p. 27). As a consequence, the effects of traumatic war experiences can be perceived and treated differently,[1] and scholars have argued that remedies to heal the "invisible wound" have always been practiced by ancient cultures worldwide (Tick, 2014).

This chapter focuses on how Italian WWII veteran Mario Rigoni Stern (1921–2008) accounted, in memoirs, novels, and short stories, for the traumatic effects the war had on his body and mind, as well as the way in which he managed to heal himself by pursuing body-mind oriented practices that helped him make sense of the past suffering and re-establish emotional and physiological homeostasis. By examining Rigoni Stern's war narratives at the convergence between Western and Eastern perspectives on holistic practices of healing, this chapter will argue that the problem of war trauma can be approached from a holistic perspective that extends beyond clinical intervention by taking into account the body-mind implications of both trauma and healing. To achieve this, the chapter will analyse a selection of Rigoni Stern's war narratives[2] within a theoretical framework that addresses the topic of healing war trauma holistically, merging Western and Eastern approaches and practices. It is worth noting that Rigoni had no direct knowledge of the Eastern traditions of Zen meditation or Buddhism. Nonetheless, his idea that living in a sacred relationship with the natural environment of the mountains and forests is a sustainable lifestyle that enhances well-being and a healthy life[3] creates a remarkable "convergence" between his intellectual resources and Zen culture.

In Western culture the issue of war trauma began to be clinically addressed only during the First World War, with the invention of the well-known phrase "shell-shock" (Wastell, 2005, pp. 1–27). After many decades during which the notion of war trauma slowly evolved, in 1980 the American Psychiatric Association introduced the fortunate formula "Post-Traumatic Stress Disorder" (PTSD).

Over the last forty-four years, PTSD has been challenged, on the one hand, as a too-wide, all-inclusive diagnosis and, on the other hand, as a reductionist approach that may leave the patient with no other options than undergoing psychiatric or pharmacological treatment (Brooke, 2017). One relevant contribution to the debate came from the cognitive theories of the "embodied mind," which at the end of the twentieth century began to claim that the mind only exists in and with the body, implying that emotions play a crucial role in cognition and interaction with the environment (Damasio, 2006/1994, p. 88). One theory of the embodied mind that particularly fits the scope of this chapter is the one expounded by Francisco Varela, Evan Thompson and Eleanor Rosch in *The Embodied Mind*, a book that explores the nexus body-mind by challenging the Western cognitive paradigm (based on logical mathematizing of the human cognition), and by conversely approaching the Eastern practice of meditation, whose purpose is "to become mindful, to experience what one's mind is doing as it does it, to be present with one's mind" (1993, p. 23). The idea of the embodied mind implies that thought is not a mere objectification of the world (and the body) through abstraction, but an experience in itself that involves the body as well as the mind. In the wake of such an interpretation, several scholars began to consider the mind no longer in Cartesian terms, that is, detached from the body, but rather as an evolutionary product of the human brain. Many studies, therefore, explore language and the verbal organisation of experience into narratives. In *More Than Cool Reason*, George Lakoff and Mark Turner claim that the very basis of human language relies not on logical principles but on what they call the "basic metaphors," which descend from sensory perception. These metaphors are no mere figures of speech but concepts that we coined after "what we take to be our bodily experience," because "we conventionally understand these concepts not by virtue of metaphoric mapping between them and different conceptual domains but rather by virtue of their grounding in what we take to be our forms of life, our habitual and routine bodily and social experiences" (1989, p. 59). Mark Turner advocated for this interpretation, claiming that

> *We understand our experience in this way because we are built evolutionarily to learn to distinguish objects and combine them in small spatial stories at human scale in a way that is useful for us, given that we have human bodies… . Image schemas are skeletal pattern that recur in our sensory and motor experience. Motion along a path, bounded interior, balance, and symmetry are typical image schemas. (1996, pp. 15–16)*

In *Philosophy in the Flesh*, Lakoff and Johnson maintain that an actual human being has no separation of mind and body (1999). On the contrary, the human mind is embodied, which means that we can only form concepts through the body and "the structure of our spatial concepts emerges from our constant spatial experience, that is, from our interaction with the physical environment" (Lakoff & Johnson, 1980, pp. 56–57). As a consequence, the mind is subject to the body's physical laws of evolution and changes through time, adapting to the changing conditions of its environment.

The theories of the embodied mind also influenced scholarship on the narrative self. Antonio Damasio claims that the self is a construction, the nature of which can be understood in terms of evolution, adaptation, development, and mapping of the organism and the environment. The self, then, is the achievement of a complex process starting with the body and ending with the "autobiographical conscience" (2010). Similarly, Gallagher states that through language experience can be put into words and made coherent, extending our biological "minimal self" to a more extended structure that permits us to make sense of our lives (2000). The same idea was also shared by Richard Menary, who claims that "the self is constituted both by an embodied consciousness whose experiences are available for narration and narratives themselves, which can play a variety of roles in the agent's psychological life" (2008, p. 63). Joseph Carroll maintains, in turn, that the relationship between the organism and its environment lies at the origin of the mind, which uses narration as an evolutionary tool to map the world and adapt (1995, pp. 2–3). From a slightly different perspective, Katsunori Miyahara and Shiogo Tanaka explain that self-constitution is a process of embodiment, rather than self-narration, that takes into account the structure of habituation as a catalyst of evolution (2023).

THE EMBODIED MIND AND THE TREATMENT OF PTSD

The idea of the embodied mind has been applied to understanding the relationship between physical trauma and its effects on the mind. Because traumatic experiences and stress involve the emotions and their processing (Sapolski, 1992), the reaction to such experiences has been increasingly described in terms of adaptation (Wastell, 2005, pp. xvi–xix and 60–61). Thus, more than one scholar has claimed over the last fifteen years that one promising approach to healing war trauma consists in the holistic approach that includes practices of well-being enhancement, among which art-therapy and, more recently, yoga and meditation. These approaches integrate "the cognitive, emotional and physiological memory towards positive adaptive functioning" (Talwar, 2007, p. 26), blending emotional and analytical cognitive processes. Artistic performance, inward-oriented tasks, and relaxation techniques imply verbal and non-verbal elaboration of the sense of control and safety, which in turn affects one's perception of stress and influences the biochemistry of the limbic system and the consequent reaction of the immune system.[4] In other words, as Hass-Cohen has it, "people can intentionally influence the body mind connection .... The way we make autobiographical meaning of what happens to them has an effect on physiological outcomes. Physiological outcomes impact autobiographical meaning making" (Hass-Cohen, 2003, p. 29).

Particularly relevant for the context of this chapter are the meditation-based approaches to treating trauma and PTSD caused by war because they lay a bridge between two different methods, namely the Western (analytically and phenomenologically oriented towards isolating symptoms and tackling trauma as a syndrome that negatively affects the individual's self-perception) and the Eastern (holistically and spiritually oriented towards pursuing the individual's well-being in terms of body-mind balance).

HEALING WAR TRAUMA AT THE CROSSROADS BETWEEN WEST AND EAST

As Micale and Pols have it, "the way Westerners experience trauma is not necessarily the same as it is experienced elsewhere; interpretations of trauma and its effects on individual well-being vary across cultures as well" (2021, p. 3). This should encourage a transcultural approach to understanding trauma and healing by starting from the environmental circumstances in which such concepts are to be applied, rather than adopting a reductionist point of view based on cognitive, psychological and physiological symptom-assessment:

> *Asian mental health professionals and lay counselors have adjusted medical and psychotherapeutic approaches to suit local approaches, thereby implicitly or, at times, explicitly critiquing Western psychiatry. Systematic critique of the globalization of PTSD has thus far been fairly circumscribed within Western psychiatric medicine itself; instead, the strongest criticisms have been formulated by anthropologists and sociologists, operating from a wide range of national backgrounds. They have noted that diagnostic categories conceived by and contained in Western psychiatric textbooks capture specifically Western behavioral and mental conditions, despite their aspirations to universality. Psychological trauma, they insist, is culturally and historically situated and cannot be extracted from its complex social, cultural, and political contexts .... Experiences of trauma vary substantially across place and time. The way individuals and communities experience traumatic events, how anguish is expressed through mental or somatic symptoms, and how emotional pain is interpreted in local frameworks of meaning depend on a variety of political, social, and cultural factors. Similarly, both personal and communal rituals and strategies for coping with and overcoming trauma vary across the world and are not necessarily compatible with individualized, Western-style treatment modalities. (p. 4)*

In light of these observations, it is noteworthy that Western practitioners and scholars have begun to look at non-Western holistic approaches since the 2010s to find new ways of treating PTSD. In 2011, a team of researchers stated that "a portable practice of repeating a mantram—a sacred word or phrase—has been shown to reduce the severity of PTSD symptoms in veterans with military trauma" (Bormann et al., 2012, p. 496), introducing the Western scientific community to the idea that "attending to spirituality in individuals who have experienced traumatic stressors might be an important tool for coping with the aftermath of those experiences" (p. 497).

Two years later, another team hypothesised that "mindfulness-based interventions may be similarly useful in treatment of [PTSD], and combat-related PTSD in particular" because "such techniques stand opposed to the psychological processes of avoidance and suppression of painful emotions and memories, which are thought to contribute to symptom maintenance in PTSD" (King et al., 2013, p. 639). The study saluted mindfulness-based group therapy as a "potentially effective novel therapeutic approach for PTSD" (p. 642), representing the pursue of an innovative approach that would need further support from other similar studies. The main benefits of this approach are that

> *Mindfulness-based therapies provide a strategy that encourages active engagement without explicit cognitive restructuring or exposure to trauma memories, are relatively easy to learn, and can be administered in an efficient group format. Increased ability to actively attend to, and generate nonjudgmental acceptance of, traumatic memories and physiological responses may help prepare individuals for trauma-focused therapies, such as prolonged exposure. (p. 644)*

The same path was trodden by another research team that one year later published the result of a similar research involving breathing-based meditation for the treatment of PTSD. Like the previous one, this study started with acknowledging that "results of pharmaceutical treatments are mixed … whereas substantial residual symptoms remain after psychotherapy … suggesting a critical need to evaluate alternative or supplementary approaches to treating PTSD" (Seppälä et al., 2014, p. 397). This assumption, alongside the "growing body of evidence [suggesting] meditation-based interventions have the potential to reduce symptoms and improve well-being" (p. 397), urged the research team to demonstrate that "breathing-based meditation practices may be particularly beneficial for PTSD given that it is a stress disorder characterized by hyperarousal, autonomic dysfunction, negative affect, and difficulties with emotion regulation" (pp. 397–398). The study resulting in reduced PTSD symptoms, anxiety, hyperarousal and startle, suggested that "by activating both the parasympathetic and sympathetic system, the breathing exercises may produce a state of both alertness and calm" (p. 403).[5] Therefore, the team claimed that Sudarshan Kriya yoga used in the study "may reduce trauma by decoupling the stimulus (i.e., recalled memories) from the fear response: Participants reported reexperiencing traumatic memories while in a breathing-induced, relaxed, physiological state. After the intervention, they reported that these traumatic memories no longer impacted them as strongly" (p. 403).

Further support to this trend came in 2018 from another study that applied yoga to a group of veterans diagnosed with PTSD who, after the treatment, reported decreased insomnia, anxiety and depression. This study explicitly adopted CAM (complementary and alternative medicine), acknowledging that such treatments are not standardised and thus hard to reproduce. Nonetheless, the team advocated for their approach by claiming the positive effect of yoga on the parasympathetic nervous system:

Slow rhythmic breathing that is synchronized to the body movements of yoga can help activate the parasympathetic nervous system and stimulate vagal activity.[6] *The parasympathetic nervous system is the rest-and-digest portion of the autonomic nervous system; it has important functions in decreasing the heart rate and blood pressure, speeding up digestive functioning, and normalizing stress hormones. Yoga may be beneficial to veterans and service members with PTSD by activating the parasympathetic nervous system to tamp down the hyperarousal cluster of symptoms. Studies have shown that yoga can also reduce levels of the stress hormone cortisol and help restore balance in the hypothalamic-pituitary-adrenal axis. (Cushing et al., 2018, p. e224)*

Finally, one more study from 2018, devoted to investigating compassion as one contributing factor in the treatment of PTSD, is worth mentioning: in this particular case, one aspect of war-related trauma to consider is the so-called "moral injury," that is, the feeling of being betrayed by one's leaders or having let down one's friends and comrades. Moral injury may occur when one fails to prevent unnecessary killing, wounding or cruelty or fails to protect friends and comrades from being wounded or killed, or because one takes part in or stands by actions that clash with one's moral principles. And because recalling these experiences challenges one's self-perception in terms of morality, it also triggers intrusive thoughts, nightmares, and reactions of anger, self-deprecation, avoidance and emotional numbing. The methodology relies on Buddhist meditation, for mindfulness reduces rumination (Litz & Carney, 2018, pp. 205) and encourages non-judgemental compassion by making one aware of universal suffering, appreciating common humanity, and cultivating kindness in everyday life. Such an approach is promising but impervious to practise, and yet, unlike other interventions (e.g. pharmaceutical), it might secure long-lasting positive effects (pp. 207 and 209).

So far, an attempt has been made to sketch how Western scholarship and practitioners have tried and developed their approaches to PTSD and war-related trauma by including non-Western traditional holistic techniques and expertise in their methodologies.[7] Zen entails meditation practices that have a connection with war-related experiences, and precisely with the education of the samurai in pre-modern Japan. In Nitobé's words, Buddhism was one of the sources of Bushidô, the code of moral principles that the samurai were taught and required to observe, and it provided the warrior with "a sense of calm trust in Fate, a quiet submission to the inevitable, that stoic composure in sight of danger or calamity, that disdain of life and friendliness with death" (1908/1904, p. 7). Nitobé idealised the educational system of the samurai by suggesting that it significantly imprinted Japanese culture as a repository of maxims aimed at shaping the spirit of the individual in terms of loyalty, rectitude, courage, benevolence, politeness, truthfulness, honour, and self-control. All these are symbolised in the art of swordsmanship because "the very possession of the dangerous instrument imparts to [the samurai] a feeling and an air of self-respect and responsibility" (p. 35).[8]

Another influential Japanese scholar who successfully introduced his culture to Western audiences, Daisetz Suzuki, presents Bushido in similar terms of "loyalty, filial piety, and benevolence" and above all as "readiness to face death" without putting too much thought on it (1993, p. 70). Such an attitude requires a mind-set that is essential to Zen, namely the "no-mind" or "doing by not doing": the "no-mind" is not an empty mind devoid of thoughts and feelings, but one that is not disturbed by its content because it does not linger on it, "is always flowing, it never halts" and therefore is not stuck on preoccupations and affects (p. 111). From the perspective of Zen, "doing by not doing" means surrendering the illusion of conscious control and identifying oneself with the activity one is performing: thus, the mind "follows its own course like water" (p. 144).[9] These ideas connect with those of simplicity (*wabi*) and unpretentiousness (*sabi*), that in turn involve a profound and complex relationship with the environment that includes compassion, tranquillity, and the awareness that everything that exists occupies its place in a complex relation with everything else (pp. 31–32).[10]

Suzuki insists on swordsmanship as the art of self-cultivation and a school of discipline and virtue, for the sword is "an instrument of spiritual self-discipline" (74). Paradoxically, the sword is not designed to bring death but to preserve life (Munenori, 2012), which means that a self-disciplined warrior avoids quarrelling and pursues compassion over violence, being well-aware that the use of the weapon will be lethal: thus, "when it is properly handled, [the sword] helps us in an efficient way to contribute to the cultivation of the mind and spirit" (Suzuki, 1993, p. 132). This is summarised in the rejection of the logical (intellectual) contraposition between life and death, whereas the former is the object of positive desire and the latter the object of negative fear and preoccupation: "He who transcends the dualistic idea of life and death goes on living, in the genuine sense of the term. When there is the thought either of life or of death, negatively or positively, this will surely prove to be a stumbling block in the way of life" (142).[11]

As claimed, Zen meditation (*zazen*) is essential to the samurai's well-being because it permits the individual to feel emotions by remaining detached and accepting them. That is an aspect Buddhism shares with one of the most influential Western ancient philosophies, Stoicism (especially in its late Roman version): "Though the philosophies are very different, both aim to curb our ego and control our negative emotions. Both Stoicism and Buddhism are, at their roots, methods for practicing wellbeing" (García & Miralles, 2017, p. 106). In both philosophies, we should enjoy things right now and here, being mindful of our surroundings in a state of "quiet alertness" (*zanshin*) and not worrying about the past and the future because the present is all that exists and is the only thing we can control. The aim of the two philosophies is therefore to pursue a state of serenity, and "to become aware of our desires and emotions and thereby free ourselves from them" (p. 108). Zen reaches this purpose through meditation, the aim of which is not to expel thoughts from the mind or objectivize them but rather the opposite: meditation "is not simply a question of keeping the mind free of thoughts but instead involves observing our thoughts and emotions as they appear, without getting carried away by them" (p. 108). Tranquillity stems from the consideration that nothing in nature lasts forever or can go through time unchanged:

> *In addition to living in the here and now, the Stoics recommend reflecting on the impermanence of the things around us. The Roman emperor Marcus Aurelius said that the things we love are like the leaves of a tree: They can fall at any moment with a gust of wind. He also said that changes in the world around us are not accidental but rather form part of the essence of the universe—a rather Buddhist notion, in fact. (García & Miralles, 2017, p. 108)*[12]

One notable difference between Stoicism and Zen is that the former relies on reason and logic, while the latter insists on the importance of practical life. Thus, if stoic meditation generally occurs in the form of spiritual exercise or logical analysis of one's thoughts, aimed at grasping the truth and meaning of life through reasoning, Zen meditation can basically consist of any activity, from drinking tea to practising swordsmanship, from gardening to cleaning one's house, and so on: "In all things, it is important to forget your 'mind' and become one with the work at hand" (Suzuki, 1993, p. 114).[13]

The theoretical perspectives sketched above encompass a holistic attitude towards the issue of war trauma based on practical and spiritual interaction with one's surroundings, environment and, at large, nature as the whole of which we are parts. One example of how the principles of Zen philosophy blend with Western culture, more focused on a self-centred perspective, can be found in the poetics and practical life of WW2 veteran Mario Rigoni Stern.

HOLISTIC HEALING IN WW2 VETERAN MARIO RIGONI STERN

The haunting memory of trauma

Mario Rigoni Stern was born in North-East Italy in 1921. His hometown, Asiago, endured massive destruction during the Great War, and the whole surrounding Alpine landscape bore the marks and scars of the heavy fighting that occurred in that area between 1916 and 1918. Mario Rigoni Stern often recalled how the abandoned trenches were an eerie playground to him and his friends in the 1920s. Young Mario never embraced Fascism, but in 1938 volunteered to join the Italian Mountain Infantry Corps (*Alpini*), seeking juvenile adventure, and in 1940 was dispatched to the front. Thus, he fought in the Italian military campaigns against France (1940), Greece (1940–1941), and the USSR (1941–1943), and in September 1943, after Italy had signed the armistice with the Allies, he was taken captive by the Germans and spent the rest of the war in concentration camps until April 1945, when he managed to escape and went back home on foot.

Rigoni Stern accounts for his war experiences in most of his books—the first of which appeared in 1953 (*The Sergeant in the Snow*)—and represents the traumatic legacy of war in almost all of his stories (Cinelli, 2022, p. 99). Rigoni Stern believed that war hurts humans, plants, and beasts. His rejection of war depends on the fact that war affects nature at large, inflicting wounds on the environment and scarring the landscape, which led him to define war as an "act of violence on everything that exists in the universe" (Motta, 1982, p. 6). Rigoni Stern talks about trauma not in theoretical terms but as a storyteller, by focusing mainly on his autobiographical experiences, two of which particularly affected him over the years causing PTSD: the catastrophic defeat of the Italian troops in Ukraine in January 1943, and the months of captivity spent in German concentration camps, enduring hunger, humiliation, and forced labour.

At the core of these experiences lies a cluster of traumatising factors: the death of friends and comrades (most of all occurred during the retreat from Ukraine), the moral injury of having participated in a criminal war of aggression, and being the victim of violence as a POW. Of all these experiences, captivity represents the most traumatising: in Rigoni Stern's books, the Lager is a place of promiscuous solitude that causes men to grow mean, indifferent and callous. The Lager inspires anger, sadness and desperation, affecting the veteran for many years after the war. About the difficulties of resuming his life as a civilian after 1945, the author said in an interview:

> *I came back broken. Obviously, my physical abjection must have influenced my morale, it's logical. I was very skinny, always feverish, and struggled to resume my normal life .... As I tried to tell my story, nobody believed me. People wanted*

to change the subject of the conversation .... It's in those moments that desperation takes the upper hand. (Milani & Rigoni Stern, 2008, p. 38)[14]

The veteran fails to resume his life because the prolonged exposition to physical and mental strain in combat and captivity still affects him. But what risks unhinging his mind is the indifference of the community to which he returns. Solitude is an alienating existential state because the survivor feels like a stranger surrounded by people who refuse to listen to his story and he isolates himself in depression (Stein, 2017, p. 123): "I felt a deadly weariness and bleak greyness as if the time of the Lager wrapped me now that I had come home and was free again, and the strength I once had seemed gone, as if it had remained entangled in the barbed wire" (Rigoni Stern, 2004a, p. 264). As he wrote in another story, the Lager "should have remained far behind"; on the contrary, the memory of Lager lingers on and wraps the survivor "like a dress" (Rigoni Stern, 2004c, p. 274). And with the first autumn snow surface the memories of the war in Ukraine, and melancholia sits in so that every time "it feels like dying a little" (Rigoni Stern, 2004b, p. 279).

Healing through the ethical compensation

Rigoni Stern slowly managed to cope with his past and began finding peace of mind by pursuing ethical compensation and reconnection with nature. Ethical compensation constitutes one of the ways of elaborating mourning amongst survivors and often consists of thinking about how many lives one saved: "Much probably, I must have killed [but] I did it out of survival instinct aroused by the war. However, whenever I was commanded to kill in cool blood, I refused. I do not regret that, even if it meant disobeying orders: I do not regret having disobeyed" (Rigoni Stern, 2014, p. 117). Moral responsibility, thus, lies at the core of ethical compensation and shapes the moral awareness of the veteran who abided by principles of justice and compassion. The memory of self-restraint, discipline, and loyalty to one's duty make the veteran aware of his state of moral satisfaction when he remembers that saving the men of his platoon was the "most difficult moment" of the war but also "his best deed ever" (p. 115).

The other facet of this ethical compensation consists in the awareness of having exchanged displays of compassion with his former foe. During the retreat in the dead of winter, Ukrainian women more than once helped Rigoni Stern by offering him shelter at night and some food. He also remembered, in *The Sergeant in the Snow*, an extraordinary episode of fraternisation that occurred in the middle of heavy fighting. On 26 January 1943, while the Italian troops were desperately fighting to break the Red Army's encirclement, Rigoni Stern sought a moment of relief, knocked at the door of a hut and got in. However, the hut was full of Russian soldiers, who stood around the table sipping hot soup from a cauldron. One of the peasant women in the hut offered the Italian soldier, too, a bowl of soup:

> *Time doesn't exist any more. The Russian soldiers look at me. The women look at me. The children look at me. No one breathes a word. The only sound is of the spoon in my plate; and of each of my mouthfuls. "Spaziba," I say when I've finished. And the woman takes the empty bowl from my hands. "Pas austa," she replies simply. The Russian soldiers watch me go out, without moving .... That's how it happened, this incident. Now, thinking it over, I don't find it at all strange, but natural—with that naturalness there must have been between all men at one time. After the first surprise all my gestures were natural. I didn't feel any fear, or any wish to defend myself or to offend them. It was very simple. The Russians were like me too, I felt. In that isba there'd been created between me, the Russian soldiers, the women and the children a harmony which wasn't just a truce. It was something much more than the respect which animals in the forest have for each other. Circumstance, just for once, had helped men to remain human. (Rigoni Stern, 1967, p. 396)*

The words "naturalness," "simple," and "harmony" recall the basic components of the Zen lifestyle: the scene speaks of unexpected and almost surreal humanness and kindness in the midst of bloodshed, self-restraint, simplicity, and tranquillity. The rhetoric of simplicity mitigates the sharp contrast between these two contexts: the characters reveal their peaceful intentions through their bodies, and the only words uttered mean kindness: "thank you" and "you're welcome." Although all the soldiers in the hut are armed, their weapons remain slung on their shoulders, and they use their hands to perform the pacific action of eating. In simplicity, they resume their sacred humanity for a moment, turning the hut from being a dangerous place on the frontline of the battle into a "safe space" where the warriors can restrain themselves from fighting for a while and rediscover an instant of peaceful cohabitation.

Many years after the war, this feeling of compassion further expanded into universal friendship and brotherhood with the population of Ukraine. In 1971, after retirement, Rigoni Stern survived a cardiac arrest and decided to visit the places where he had fought in 1943 to honour the memory of his lost friends and comrades. The account of that journey was published one year later with the title "Return to the Don River" (1972). With that journey, Rigoni Stern wanted to "show his gratitude to the people of the villages" that were kind to him during the war: he never called the Russians "enemies" and remembered them as "worth his respect and awe," for he believed they deserved the apology of those who had invaded their land (2004b, p. 292; 2014, p. 113). The awareness of having taken part in an imperialistic war was a moral burden, but the awareness of having restrained himself from being gratuitously violent and plundering the homes of civilians sooths the conscience and makes it possible to restore friendship and mutual respect after the war.

The ethical compensation includes the cult of the dead:[15] in "Return to the Don River" Rigoni Sterns claims that each fallen soldier has a story: "Who could say everything? No one. No one will ever know. And for each of them, there is one different story. And we were many" (2004b, p. 304). The land that was once devastated by war has meanwhile become "the most tranquil place in the world" where reign "deep peace, profound silence, and infinite tenderness" (p. 317). "Tranquillity," "peace," and "silence" remind us, once again, of the Zen approach to nature and landscape: the outer world reflects what one feels inside, and reconciliation with one's past produces, in this case, inner peace and serenity. At the core of this process lies awareness, which also occupies the central place in Zen meditation.

Healing by reconnecting with the natural environment

By revisiting his war experiences, Rigoni Stern realises that war reveals people for what they are (2014, p. 126): "The soul of a man is a microcosm" (Sacco & Rigoni Stern, 2008, p. 92) capable of mirroring the whole universe. Therefore, to reconcile with his past, the veteran must acknowledge, accept, and welcome the bad and the good memories as momentary lapses of the broader biographical continuity. However, this continuity is no close and isolated monad: it should be looked at from the perspective of the interconnection between the individual and all other beings and things existing in the world. Thus, ethical compensation must include reconnection with nature. In the short story "The Axe", Rigoni Stern represents this transit from loss to recovery using a small parable:

> *At night, I screamed in my sleep. By day, I wandered in the forests but wouldn't hear the finches, see the deer's footprints, or smell the elder tree. Nor did I look for anyone. One morning, I listened to the axe beating on the slope of the mountain: it was a novel sound. It was the axe of the lumberjack, not a machine gun, and I was aware of that. I walked that way, almost running to reach that sound, and when I came closer, I stopped. Raising his head, he saw me standing there, watching at him. He greeted me with a smile. He took his canteen from a bough, poured some water, and offered it to me: "You thirsty?" he said. (2004c, p. 275)*

The short story "The Axe" exemplifies how solidarity and simplicity can reconnect a wounded soul with the world. Such reconciliation takes the form of *vita activa*,[16] which in another story entitled "[...]" occurs as a "silent dialogue" with nature: "I started tending my vegetable garden and chopping wood, but always alone and silently. One day I realised the birds were still singing and flowers were blossoming on the grazes" (Rigoni Stern, 2003a, p. 72).

Paradoxically, one of the ways by which Rigoni Stern managed to reconnect with nature was hunting: in chasing and killing prey, he acknowledged an act of sacred violence and a spiritual connection with the beast in its natural environment. Killing the animal meant not only increasing the possibility of eating protein and fat (Rigoni Stern, 2014, p. 23) but also creating a profound and grateful bond with the animal that, by its death, permits the hunter to survive.[17] To Rigoni Stern, hunters ought to be "nature keepers" rather than "consumers" because hunting means "harvesting, not wasting: to pick fruits, one need not cutting down the tree!" (Rigoni Stern, 2014, pp. 13–14). Moreover, the forest is "something one should not defile" (p. 27) because it is "the portrait of the God that is continuously born anew in humans and for the humans" (p. 84). Hunting, as an "ancestral need," is the opposite of the killing at war, which is destructive and unnatural. Hunting is a sort of duel between two beings struggling to survive, and in such a view, the killing is purposeful: the aware hunter does not kill for the sake of killing but to collect food and contribute to the demographic growth of animals that may become too numerous and therefore harmful to their environment. Thus, Rigoni Stern managed to re-establish a harmonic relationship with the environment of the forest and its living creatures, as he writes in the short story "The Dog I Saw Cry": "I often remember the post-war years when hunting a grouse in the mountains saved me from my Lager-bound desperation" (Rigoni Stern, 2004e, p. 121).

Hunting and foraging constitute primeval human activities developed over millennia of evolution: the human being who learns to adapt and borrows from nature what is needed to survive leads a healthy and balanced good life of harmonic well-being. The prehistoric and modern humans are different only superficially:[18] if observed more closely, they reveal that humankind depends on nature as a guest that, in order to survive, should harvest without destroying (Rigoni Stern, 2014, pp. 14, 23, 75 and 172).

The concept of harmony

The concept of harmony is key to understanding how Rigoni Stern deals with war trauma. Deriving from the Greek word *ρμον α*, meaning the balanced connection of the parts in an organism, harmony is a characteristic of nature, for all things exist interrelated, and the opposite forces and vital principles coexist in equilibrium. In Rigoni Stern's opinion, one ought to seek harmony in the relationship between humans and nature with "respect, intelligence, and care" (p. 89). This respectful care for nature consists in the sense of the limit that "makes one aware of reality" (Rigoni Stern, 2004f, p. 144), and is inspired by the active connection with nature that "promises life will go on also once you've gone" (Rigoni Stern, 2014, p. 43). Like in Zen philosophy, this enlightenment permits one to attain inner peace and concentrate on the present, when life flows and the memory of the past appear not as a detached reality but as a part of life as a whole, which returns to itself in circles of life and death. Like the wise who practices Zen, Rigoni Stern found relief from his war trauma in reconnecting with nature (*shizen*) and simplicity (*shimpuru-sa*), for this view of life frees one from the fear of death and helps one to focus on the present and its value. One example of that attitude can be found in the words the veteran used to explain the fear of death to a group of schoolboys:

> *Death is a fact of nature, for all that lives must die. Suffering, though, is ugly and hard to overcome and bear. But death is welcome. I had some moments in which I held my breath when I heard the bullets whiz before my nose .... I held my breath as though retaining some air in my lungs could prolong my life a bit, at least for those few moments I could not breathe. I did so, waiting to die. Nothing more. (pp. 121–122)*

To Rigoni Stern, inner peace is not synonymous with ascetic inaction. Everyone can find it by cultivating respect and compassion. There is the key to healing from the traumatic experience of destructive violence endured at war.

As mentioned before, Zen advocates for an attitude towards nature that can be summarised as being aware of the present moment, appreciating the impermanence of all things, pouring one's effort into what one does without overthinking, and remembering that we are part of the whole, interconnected with everything else. This attitude may seem detached and apathetic, but it is actually mindful and balanced, as Shintō priest Katō Taishi convincingly claims, reflecting on the centrality of *kami* in Shintō:[19]

> *Both being and emptiness show an affinity with the phenomenon of kami in several respects. They are realities that are in some sense manifest, always present, yet at the same time elusive, impossible to pin down. They are perpetually there, unchanging, yet at the same time "dynamic" and "active" in some sense. They transcend individual things and figures, opening up a space in which the true presence or "sacredness" of things can come to be fully realized. (Taishi, 2018, p. 14)*[20]

According to Shintō, every living and inorganic thing has a "soul" that participates in the whole of nature,[21] for "everything is a reflection of the other: the Universe can be understood through a stone and the stone through the Universe" (Kalland, 2002, pp. 150). Rigoni Stern shares a very similar conception of nature as the home the humans dwell as guests for a limited lapse of time, a place they must inhabit with care and gratitude. War subverts the terms of this ethical relationship through exploitation and devastation, cutting off the humans from the whole and causing them to lose their balance and sense of belonging. Thus, reconnection to nature is one thing with reconnection with oneself.

CONCLUSIONS

War trauma remains to date a tricky problem to tackle both in the West and the East, regardless of its being related to past or present conflicts. The "invisible wounds" of war continue to affect those who experience the violence and suffering caused by war, and there is seemingly no exhaustive theory, approach, or doctrine capable of outlining the ideal way of treating war trauma. That is primarily because different cultures may perceive and define the very notion of trauma in diverse ways.

In the West, the treatment of traumatised war veterans mainly consists of clinical intervention, mainly based on psychotherapeutic (to ease the psychological burden of trauma and possibly suppress it) and pharmacological (to tackle the symptoms of PTSD). However, as many scholars and practitioners have argued in recent years, such interventions may fail to achieve full recovery because they focus on the mind and the body separately. That has convinced Western practitioners to include diverse approaches into their "toolboxes"—e.g. meditation—drawing inspiration from Zen and other non-Western traditions such as the Indian *Vipassana*, or *Chan* Buddhism. These philosophies have traditionally approached well-being from a holistic perspective based on the body-mind balance and pursue a harmonic connection with one's environment and nature. Reconciliation, atonement, forgiveness, and responsibility are fundamental to healing trauma. However, healing trauma is a bottom-up process that begins with a healthy connection between the traumatised and their physical, cultural, social and moral environment. An approach to life as the one taught by Zen facilitates healing because it reconnects people with simplicity, emphasising the importance of the present moment instead of rumination on the past, which permits one to absorb past bad memories in the tranquillity of self-awareness. Therapy, especially one that combines clinical and holistic approaches, is viable in helping veterans find their way back.

The case of Mario Rigoni Stern offers an example of such a fruitful encounter between Western and Eastern cultures by practising two ways of healing: one is based on *vita activa* and entails several aspects of the virtuous lifestyle pursued by Zen philosophy.[22] As Rigoni Stern claimed that people reveal themselves in what they do, he also reassessed his past non-judgmentally, thus re-establishing an ethical relationship with his former foes and facilitating the healing of the effects of traumatic memories of violence. Moreover, by reconnecting physically and ethically with nature, cultivating simplicity, attending work, hunting, and gardening, Rigoni Stern recognises nature as the spiritual, ancestral home where every wounded person can find consolation and relief:

> *I believe things should be done well, because there is no greater satisfaction than a well-done job. A well-done job, any job that one does not for profit but for personal enrichment, whether manual or intellectual, is a source of great*

satisfaction. I tend my vegetable garden, and when I see the flowerbeds neatly trimmed with manure spread and the soil leveled, I feel fulfillment as when I finish writing a good story. And I add: a solid pile of logs, well aligned and square, one that won't fall over, is beautiful. (Mazzacurati & Paolini, 2006, pp. 78–79)

The other way of healing consists of storytelling, which is more characteristically rooted in the Western tradition of autobiographical self-representation and self-understanding through language and discourse. By storytelling, Rigoni Stern can share his wisdom and experience with those who do not know war directly, especially the younger generations, thus transmitting his view about a sustainable lifestyle in which humans lead good lives in balance with their environment and others by respecting different cultures and bearing responsibility for their actions. This blending of diverse approaches to a lifestyle based on awareness, activity, harmony, and compassion paves the way to individual well-being, reminding us of the need to transcend the cultural borders of nationalism to recognise that humans can meet each other by sharing their world in the present and with simplicity: "There are moments in war and peace when humans discover their real points of contact, concealed in what they do. Spanish and Russian shepherds or German and Sicilian blacksmiths find communion in their experiences" (Visetti, 2003, p. 27). Rigoni Stern claimed that the wounded find comfort and consolation in nature, but one can add that they can be found in the awareness by which one attends the daily tasks and duties of life, sharing such a vision with others, and pursuing compassion and mutual understanding.

REFERENCES

Arendt, H. (1998). *The Human Condition*. The University of Chicago Press.

Bormann, J., Liu, L., Thorp, S., & Lang, A. J. (2012). Spiritual Wellbeing Mediates PTSD Change in Veterans with Military-Related PTSD. *International Journal of Behavioral Medicine*, *19*, 496–502. DOI: 10.1007/s12529-011-9186-1 PMID: 21874605

Brooke, R. (2017). An Archetypal Approach to Treating Combat Post-Traumatic Stress Disorder. In Downing, D., & Mills, J. (Eds.), *Outpatient Treatment of Psychosis. Psychodynamic Approaches to Evidence-Based Practice* (pp. 171–195). Karnak.

Cinelli, G. (2022). *Le guerre di Mario Rigoni Stern. Trauma, racconto, guarigione* [The Wars of Mario Rigoni Stern. Trauma, Narrative, and Healing]. Morlacchi.

Cushing, R., Braun, K., Alden, S., & Katz, A. (2018). Military-Tailored Yoga for Veterans with Post-traumatic Stress Disorder. *Military Medicine*, *183*(5/6), e223–e231. PMID: 29415222

Daizen Victoria, B. (2006). *Zen at War*. Rowman and Littlefield.

Damasio, A. (2006). *Descartes' Error. Emotion, Reason and the Human Brain*. Vintage. (Original work published 1994)

Damasio, A. (2010). *Self Comes to Mind. Constructing the Conscious Brain*. Pantheon.

Gallagher, S. (2000). Philosophical Conceptions of the Self: Implications for Cognitive Science. *Trends in Cognitive Sciences*, *4*(1), 14–21. PMID: 10637618

García, H., & Miralles, F. (2017). *Ikigai. The Japanese Secret to a Long and Happy Life*. Penguin.

Hashimoto, A. (2015). *The Long Defeat. Cultural Trauma, Memory, and Identity in Japan*. Oxford University Press.

Hass-Cohen, N. (2003). Art Therapy Mind Body Approaches: Some Applications of Relational Neuroscience to Art Therapy. *Progress: Family Systems Research and Therapy*, *12*, 24–38.

Kalland, A. (2002). Holism and Sustainability: Lessons from Japan. *Worldviews: Global Religions, Culture, and Ecology*, *6*(2), 145–158.

King, A., Erickson, T., Giardino, N., Favorite, T., Rauch, S., Robinson, E., Kulkarni, M., & Liberzon, I. (2013). A Pilot Study of Group Mindfulness-Based Cognitive Therapy (MBCT) for Combat Veterans with Posttraumatic Stress Disorder (PTSD). *Depression and Anxiety*, *30*, 638–645. PMID: 23596092

Lakoff, G., & Johnson, M. (1980). *Metaphors We Live By*. University of Chicago Press.

Lakoff, G., & Johnson, M. (1999). *Philosophy in the Flesh. The Embodied Mind and its Challenge to Western Thought*. Basic Books.

Lakoff, G., & Turner, M. (1989). *More Than Cool Reason. A Field Guide to Poetic Metaphor*. University of Chicago Press.

Litz, B., & Carney, J. (2018). Employing Loving-Kindness Meditation to Promote Self- and Other-Compassion Among War Veterans With Posttraumatic Stress Disorder. *Spirituality in Clinical Practice*, *5*(3), 201–211. DOI: 10.1037/scp0000174

Luchetta, S. (2020). Dalla Baita al Ciliegio. La montagna nella narrativa di Mario Rigoni Stern [*From the Baita to the Cherry-Tree. Mountain in Mario Rigoni Stern's narrative*]. *Mimesis*.

Marcus Aurelius. (1907). *To Himself*. MacMillan.

Marsilio, M. (2021, May 19). Arboreto salvatico: lo sguardo "ecocritico" di Mario Rigoni Stern [Wild thicket. Mario Rigoni Stern's "ecocritical" glance]. *La letteratura e noi* [Literature and us]. Retrieved September 5, 2025, from https://laletteraturaenoi.it/2021/05/19/arboreto-salvatico-lo-sguardo-ecocritico-di-mario-rigoni-stern/

Mazzacurati, C., & Paolini, M. (2006). *Ritratti. Mario Rigoni Stern* [Portraits. Mario Rigoni Stern]. Biblioteca dell'immagine.

Menary, R. (2008). Embodied Narratives. *Journal of Consciousness Studies*, *15*(6), 63–84.

Milani, G., & Rigoni Stern, M. (2008). Intervista a Mario Rigoni Stern. [Interview with Mario Rigoni Stern] In Milani, G. (Ed.), *Mario Rigoni Stern, Hermann Heidegger. Ritorno sul fronte* (pp. 9–38). Transeuropa.

Miyahara, K., & Tanaka, S. (2023). Narrative Self-Constitution as Embodied Practice. *Philosophical Psychology*, *38*(4), 1731–1755. DOI: 10.1080/09515089.2023.2286281

Miyamoto, I. (1974). The Real Value of Tied Aid: The Case of Indonesia in 1967-69. *Economic Development and Cultural Change*, *22*(3), 436–452.

Motta, A. (1982). *Mario Rigoni Stern*. La Nuova Italia.

Munenori, Y. (2012). *The Life-Giving Sword. Secret Teachings From the House of the Shogun*. Shambahla.

Nakamura, E. (2016). "Invisible" War Trauma in Japan: Medicine, Society and Military Psychiatric Casualties. *Historia Scientiarum, 25*(2), 140–160.

Nelson, J. (2003). Social Memory as Ritual Practice: Commemorating Spirits of the Military Dead at Yasukuni Shinto Shrine. *The Journal of Asian Studies, 62*(2), 443–467.

Nitobé, I. (1908). *Bushido. The Soul of Japan*. The Project Gutenberg eBook (13th ed.) https://www.holybooks.com/ (original work published 1904)

Okakura, K. (1906). *The Book of Tea*. Putnam.

Ono, S. (1962). *Shinto. The Kami Way*. Tuttle.

Pols, H., & Micale, M. S. (2021). History, Trauma, and Asia. In Micale, M. S., & Pols, H. (Eds.), *Traumatic Pasts in Asia. History, Psychiatry, and Trauma from the 1930s to the Present* (pp. 1–34). Berghahn.

Raikar, S. (n.d.). Limbic System. In *Encyclopedia Britannica*. Retrieved September 3, from https://www.britannica.com/science/limbic-system

Rigoni Stern, M. (1967). The Sergeant in the Snow. In *R. Biason, M. Tobino, & M. Rigoni Stern, The Lost Legions. Three Italian War Novels by Renzo Biason, Mario Tobino, and Mario Rigoni Stern* (Colquhoun, A., & Cowan, A., Trans.; pp. 303–412). Knopf.

Rigoni Stern, M. (2003a). […]. In *Sentieri sotto la neve* [Pathways under the snow] (3rd ed., 67–72). ed. Einaudi.

Rigoni Stern, M. (2004a). Un ragazzo delle nostre contrade. [*A boy from our hamlet*] In *Il sergente nella neve – Ritorno sul Don* [*The sergeant in the snow – Return to the Don river*]. 17th ed., pp. 249–268). Einaudi.

Rigoni Stern, M. (2004b). Ritorno sul Don [Return to the Don river]. In *Il sergente nella neve – Ritorno sul Don* (17th ed. 277–317). Einaudi.

Rigoni Stern, M. (2004c). La scure [The axe]. In *Il sergente nella neve – Ritorno sul Don* (17th ed. 269–275). Einaudi.

Rigoni Stern, M. (2004e). Il cane che vidi piangere. [The dog I saw cry] In *Aspettando l'alba e altri racconti* (pp. 120–125). Einaudi.

Rigoni Stern, M. (2004f). Piccola cronaca del blackout. [A small chronicle of the blackout] In *Aspettando l'alba e altri racconti* (pp. 142–144). Einaudi.

Rigoni Stern, M. (2014). *Il coraggio di dire no. Conversazioni e interviste 1963–2007* [The courage of saying no. Coversations and interviews]. Einaudi.

Rots, A. (2013). *Forests of the Gods. Shinto, Nature, and Sacred Space in Contemporary Japan*. Doctoral Thesis. University of Oslo.

Saito, H. (2017). *The History Problem. The Politics of War Commemoration in East Asia*. University of Hawai'i Press.

Salzberg, S., & Kabat-Zinn, J. (1997). Mindfulness as Medicine. In Goleman, D. (Ed.), *Healing Emotions. Conversations with the Dalai Lama on Mindfulness, Emotions, and Health* (pp. 107–144). Shambhala Publications.

Sato, S. (1981). *Two Moons. Short Zen Stories*. Dai Nihon.

Senzaki, N., & Reps, P. (1957). *101 Zen Stories*. Charles Tuttle.

Seppälä, E., Nitschke, J., Tudorascu, D., Hayes, A., Goldstein, M., Nguyen, D., Perlman, D., & Davidson, R. (2014). Breathing-Based Meditation Decreases Posttraumatic Stress Disorder Symptoms in U.S. Military Veterans: A Randomized Controlled Longitudinal Study. *Journal of Traumatic Stress*, *27*, 397–405. PMID: 25158633

Stein, J. (2017). The Meaning of "Loneliness" for Traumatized Veterans: A Semiotic Investigation of Veterans' Written Narratives. *Journal of Veterans Studies*, *2*(2), 121–139. DOI: 10.21061/jvs.v2i2.19

Suzuki, D. (1993). *Zen and Japanese Culture*. Charles Tuttle. (Original work published 1959)

Taishi, K. (2018). The Universality of Shintō, Clarified by Some Buddhist Concepts. *Japan Mission Journal*, 10–18.

Talwar, S. (2007). Accessing Traumatic Memory through Art Making: An Art Therapy Trauma Protocol (ATTP). *The Arts in Psychotherapy*, *34*, 22–35.

Tick, E. (2014). *Warrior's Return. Restoring the Soul after War*. Sounds True.

Trefalt, B. (2017). Collecting Bones: Japanese Missions for the Repatriation of War Remains and the Unfinished Business of the Asia-Pacific War. *Australian Humanities Review 61*, 145–159.

Tsai, C. C. (1994). *Zen Speaks*. Doubleday.

Turner, M. (1996). *The Literary Mind. The Origins of Thought and Language*. Oxford University Press.

Varela, F., Thompson, E., & Rosch, E. (1993). *The Embodied Mind. Cognitive Science and Human Experience*. MIT Press.

Visetti, G. P. (2003). Intervista a Mario Rigoni Stern [Interview with Mario Rigoni Stern]. *La Repubblica* (15 Dec.), 27.

Wastell, C. (2005). *Understanding Trauma and Emotion. Dealing with Trauma Using an Emotion-Focused Approach*. Allen & Unwin.

Watts, A. (1989). *The Way of Zen*. Vintage.

Wilde, L. (2020). Trauma Across Cultures: Cultural Dimensions of the Phenomenology of Post-Traumatic Experiences. *Phenomenology and Mind, 18*, 222–229. DOI: 10.17454/pam-1816

Zwigenberg, R. (2018). Nuclear Minds: Japanese Psychiatry's Encounter with the Atom. *Jinbun, 49*, 93–101.

ENDNOTES

1 "Western conceptions and therapeutic initiatives are not always congruent with local approaches dealing with disaster, disruption, and trauma" (Pols & Micale, 2021, p. 2). Japanese psychiatrists of the twentieth century "were not sympathetic to the idea of long-term trauma" (Zwigenberg, 2018, p. 94), and if "military doctors tended to downplay symptoms and tried to return shell-shocked soldiers to their units as far as possible," civilian doctors, too, "generally preferred physical and somatic evidence to mental evidence and were generally hostile to trauma" (p. 96). As a consequence, the general approach to war-related trauma during the Second World War in Japan consisted, not unlike the early attitude of Western military psychiatrists during the Great War, in blaming the spiritual weakness, lack of resilience and even the moral degeneration of traumatised soldiers, mainly treated by coercive methods (Nakamura, 2016, pp. 155–156). It is no by chance, then, that the APA's formula of PTSD began to circulate in Japan only after the devastating earthquake of 1995.

2 The selected works are (listed chronologically): *Il sergente nella neve* [The sergeant in the snow] (1953), *La scure* [The axe] (1972), *Un ragazzo delle nostre contrade* [A boy from our hamlet] (1972), *Ritorno sul Don* [Return to the Don river] (1972), *Rito sull'Altipiano* [A rite on the Plateau] (1986), *[…]* (1998), *Il 21 di marzo* [21st of March] (2004), *Il cane che vidi piangere* [The

dog I saw cry] (2004), and *Piccola cronaca del blackout* [A small chronicle of the blackout] (2004). Since the Italian titles have been provided here, the works will be quoted only in English in the text. *The Sergeant in the Snow* has been quoted from the English translation of 1967.

3 In his works *Arboreto selvatico* [Wild thicket] (1991) and *Uomini, boschi, api* [Men, woods, and bees] (1980), Rigoni Stern considers the symbiosis existing among humans and other living creatures, a sacred, practical, and symbolic relationship that has since ever fuelled myths and legends concerning animals and trees. See Luchetta (2020, p. 44) and Marsilio (2021).

4 The limbic system refers to the part of the brain responsible for processing emotions (Raikar, n.d.).

5 The parasympathetic and sympathetic system includes components of the nervous system, relating to involuntary, pre-reflective, and uncontrolled physiological responses. See Editors of the Encyclopaedia Britannica (2025).

6 Vagal activity, or vagal tone, is the regulation of nervous functions of the vagus nerve. This is "a crucial component of the parasympathetic nervous system, facilitating communication between the brain and various organs, including the ears, heart, lungs, pancreas, spleen, and gastrointestinal tract" (Ma, Wang and Hashimoto, 2024).

7 "Although meditation techniques have a long history of use in the context of spiritual training, it is only recently in the West that these methods have begun to be systematically applied and studied as part of a medical and psychological treatment regime" (Salzberg & Kabat-Zinn, 1997, p. 107).

8 Takuan Sōhō defined the mind-set of the samurai in the 17th century in terms of loyalty, diligence, discipline, filial love, and austerity (1990, p. 41). One should also bear in mind that Bushido, as a set of principles and rules, was subject to change accordingly with the political circumstances. Although Buddhism greatly influenced Bushido, this was also a way of controlling the restless samurai especially between the 15th and the 17th centuries, during the period of intense fights and political struggle for the unification of Japan. Moreover, Budo/Bushido not only refers to swordsmanship but also to archery (*Kyudo*), and other forms of martial arts connected by the same principles such as judo, aikido or karate. See also Miyamoto (1974). I am grateful to Andrei Teodorescu for his precious advice that helped me understand complex aspects of Japanese culture with a "beginner's mind" (*sho shin*).

9 The same idea was expressed in the 17th century by Takuan Sōhō in his writings by which he addressed the sword masters to teach them the way of Bushido. The "unfettered mind" (or no-mind) is "unmoveable" in Sōhō's words, for it glances at things without being stopped by them (1990, pp. 21–24).

10 Kazuko Okakura (1906) mentions the Japanese "natural love for simplicity" (p. 155) opposed to Western proneness to complexity and the ornamental (p. 93), which would make the tea room a place or "pureness and simplicity" apt for the practice of meditation (p. 79). Not unlike Suzuki, Okakura nuanced an idea of moral and spiritual superiority of the Eastern (namely Japanese) culture over Western materialism.

11 It is worth mentioning that Suzuki was criticised for his proneness to Japanese imperialism during the 1930s when Zen, Buddhism and the so-called "State-Shinto" were strategically used to legitimate the Japanese military expansion in continental Asia. See Daizen Victoria (2006, pp. 96 and 147).

12 Marcus Aurelius claims that "everything is in change. You yourself are undergoing continuous variation, and piecemeal destruction. So is the world at large" (1907, pp. 114–115).

13 Zen meditation does not exclude the intellectual practice of listening to short stories, often narrated by monks or attributed to famous monks and aimed at challenging one's common sense and enhancing one's ability to reflect on paradoxical parables to extract maxims and teachings of wisdom, compassion, and spirituality. Such stories are often mentioned in books about Zen (e.g. Watts, 1989, and Suzuki, 1993) and have been collected in anthologies, two famous examples of which are *101 Zen Stories* (Senzaki & Reps, 1957), *Two Moons* (Sato, 1981), and *Zen Speaks* (Tsai, 1994) in the format of comics.

14 All translation from Rigoni Stern and other works written in other-than-English languages are mine unless otherwise stated.

15 All societies honour their dead, especially those who fell in battle to defend the community. However, while on the one hand, this tribute facilitates closure and pacification among the mourners, it also raises, on the other hand, controversial concerns because nationalist commemoration "eliminates ambiguities from historical facts" (Saito, 2017, p. 5). Moreover, such "one-sided stories ... help anchor and stabilise individual and collective identity while repairing biographical wounds, and avoid threatening political entanglement with the outside world" (Hashimoto, 2015, p. 47). In Japan, to remain within the framework of a West-East comparison, this aspect became a matter of political controversy around the commemoration of the spirit of the war dead

at the Yasukuni Shinto Shrine, where millions of fallen soldiers are also enshrined, among whom even some war criminals. See Saito (2017, pp. 31, 61, and 109–110); and Nelson (2003). The cult of the dead can also concern the collection of the bodily remains of fallen soldiers, which is also problematic due to the ethical and political implications of such activity. See Trefalt (2017).

16 "The *vita activa*, human life in so far as it is actively engaged in doing something, is always rooted in a world of men and man-made things which it never leaves or altogether transcends .... All human activities are conditioned by the fact that men live together" (Arendt, 1998, p. 22).

17 Such a conception of hunting as a practical and spiritual relationship with wilderness is not alien to other cultures, especially traditional ones in which hunters still remember the ways of their ancestors. One notable example in Japan is the Ainu culture on the island of Hokkaido, to which NHK broadcasting company devoted the documentary *Ainu Cultural Advocate: Monbetsu Atsushi* on 26 June 2024: https://www3.nhk.or.jp/nhkworld/en/shows/2103019/.

18 Ötsi the Iceman "is a modern man like us, but more aware and better than us able to adapt .... Who could start a fire today in a wood under the rain? Almost no one .... If I had not been able to start a fire, I would have died" (Rigoni Stern, 2014, p. 46).

19 Without attempting any general contextualisation of Shintō in the limited space of this chapter, it is however worth mentioning that this religion is specific to Japan and is mainly based on the idea that in every object and living creature a sacred spirit resides. Therefore, Shintō venerates nature as the realm of the sacred made visible and tangible in its changing and impermanent physical forms. These sacred entities are called *kami* and could be any natural object (a rifer, a stone, or a tree) or an animal. Even worthy humans can become *kami* after their demise: "In Shinto there is no absolute deity that is the creator and ruler of all. The creative function of the world is realized through the harmonious cooperation of the kami in the performance of their respective missions" (Ono, 1962, p. 27).

20 It is worth mentioning that Taishi presented this text in an international conference on interreligious dialogue, trying to show the universality of such a concept as that of *kami* to bridge between the Western and Buddhist conceptions of emptiness (p. 12).

21 Such an approach has been idealised and even turned into ideology during the Late nineteenth and the first half of the twentieth century by creating the myths of the "sacred forest," innate Japanese "love of nature," and an attitude

towards nature that would ideally voice the "soul of Japan." See Rots (2013, pp. 160, 163 and 174–175).

22 Rigoni Stern, as already mentioned, was not acquainted with the Eastern spiritual traditions, but he participated in ancient traditions handed down in his native homeland in the Alps that advocated for a spiritual symbiosis between the humans and nature. See, for example, the short stories *A Rite on the Plateau* (2003b) and *March 21st* (2004d).

Chapter 5
"I Looked at Myself, Smiled at Myself": Repairing Mental Well-Being Through Subaltern Ekphrasis

Alessandro Toma
http://orcid.org/0009-0005-0503-9785
Durham University, UK

ABSTRACT

The escalation of collective traumata, hegemonic oppression, and growing limitations on civil rights continue to exacerbate the precarious mental well-being of marginalised communities. The systemic mutism to which these groups are subjected makes it imperative to investigate the potential of the arts to heal traumatised and subaltern subjects. Ekphrasis, among the various media and rhetorical devices employed in the Humanities, appears to be a congenial dialogical instrument for researching this topic. This chapter aims to disentangle ekphrasis from its classical representational understanding as a means for translating a (visual) medium into another (verbal) (Heffernan, 1993). Drawing on the theories of Melanie Klein, Silvan S. Tomkins (1962-1991), W.J.T. Mitchell (1994), and Elena Ferrante's poetics ekphrasis is reevaluated—using Ferrante's Troubling Love (1992) as a case study—as a powerful tool for subaltern groups to become aware of their status and traumata, thereby opening a path towards psychological recovery.

INTRODUCTION

Solo a chi ama il Diverso accende i suoi splendori.

DOI: 10.4018/979-8-3373-3521-6.ch005

Elsa Morante, Alibi (1958)[1]

Ekphrasis has been the subject of intense debate in the history of literary criticism. Nevertheless, at the beginning of the 1990s, scholars attempted to confine the definition of ekphrasis to that of a rhetorical device primarily used to convey a work of plastic art in literature (Cometa, 2024, p. 26). Since then, the widespread academic consensus has been based on James A. W. Heffernan's formula: ekphrasis is "the verbal representation of visual representation" (Heffernan, 2015, p. 18).

The increasing presence of digital and hyperlinked images, however, strengthened by the advent of the internet, asked researchers to consider whether past theories of intermediality need to be reevaluated (see Jansson, 2018; Lindhé, 2013). On this point, Liliane Louvel highlights the need to further explore the digital evolution of this rhetorical device "since [the phenomenon] is no longer confined to books" (2018, p. 245). As a consequence, it also becomes necessary to review "the [contemporary] relation between word and image in general and of the [literary] figure of ekphrasis in particular" (Louvel, 2018, p. 245).

Another growing interest in the humanities is the study of the influence of affect on human beings, their agency, and their mental well-being (Clough, 2007, pp. ix–xiv). Indeed, psychotherapy, psychology, and philosophy have provided valuable insights into the power of affect to contribute to well-being since antiquity—for example, the concept of enargeia, which was the psychological characteristic of ekphrasis in ancient rhetoric (Webb, 2009, p. 5). In the last century, Silvan Tomkins outlined one of the most detailed modern systematisations of the affective phenomenon in his *Affect Imagery Consciousness* (1962-1991).[2] Building upon his ideas, cultural theorists have further elaborated his system emphasising how the study of affect could help understand the influence of societal structures on humans' agency (see Ahmed, 2020; and see Sedgwick, 2003). Literary studies are also showing increasing interest in the potential that affect theory offers to approach texts, genres, and rhetorical devices to better understand the influence literary production has on individuals (see Ahern, 2024).

These growing academic interests provide considerable impetus for investigating the potential of ekphrastic writing to articulate how humans achieve a new state of mental well-being. Indeed, affect theory, psychoanalysis, and literature offer valuable insights into the influence of imagery on the human mind. As Tomkins remarks on the relation between affect, imagery, and consciousness: "there isn't any way to separate the three interlocked concepts. Affect produces attention that brings its trigger into consciousness, and the world we know is a dream, a series of images colored by our life experience" (Tomkins, 2008, p. xi). Psychotherapist Melanie Klein also provides illuminating insights into the power of affect, phantasy and the worlds created by the human mind to foster an individual's psychological well-being. In literary study, Elena Ferrante's non-fictional works offer valuable elements for enquiring into the theoretical foundations of this chapter. In *Frantumaglia: A Writer's Journey*, Ferrante lists the psychoanalysts that most influenced her novels and she remarks, "I read Melanie Klein passionately" (2016a, p. 122; 2007; see De Rogatis, 2018, p. 100; Wehling-Giorgi, 2016).[3] Furthermore, the author repeatedly stresses the central role of imagery in her *oeuvre* (Ferrante, 2021, pp. 50–52), around which, in a *vortex of affect*, she constructs the plot of her stories (2016a, p. 108).

The individuals under examination in these pages are to be considered as the result of systematic subjection to hegemonic power structures. Philosopher Antonio Gramsci offers a compelling explanation of the formation and influence of said structures on what he calls the subaltern. According to him, hegemony is not only a political, juridical and economic power, but it is also the process of formation of a leading class, which influences people on a cultural and moral level before and after coming to actual power (Gramsci, 1992, p. 182). These influences, though, are not only forced upon the subaltern. The interests of subaltern groups are also, to some extent, considered in the formation of the ruling hegemony. In Gramsci's words,

> *The life of the State is conceived of as a continuous process of formation and superseding of unstable equilibria [emphasis added] ... between the interests of the fundamental group and those of the subordinate groups—equilibria in which the interests of the dominant group prevail, but only up to a certain point." (1992, p. 182)*

Furthermore, the subaltern, as a result of hegemonic subjection and violence, lives in a constant state of eroded mental well-being. As E. Virginia Demos remarks, this results as the deprivation of "the two most biologically based essentials in life" (2019, p. 228), which are the ability of signifying and asserting agency over one's world. As a consequence, the lack of these two foundational elements engenders traumata in the individual's psyche, since the subject is not able to articulate—and to a certain extent comprehend—their condition. Nevertheless, a subaltern individual shares a violation of their biologically based essentials with the subordinate group to which they belong. Thus, given this communal violation of basic needs, the subaltern, besides their own, inherits also a series of traumatic experiences rooted in their community, which eventually results in a transgenerational trauma.

Building on Tomkins's affect theory, Kleinian psychoanalysis, Elena Ferrante's poetics, and theories of ekphrasis, this chapter considers ekphrastic writing as an ideal *locus* for articulating the subaltern subject's process of becoming aware of their condition. The ekphrasis of the subaltern or subaltern ekphrasis, thus, becomes the speaking interstice in unstable societal equilibria, thanks to which the subaltern, transgenerational traumatised individual is finally able to regain mental well-being.[4]

Given the centrality of Kleinian theories, affect, and imagery in Ferrante's poetics, her debut novel *Troubling Love* (2006) presents a compelling case study for examining subaltern ekphrasis. Ferrante's novel recounts the healing process of Neapolitan comics illustrator Delia. This process, which begins after her mother Amalia's suicide, not only helps the protagonist accept the loss she suffered. It also enables her to recover from her childhood trauma, to fully acknowledge the role Amalia played in the development of her personality, and the societal abuses they both suffered. In the novel, this mental rehabilitation is depicted through a compound of several ekphrases. From the opening scenes to the final line, Delia's story unfolds through *encounters* with various objects—pictures, paintings, dresses, reflections, etc.—which mark key episodes of the novel, all through the rhetorical device of ekphrasis. To use Stiliana Milkova's words, "Ferrante's writing is entirely ekphrastic" (2016, p. 161), and Delia's story can be considered a novel-length ekphrastic experience.

In what follows, after an account of some classical theories of ekphrasis, I will delineate the methodological premise of the study. I will then outline a theory of ekphrasis through the redefinition of three key aspects of this rhetorical device: the ekphrastic gaze, the ekphrastic object, and the moments of ekphrastic fascination. Ferrante's poetics and her novel *Troubling Love* will provide invaluable insights into the functioning and form of subaltern ekphrasis throughout the chapter.

CRITICISING FROM WITHIN: ON THEORIES OF EKPHRASIS

As mentioned in the previous section, Heffernan's formula of ekphrasis as "the verbal representation of visual representation" has been accepted as the standard definition of this rhetorical device since the early 1990s (Heffernan, 2015, p. 18). However, this formula does not account for the full range of possibilities in ekphrastic writing.[5] In recent years, the maxim has been challenged in its theoretical assumption, for instance, concerning its representationalism (Kennedy, 2016, pp. 7–14; and see Kennedy & Meek, 2018, pp. 13–14). Indeed, the implied basis of the ekphrastic praxis revolves around the idea of a transposition from one kind of representational sign (visual) into another (verbal). Even though this may be true for the majority of ekphrases, it becomes questionable when non-representational media are considered. To use William J. T. Mitchell's words,

> *there is no essential difference between texts and images and thus no gap between the media to be overcome by any special ekphrastic strategies. Language can stand for depiction and depiction can stand in for language. ... It would be very difficult to account for the existence of pictographic writing systems if pictures could not be employed as the medium for complex verbal expression. (Mitchell, 1994, pp. 160–161)*

The approach presented in this paper contrasts with the classical representational tradition of ekphrastic theory. Dating back to the early modern period, this tradition pitches these two art forms against one another, in *paragone*, a struggle for artistic pre-eminence.[6] David Kennedy and Richard Meek have already demonstrated that the term *paragone* and the idea of a fight between arts have been linked only *a posteriori* to this academic discourse (Kennedy & Meek, 2018, pp. 5–6). It was indeed the Horatian tenet of "*ut pictura poësis* [that] was even more influential and ubiquitous than the *paragone* in the early modern period" (Kennedy & Meek, 2018, p. 5).[7] For instance, different paintings from the Renaissance validate the idea of a discourse on ekphrasis founded on a reciprocal enhancement between the two art forms. An exemplar piece is *Pittura e Poesia* by Francesco Furini (1626). The canvas portrays two figures, Poetry and Painting, displayed hugging, mirrored-like, in a sapphic kiss, which stresses the ideas of similarity and complementarity by depicting a peaceful relationship between the two arts (Figure 1). On top of that, Poetry holds a scroll with a Latin inscription "CONCORDI LVMINE MAIOR"— Furini's addition to the Horatian maxim—to stress that the sister arts elevate themselves only if invested by the same light, by the same prestige (Bisceglia, 2023).

Figure 1. Pittura e Poesia (Palazzo Pitti, Galleria Palatina, Sala di Berenice) [Oil painting on canvas] (Furini, 1626)

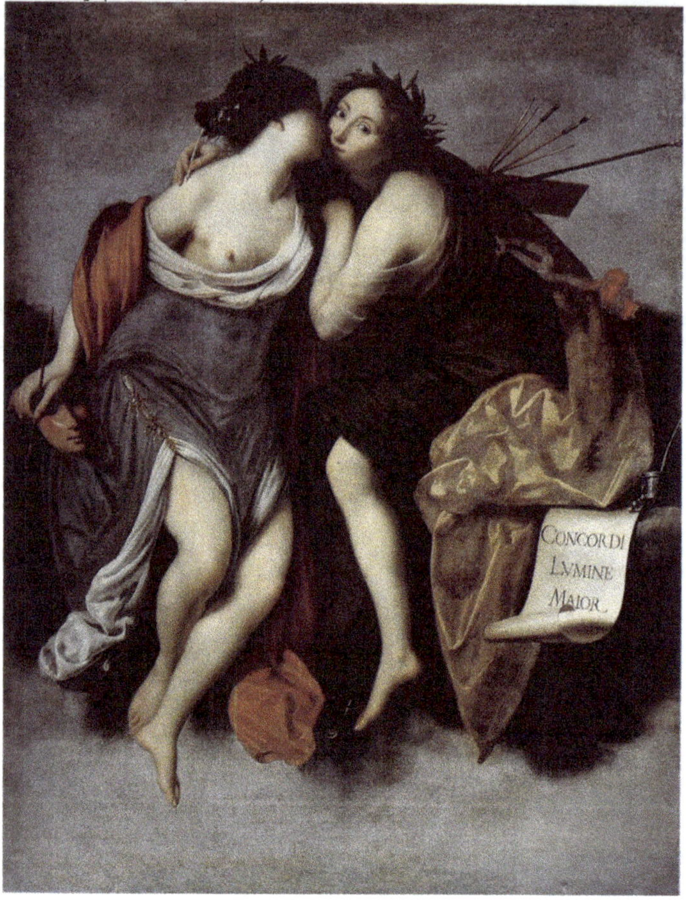

A final preliminary question is to what extent the theory of ekphrasis outlined in this chapter is indebted to Mitchell's *Picture Theory* (1994), given the relevance of the scholar's model in contemporary academic discourse. These pages will borrow some terms from Mitchell's system. For example, the concept of ekphrasis as a fascination that unfolds "in three phases or moments of realization" (Mitchell, 1994, pp. 152–156). Mitchell names these three phases: ekphrastic indifference, ekphrastic hope and ekphrastic fear. The scholar contends that the first one "grows out of a commonsense perception that ekphrasis is impossible"; the second one "is the phase when the impossibility of ekphrasis is overcome in imagination or metaphor"; the third one "is the moment of resistance or counterdesire that occurs when we sense that the difference between the verbal and visual representation might collapse" (Mitchell, 1994, pp. 152–154). Furthermore, Mitchell's conception of the ekphrastic object as the "resident alien" (Mitchell, 1994, p. 157), i.e., a fictional object "to be found only in the text" (Mitchell, 1994, p. 157), will offer valuable for the theorisation of subaltern ekphrasis.

Mitchell also provides a thought-provoking reading of Gotthold Ephraim Lessing's *Laokoon* (1766). In his interpretation of the latter, the scholar highlights the implicit connections between gender, ekphrastic writing, and the ekphrastic object, as well as the power structures they signify. Building on these considerations, Mitchell contends that, in Lessing's model, the commonly male-identified subject fears being emasculated by the feminine-identified ekphrastic object (see Mitchell, 1986, pp. 109-110). Although Lessing never explicitly states this gendered opposition between the viewer and the object, some passages of his treatise eloquently demonstrate this fear of morphing into a subaltern other.[8] Indeed, to gender the parties in theories of ekphrasis was common until the 1990s (see Kennedy & Meek, 2018, p. 10), and to some extent it is also present in Heffernan's work (Heffernan, 1993, pp. 3–5). The gendered dimension of this rhetorical device is worth bearing in mind. Indeed, the articulation of subalterns' ekphrastic experiences brings about, in authors like Ferrante, not only a character's path to mental well-being but also a critique of hegemonic discourses and biases in literary theory and praxis (see Milkova, 2016, p. 161; 2021, p. 24).

THE POWER OF DEPRESSION: PREMISE OF A METHOD

One of the most recent theories of ekphrasis is that of David Kennedy. Kennedy describes ekphrasis as the rhetorical device used

> *to convey the experience of a person, a place or an object to an audience. Conveying this experience involves not only the careful description of telling details but also a sense of what encountering [emphasis added] the person, place or object felt like. (Kennedy, 2016, p. 24)*

Building on Kennedy's conceptualisation of the rhetorical device, subaltern ekphrasis is regarded as the articulation of an encounter between the subject and the object seen/the other. During this encounter, which occurs in the interstice of unstable societal equilibria, the subaltern gazer gains a newfound awareness of their status and, consequently, can work towards mental well-being.

It is worth highlighting that the outlined theory does not claim a universal character. Indeed, only some authors and some texts are suitable for this approach. It is primarily the ekphrastic experiences voiced by subaltern lyrical 'I's and first-person narrators that prove more suited for this reading. In *In the Margins: On the Pleasures of Reading and Writing* (2021), Ferrante expounds on this potentiality of first-person narrators to subvert imposed narratives and to bring about, through the interplay of strong affects and imagery, novel realisations about themselves, "I developed a first-person narrator who, excited by the random collisions between her and the world, deformed the form that she had been laboriously given, and from those dents and distortions and injuries squeezed out other, unsuspected possibilities" (2022, section "Aquamarine", para. 17).[9]

To understand how subaltern ekphrastic experiences function, the methodological foundations of this process must first be outlined. The underlying methodology of the chapter is built upon Klein's concept of phantasy, her description of the psychological paranoid and depressive positions in the early stage of life (1984, pp. 14–16), and the affect theory of Tomkins. Furthermore, elements of Ferrante's poetics will help elucidate the functioning of subaltern ekphrasis.[10]

The starting point of the approach outlined in these pages is Klein's conceptualisation of phantasy, i.e., the mental representation of body sensations, affect and relationships with objects (Spillius & Hinshelwood, 2011, p. 3). According to Klein, phantasy is not only the realm of made-up thoughts and stories, but also the subconscious place in which the subject confronts their self with external objects. These objects of confrontation are projected onto the individual's psyche and are associated with split parts of the individual's ego, becoming then internal objects. As such, they exercise a profound influence on the subject's character and thoughts. In Klein's words,

> *the phantasies and feelings about the state of the internal object influence vitally the structure of the ego. ... The effect of this phantasy is a very real one, because it leads to feelings and relations (and later on thought processes). (Klein, 1946, p. 101)*

The psychoanalyst's emphasis on the influence that humans' phantasies have on feelings and thought processes strengthens the pivotal role of her theory in understanding subaltern ekphrasis. If the objects humans see profoundly influence an individual's psyche, then subaltern ekphrasis, as the encounter between a viewer and an object, will be regarded as a Kleinian thought process that engenders, through feelings and relations to things, those unsuspected possibilities for the self mentioned by Ferrante (2022, sec. "Aquamarine", para. 17).

Another defining characteristic of Kleinian phantasy is its temporal rather than spatial dimension. Instead of being located in a definitive space, objects are in a constantly moving and changing relation with the subject's psyche (Klein, 1946, p. 101). This last trait of humans' phantasy perfectly introduces the foundational element of the approach outlined here, i.e., Klein's concept of position. The psychoanalyst emphasises with this idea

> *a model of development in which anxieties, defences, impulses and object relations are grouped together in constellations ... that are both overlapping and*

fluctuating. The idea of position conveys a … flexible to-and-fro process [emphasis added] [with said objects]. (Spillius & Hinshelwood, 2011, pp. 449–450)

Thus, a position becomes an individual's affectively driven posture towards an object that, through time, influences and changes the subject's mind. In the case of subaltern ekphrasis, the subject then finds themselves in a temporal, affectively driven thought process. It is as a result of this process that the subaltern, alternatively changing psychological positions and consequently, disrupting vicious patterns, faces the possibility of regaining mental well-being. In *Frantumaglia: A Writer's Journey*, Ferrante helps expound the way in which moments of realisation, by disrupting imposed temporal dimensions through affects, engender in the subaltern a consciousness about transgenerational traumata and consequently, awareness of their status. In her words,

For a better understanding, we should speak of how suffering modifies the image of time. The eruption of suffering cancels out linear time, breaks it, makes it into whirling squiggles. The night of time crouches at the edges of the dawn of today and tomorrow. Suffering casts us down among our single-celled ancestors, among the quarrelsome or terrorized muttering in the caves, among the female divinities expelled into the darkness of the earth, even as we keep ourselves anchored … to the computer we're writing on. Strong feelings are like that: they explode chronology. An emotion is a somersault, a tumble, a dizzying pirouette. (Ferrante, 2016a, pp. 107-108)[11]

As introduced above, Klein ascribes two distinct positions to the realm of phantasy: the paranoid and the depressive ones. During the paranoid position, the subject splits parts of their self into an object of relation and is unable to reconcile with these smaller pieces, consequently failing to repair their fragmented ego. This state of mind brings about fears of persecution, guilt, and mourning that impede the process of development of the individual's mind (Klein, 1946, p. 104). As a consequence of these negative emotions, the subject experiences "a momentary impairment of logical thinking which amounts to thoughts being cut off from one another and situations being split off from one another; in fact, the ego is temporarily split" (Klein, 1946, p. 104). Thus, those thought processes typical of the realm of phantasy are not ignited, and the subject does not reach a new awareness of their status and a reparation of their split psyche. On the other hand, the depressive position is a state of mind in which the subject becomes capable of repairing the split parts of their self and the world around themselves into a new enhanced whole (Garvey, 2023, p. 54; Klein, 1946, p. 105). According to Klein, this process of reparation leads to

feelings … [which have] the effect of further integrating the ego, because it makes for an increased understanding of psychic reality and better perception of the external world, as well as for a greater synthesis between inner and external situations." (Klein, 1946, p. 105)

Consequently, in the depressive phase, the individual surpasses negative feelings of fear and guilt and, through positive and powerful feelings of love, trust, and joy, eventually repairs their split self (Klein, 1946, p. 106).

In theorising subaltern ekphrastic experiences, the most relevant splitting modes of the paranoid positions is the fragmentation process of a subject's self. Klein describes fragmentation as the splitting of an extremely weakened self as a consequence of anxieties and suffering from birth onwards. The individual in question

> *cannot—for internal or external reasons—cope with the impact of depressive anxieties, a vicious circle arises. For if persecutory fear, and correspondingly schizoid mechanisms, are too strong, the ego is not capable of working through the depressive position. (Klein, 1946, p. 105)*

In the cases under examination, the extreme fragmentation of the subaltern self is caused by external reasons such as transgenerational trauma, the suffocating influence of hegemonic discourses and their systematic violence. Subaltern ekphrasis serves as a tool to overcome the vicious circle of fragmentation. In *Frantumaglia: A Writer's Journey*, Ferrante describes the mental development of her characters as the consequences of an ekphrastic experience, of an act of surveillance. According to the author, surveillance does not comprehend control over an enemy. It rather means to watch over one's own body, to determine themselves against hegemonic discourses, to engender change of one's status through the power of emotion: "surveillance is, if well understood, more an emotional tendency of the whole body, an expansion and an inflorescence on and around it" (Ferrante, 2016a, p. 104).[12] Therefore, Ferrante's concept of surveillance highlights the centrality of the inward gaze to engender a change in the subaltern's state of mind. Consequently, through moments of ekphrastic fascination, the subaltern moves from a paranoid to a depressive position, gaining a better understanding of their conditions.

Eve Kosofsky Sedgwick offers valuable tools for delineating the theoretical frame of subaltern ekphrasis by connecting Tomkins's affect theory to Kleinian psychoanalysis. In *Touching Feeling: Affect, Pedagogy, Performativity*, Sedgwick describes what a "reparative reading" stance entails (2003, p. 146). According to the scholar, this reading method must be viewed as the application of Melanie Klein's concept of the "depressive position" to the development of both reading practices and, more broadly, theories (Klein, 1946, p. 105). Reparative reading rests on an "additive and accretive" impulse to "assemble and confer plenitude on an object that will then have resources to offer to an inchoate self" (Sedgwick, 2003, p. 149). Consequently, a repaired theory has its foundations in existing systems, yet arises from the desire to provide new tools for selves whose amorphism is produced by the systemic oppression of hegemonic cultures, enabling them to articulate their own voices (Sedgwick, 2003, pp. 150–151). Building on this methodology, it is then possible to offer a repaired theory of ekphrasis by assembling split parts of existing theories into a new system. In this way, a model is developed that accounts for that kind of ekphrastic writing whose meanings are otherwise overlooked by classical theories—labelled as "paranoid" by Sedgwick (Sedgwick, 2003, pp. 125–126). The proposed theory must not be considered solely a reparative one, though. Indeed, Sedgwick stresses that the intertwining between paranoid and reparative features in a theory is difficult to escape (2003, pp. 145–147).

Sedgwick highlights two other features of paranoid and reparative models using Tomkins's definition of strong and weak affect theories. According to Tomkins, strong theories are those that aim to recount "a wide spectrum of phenomena" under the same set of rules (Frank & Wilson, 2020, pp. 93–95; Tomkins, 2008, p. 519). The goal of this kind of affect-driven theory is to describe how humans, in a snowball-like process of mistakes over mistakes, learn to avoid bad situations (Tomkins, 2008, pp. 458–461). As a result, such theories tend to operate deductively, prioritising generalisable systems over attention to the specificity of individual cases. The similarity with the paranoid position is evident. Indeed, during this phase, the individual cannot confront their fears and guilts, but rather complies with the external forces that fragment their self. Thus, they are unable to realise the extent of their eroded mental condition. On the other hand, a repaired theory corresponds to Tomkins's "weak" theory, which is a system that accounts only for the "description of the phenomena which it purports to explain" (Tomkins, 2008, p. 519). Consequently, while strong affect theories impose their explanatory systems top-down, weak theories emerge bottom-up from their objects of analysis. Accordingly, in the cases examined in this chapter, the condition of subaltern individuals informs the nature of subaltern ekphrasis. Indeed, during reparation, the fragmented subject escapes the influence of external forces and emerges with a new self, characterised by an enhanced awareness of the world around them and their own nature.

To sum up: subaltern ekphrasis is an affect-driven weak, repaired approach to ekphrastic writing. Considering the influence of phantasy on human life, this theory describes the process of a subaltern subject's awakening. In a temporal dimension, a subaltern, traumatised, and extremely fragmentated individual moves from a paranoid to a depressive position. During the paranoid posture, the individual gazes at their object of relation, i.e., the *encountered* object, with fears of merging with it. Consequently, they cannot recognise and reconcile with the parts of their self projected on the object. The subaltern's thought process is impeded; a real change in their mental well-being cannot occur. Once the subject reaches the depressive position, they eventually recognise the scattered parts of their self in the encountered object. Working through feelings and thought processes, the subject's psyche can now produce a new, repaired object. Through this last encounter, the subaltern finally reaches a better awareness of their status and regains mental well-being.

ENCOUNTERING THE OTHER: A REPAIRED APPROACH TO EKPHRASIS

In this section, I will outline the repaired approach to ekphrastic writing under examination in this chapter, focusing on:

- The ekphrastic gaze, building on Claus Clüver's idea that "the observer's gaze ought to be the central concern of the discourse on ekphrasis" (Clüver, 2018, p. 240).
- The ekphrastic object, as some details about its role still need to be outlined.
- The three ekphrastic moments, for which I will take Mitchell's schema as a starting point, accepting in this study only ekphrastic hope and fear, and adding a third, new phase to the encounter: ekphrastic joy.

In the previous section, subaltern ekphrasis has been defined as a system characterised by its intertwining of a paranoid strong theory and a reparative weak one. This helps in understanding the reason subaltern ekphrasis cannot accept all three moments of Mitchell's theory. A strong theory perfectly mirrors the three ekphrastic phases that the scholar ascribes to this rhetorical device. More precisely, the main characteristic of ekphrastic indifference, hope, and fear is the collection of a set of mistaken interpretations, which results in a paranoid signification and eventually in the repulse of the object of fascination. Instead of favouring a change in the subject's ego, this reinforces the viewer's compliance with hegemonic discourses. Furthermore, the universal nature of Mitchell's system cannot offer a detailed account of the potential some ekphrases have, since it does not provide adequate tools to enquire into underrepresented ekphrastic experiences. Therefore, the introduction of a weak and reparative component in subaltern ekphrasis outlines how some viewers access meanings otherwise obscured by a strictly paranoid and strong theory (see Sedgwick & Frank, 1995, pp. 518–519; and see Tomkins, 1995, p. 170).

Moreover, Mitchell's first ekphrastic moment, that is, ekphrastic indifference, "grows out of a commonsense perception that ekphrasis is impossible" (Mitchell, 1994, p. 152). In the case of subaltern ekphrasis, however, the traumatised subaltern subject never perceives their ekphrastic encounter as impossible. Rather, they encounter the ekphrastic object and feel it (Kennedy, 2016, p. 24). They fragment their self into it and remain in constant dialogue with it. Thus, subaltern ekphrasis is foremost a psychological experience rather than a semiotic exchange between different media. At the same time, Mitchell's moments of hope and fear, i.e., the hope of reconciliation with, and the fear of the ekphrastic object, are constituent parts of subaltern ekphrastic experiences. Indeed, these two moments required an active engagement with the object of relation. It is for this reason that the assumption of the observer's gaze as the centre of the ekphrastic practice is functional to link the strong character of Mitchell's theory to the specificity of an experience lived by a single subaltern viewer. Building on the moments of fascination outlined by Mitchell, a third, different ekphrastic moment characterises subaltern ekphrasis: the phase driven by the positive affect of joy. These three phases correspond to the Kleinian "*to-and-fro*" movement between distinct positions in the individual's mind, as outlined in the previous section (Spillius & Hinshelwood, 2011, p. 450).

The Ekphrastic Gaze

"The observer's gaze ought to be the central concern of the discourse on ekphrasis" (Clüver, 2018, p. 240), and it could not be otherwise in the approach outlined in this chapter. The conception of the ekphrastic gaze is rooted in Kennedy's idea of ekphrasis as an encounter:

I have chosen to use [the idea of ekphrasis as an encounter] not only because of its meanings of an accidental or unexpected meeting, but also because of its sense that as a consequence of such a meeting there is a change of direction. An encounter is also something that takes place as a direct "coming upon". There are also connotations of conflict or sudden clash. (Kennedy, 2016, p. 22)

Consequently, subaltern ekphrasis is considered the articulation of an accidental or unexpected meeting which prompts the viewer to a "change of direction" (Kennedy, 2016, p. 22). Given the temporal nature of the subaltern's phantasy, the subject's "engagement with the object of an intensive gaze" (Clüver, 2018, p. 247), i.e., a Kleinian object of relation, brings about a shift between the paranoid and the depressive position. Thus, the three ekphrastic moments happen during the gaze at the different objects that the subaltern encounters.

Scholar Claus Clüver contends that ekphrasis "verbalizes a real or fictive viewer's perceptions of, or reactions to, characteristic features of configurations that exist, or suggests the perceived existence of such configurations in virtual, or fictive, reality" (2018, p. 252). Elaborating on this, the ekphrastic writings by subaltern gazers are commonly employed as tools to articulate the encounter and open confrontation with characteristics that exist in the self, but are usually repressed by hegemonic discourses to the point of fragmentation and weakening of the subject's ego. Indeed, the ekphrastic process "involves an act of intersemiotic 'translation' that is structurally comparable to the conversion from traumatic into narrative memory" (Wehling-Giorgi, 2023, p. 260). Taking this a step further, it could be stated that subaltern ekphrastic writing provides the gazer with an agency to articulate their otherness once a depressive-reparative position is reached. An agency that hegemonic power structures would otherwise suppress, as Ferrante shows in her works.

In *Troubling Love*, the gaze of Delia, the first person narrator, is the core of her process of reaching a new awareness of her past traumata and, consequently, a regained mental well-being. It is, indeed, her gaze at the overwhelmingly heteronormative paintings of her father, for example, that engenders moments of reflection on the patriarchal violence her mother and she had to suffer. In her ekphrasis of the father's gipsy painting, the lack of women's facial features mirrors the deprivation and repression of identity the subaltern endures under the influence of hegemonic structures,

> *I had no doubt that the pastel sketches reproduced my mother's body. ... What he did best was the hair. He would leave those women without features but above the empty oval of the face he would skilfully draw a majestic construction, unmistakably similar to the beautiful creation that Amalia knew how to make with her long hair. (Ferrante, 2006, p. 112)*[13]

Moreover, it is Delia's gaze at her mother Amalia's and her identity card photos that evokes the first-person narrator's ekphrastic experiences throughout the story. In the novel's ending, it is also Delia's gaze at her mother's dress that brings about the main character's realisation of the sexual abuse she endured in her childhood and subconsciously repressed. I will examine these ekphrases in the following sections.

The Ekphrastic Object

Subaltern ekphrastic writings reveal a different relationship between the viewer and the object than the one theorised in classical theories of ekphrasis. Building on Mitchell's definition, the ekphrastic object is a resident alien to be found only in the text (Mitchell, 1994, p. 157), i.e., a fictional object in a fictional world. Within the dynamic of subaltern ekphrastic encounters, this resident alien acquires the position of the other as opposed to the self of the gazer. Indeed, in the case of subaltern ekphrases, the object is not a mere visual element. It rather comprises split parts of a subaltern, traumatised, fragmented self in the realm of their phantasy. Thus, the description of the object as a resident alien perfectly matches the description Klein makes of the object of relation, i.e., the representation of a real object in the individual's phantasy.

Moreover, the position of the subject in relation to the object is not a vertical hegemonic one, as outlined in classical theories of ekphrasis. Indeed, the lyrical 'I' and first-person narrators are subaltern subjects as well. Borrowing Louvel's description of the ekphrastic object,

> *the relation of word and image [is not] in terms of a vertical structure but in the mode of the rhizome, refusing the gendered separation between feminine image and male text. ... No mortal struggle is involved, but rather a fruitful collaboration and a productive encounter. (2018, p. 260)*

The object, therefore, also possesses an active role in the dynamics of the ekphrastic encounter. It is a constituent part of a play of resonances between two bodies that constantly affect and are affected, influencing each other.

Considering the praxis of ekphrasis as the articulation of a gaze at an object, i.e., the encounter of a subject with the latter, the ekphrastic text remains an articulation of a viewer's perception of the affect/effect the object has on them. As a result, the ekphrastic object becomes an autopoietic production of the viewer's mind. It is born inside the viewer's model of reality itself, and its meaning is only a construction of the viewer's perception. By autopoietic, I refer to biologists Humberto Maturana and Francisco J. Varela's concept of "autopoiesis" (Maturana & Varela, 1980, pp. 77–79), i.e., the ability of organisms to engender themselves.[14] Varela and Maturana's theory was first outlined in *Autopoiesis and Cognition: The Realization of the Living* (1980) and it was later developed in other publications. However, their first theorisation of the nature of life is helpful in further delineating the nature of the ekphrastic object. According to Maturana and Varela, once a living system generates itself, it becomes an observer of both the self and the environment in which it lives (see Maturana, 1970, p. 1). This observer, or gazer, can define only what lies in its domain of interactions, since, in Maturana and Varela's system, "the ultimate reference for any description is the observer [itself]" (Maturana & Varela, 1980, p. 8). This idea recalls Klein's definition of phantasy and object of relation, since phantasy is the *locus* of human perception of external objects of relation.

Given this autopoietic feature, the subaltern ekphrastic object is defined as a play of mirrors between parts of the subject's self. It is the representation of one's fragmented ego encountering the otherness in itself projected onto an object. As a consequence, the ekphrastic object could not be about the fear of other entities, as Mitchell argues (see Mitchell, 1994, p. 169). Instead, it is about the fear of those parts of the self, the less explored ones, the ones left unspoken by hegemonic discourses, the ones that make the I tremble in the moment of the encounter.

Troubling Love is marked by intense gazes that frequently arise from the projection of the protagonist's fragmented self onto objects—an autopoietic instance. Nevertheless, throughout most of Delia's novel-length ekphrasis, these projections are perceived as a confrontation with the other, with a fearful resident of her psyche. A peculiar example of this relation between gazed object and gazing subject is the ekphrasis of Delia's reflection in the mirror of her mother's house. In this encounter, the protagonist fails to recognise her own image; instead, she describes it as a resident alien, as the reflection of her mother Amalia to which she refuses to acknowledge any resemblance. Dismissing the similarity with contempt, Delia describes her reflection as follows

'You're a ghost', I said to the woman in the mirror. She [emphasis added] had the face of a person in her forties, she closed first one eye, then the other, drawing

a black pencil over each. She was thin, angular, with prominent cheekbones, the skin miraculously unlined. Her hair was cut very short in order to display as little of its black color as possible, although, to my relief, the black was finally fading to gray and preparing to disappear forever. I [emphasis added] put on the mascara.[15] *(Ferrante, 2006, p. 42)*

Katrin Wehling-Giorgi highlights how the figure of the ghost is usually employed to articulate systematically silenced stories (2023, p. 250). Thus, by encountering such an object of relation, Delia's ekphrasis portrays the dissociative character of trauma, which causes "the division of an individual's personality" (Wehling-Giorgi, 2023, p. 255). In the excerpt, the protagonist's dissociation becomes evident at first through her failure to acknowledge that she is looking at her own reflection. Secondly, the fragmentation of Delia's ego is marked by the combination of third- and first-person pronouns, although she is always the first-person narrator of her story. The quoted passage exemplifies how a traumatised, subaltern subject typically fails to "integrate sensory data at a cognitive or linguistic level" in the articulation of their experiences (Wehling-Giorgi, 2023, p. 255). Therefore, they must resort to the power of "ekphrastic imagery" to interpret the real meaning of the object at which they are gazing (Wehling-Giorgi, 2023, p. 254). Thanks to this, the subaltern subject will eventually repair the fragmented parts of their weakened ego into a new whole.

The Ekphrastic Moments

As introduced above, the three subaltern ekphrastic moments are ekphrastic hope, fear, and joy. These moments are driven by three distinct Tomkinsian affects. The affect of excitement characterises the moment of hope, whereas fear–terror governs the phase of fear. By contrast, the pervasive and positive affect of joy drives the third and final ekphrastic moment. This positive affect renders the theory of subaltern ekphrasis weak, since joy promotes a confrontation with the object of relation rather than its avoidance. Joy also enables the viewer to overcome the paranoid positions of the first two ekphrastic moments and to be open to change through the encounter with the unspoken parts of their fragmented self. Tomkins describes this relation between excitement, fear, and joy as a sudden reduction of stimulus density (Tomkins, 1995, p. 9). Therefore, at the basis of the affective functioning of the three moments of subaltern ekphrasis, there is a reduction from a state of continuous fear and excitement (high density affects) to the low density affect of joy. This process is easily linked to the idea of position as *to-and-fro* movement in relation to an object described by Klein.

Ekphrastic Hope

The first moment of the ekphrastic encounter is hope. In this phase, the subaltern viewer experiences a brief moment of faith in the possibility of understanding the nature of the ekphrastic object. The subject believes they could gain this "knowledge in the form of exposure" (Sedgwick, 2003, p. 138). Hope is, therefore, to be read as faith in the self's ability to reveal the other as knowledge. As a consequence, the subaltern subject starts searching for meanings, constructing a narrative about the object of intensive gaze. The theory is in its strong part. Driven by the high-density affect of excitement and in a paranoid position, the subaltern ego attempts to confine the nature of the ekphrastic object to a single, definite, and pleasing narrative through the use of a strict set of rules.

Tomkins's conceptualisation of affect experiences in scripts could help elucidate the underlying functioning of this first ekphrastic moment. A script is a set of scenes that an individual uses as a general orientation in life. The scene is the basic affective element, a relationship with an object magnified by an affect. In his account of the various kinds of scripts, Tomkins introduces the "*Limitation*-remediation scripts" (Tomkins, 2008, p. 679), which are strictly linked with hope. For Tomkins, "hope [is] the great engine of the religions of the oppressed[, in which] limitation shared becomes limitation attenuated under such circumstances" (2008, p. 680). Consequently, during the moment of ekphrastic hope, in a state of increased affective stimulus, the subaltern viewer glances, in their gaze at the ekphrastic object, the possibility of constructing a comforting narrative to cope with a situation of distress. Nevertheless, the true nature of the ekphrastic object remains inaccessible, due to the unsatisfying and imperfect scenes that characterise the script of hope (Tomkins, 2008, p. 679). The object is, therefore, overtly non-specific and perceived as alien by the subject. The subaltern's fragmented and weakened ego could not heal.

In Ferrante's novel, Delia's ekphrastic hope is evoked by her way of gazing at herself in the mirror. During this phase, as mentioned in the previous section, Delia does not want to acknowledge the resemblance between her and her mother-reflection. For instance, after the ekphrasis of her reflection, she comments, "'I don't look like you', I whispered as I put on some blusher. And in order not to be contradicted, I tried not to look at her." (Ferrante, 2006, p. 42).[16] In doing so, Delia not only refuses any similarity between her and her "ghost"/reflection/mother (Ferrante, 2006, p. 42). She also tries to construct her narrative, without gazing at the other, split part of her ego.

Another exemplary excerpt from *Troubling Love* helps introduce the passage from ekphrastic hope to ekphrastic fear. The protagonist delivers the first ekphrasis of her father's gipsy painting. During this episode, Delia avoids a confrontation with the gazed objects, which evokes a lapidary comment. The first-person narrator openly says:

I had forgotten nothing but I didn't want to remember. If necessary, I could have told myself everything, in every detail; but why do it? I told myself only what was useful, according to the situation, deciding from moment to moment on the wave of necessity.[17] *(Ferrante, 2006, p. 49)*

The articulation of Delia's subaltern gaze perfectly represents the state of her phantasy, which is constrained by the rules of a paranoid script of hope. As a consequence, she recounts only what is necessary to construct a "religion of the oppressed" (Tomkins, 2008, p. 680), a useful narrative to avoid situations of distress. Her narrative must, then, be one of subjection to the hegemonic discourse in which she is embedded, yet not a completely normative one. Ferrante perfectly represents this by choosing a painting of a woman, produced by a man in series, as Delia's object of relation. As a consequence of her excitement about exposure and knowledge, Delia not only acquires an awareness of the need to construct a narrative to protect herself from the truth. She also becomes scared of the effects a confrontation with the objects could bring on her ego. Therefore, in an increasingly paranoid position of subjection to patriarchal hegemony, the protagonist still does not manage to see and to repair the different split parts of her traumatised and fragmented self into a new whole.

Ekphrastic Fear

Fear is the paranoid moment *par excellence*. The subject cannot do anything other than show "resistance and counterdesire" to the eagerness for knowledge it had in the first part of the encounter (Mitchell, 1994, p. 154). In order to cope with the negative affect of fear, the viewer stops trying to expose the meaning of the ekphrastic object. The narratives they construct maximise their rhetorical strength by reducing "more and more remote phenomena to a single formulation" (Tomkins, 2008, p. 519). As a consequence, fear shifts the focus of the ekphrastic encounter: from excited hope to prevent harm through knowledge to a paranoid fear of the effects of seeking knowledge.

During the passage between excitement and fear, i.e., between ekphrastic hope and fear, the affect density of the subaltern subject reaches its peak. To put it in Kleinian terms, the subaltern ego is at its highest moment of fragmentation. It is so deeply paranoid and weakened that it needs to constrain the object in a prescribed narrative and form. The affect of fear, then, imprints the subject's mind. The subaltern is forced to shield themselves from the negative affect they begin to experience. The object eventually becomes a dangerous resident alien that needs to be confined by the strong accepted rules of societal hegemonic structures.

Tomkins's "paranoid posture" further elucidates the affective functioning of ekphrastic fear (Tomkins, 2008, p. 530). Following the failed exposure of the ekphrastic object during the moment of hope, the subject perceives the other as a possible source of humiliation (Tomkins, 2008, p. 528). Consequently, the individual confers a limited meaning to the other. This interpretation of the object stems from the paranoid-maniac ego's fear of humiliation that could come with a full exposure of the other as a collection of split parts of the self. In the case under examination, the subaltern subject resorts to strong theories, i.e., hegemonic discourses, in their account of the ekphrastic object. Consequently, Tomkins's paranoid posture, driven by the negative affect of "fear-terror" (Tomkins, 2008, p. 530), describes precisely the process of "an individual [that] generates and tests every conceivable strategy to avoid and escape total defeat at the hand of the humiliating bad object" (Tomkins, 2008, p. 531). In some ekphrastic encounters, this is the last stop for the subject. Thus, the viewer will avoid a confrontation with the object that goes beyond fear/paranoia, and their ego will be doomed to a state of extreme fragmentation. Rather than apprehending the otherness of the object as split parts of the self, the object is presented as the other outside the self.

If, in the first phase of *Troubling Love*'s novel-length ekphrastic experience, Delia manages to construct her ekphrastic narrative, in the second moment of fascination she can no longer do so without fearing the ekphrastic object. In the moment of ekphrastic hope, the protagonist was indeed protected by her subaltern religion and by her faith in the revealing nature of her pleasing narrative. During the moment of ekphrastic fear, though, she needs to defend herself from a highly dense and negatively affected confrontation with the true nature of the ekphrastic objects. She still cannot repair the split parts of her identity. Therefore, Delia's new paranoid ekphrasis must articulate through the use of a strong hegemonic theory a supremacy of the weakened I over a subaltern and muted ekphrastic object. Thus, the protagonist is moved by her paranoia to distance herself from the other, from the strongest projection of her traumatised split parts, i.e., the image of her mother Amalia.

Delia's ekphrasis of Amalia's altered identity card photo initiates the moment of ekphrastic fear. In describing her mother's picture, Delia indeed recounts an encounter with an uncanny, altered Amalia, an Amalia whose features have been erased. The ekphrastic object has lost the possibility of being recognised as itself. Delia-terrorised-subject must physically erase Amalia-bad-object:

> *The long, baroquely sculpted hair ... had been carefully scraped away. The white that emerged around her head had been changed with a pencil to a nebulous gray. With the same pencil someone had slightly hardened the features of her face. The woman in the photograph wasn't Amalia: it was me [emphasis added].*[18] *(Ferrante, 2006, p. 61)*

The strong final sentence, which also closes the chapter, introduces the kind of paranoid narrative that will characterise the following ekphrases. As mentioned above, the primary power of the articulation of ekphrastic fear lies in hegemonic power structures. These are used by the protagonist to silence the other, to subject them to her narrative. Delia's adherence to the rules of these structures will keep her ego split. Only in the last, positively affected moments, will she recognise the true oppressive and hegemonic nature of her paranoid narrative. This realisation will enable her to freely interface with the perceived otherness of the ekphrastic object and accept this as traumatised, split parts of her fragmented self.

Ekphrastic Joy

While some subaltern subjects remain stuck in the clutches of ekphrastic fear, there are nevertheless others who manage to overcome fear and reach the last phase of the ekphrastic encounter: the moment of joy. After a steady increment of stimulus density from the moment of excitement-hope to that of fear (Tomkins, 2008, pp. 160-162), during ekphrastic joy, the subaltern I is brought to a sudden "decreasing gradient" (Tomkins, 2008, p. 118). Indeed, Tomkins contends that the positive affect of joy counteracts negative affects—be it fear, disgust, or shame—with the help of an "ally" (2008, p. 262). Typically, this ally, especially in childhood, is the figure of the mother, which in adult life evolves into that of the peers (Tomkins, 2008, p. 263). In the case under examination, however, the subaltern subject has faced, until this moment, ekphrastic objects, which are an autopoietic split part of their increasingly weakened ego. Searching for an external ally as the adjutant of joy will be, therefore, misleading in subaltern ekphrasis; the warfare is indeed between parts of the individual's self.

Nevertheless, Tomkins's affect theory offers another congenial explanation for the functioning of subaltern ekphrasis. Indeed, the stimulus of fear can also be reduced through joy by "divesting [an] interiorized ally of all external reference" (2008, p. 264). This consists of *splitting* the self into two parts, one still under a strong hegemonic theory of fear and one without any other reference but the inner world of the self. Consequently, "the individual can tolerate or master non-optimal conditions without dependence on the actual presence of the ally" (Tomkins, 2008, p. 264). The alliance between these parts of the self is, therefore, what evokes joy and reduces fear. The action of this process lies precisely in this newly gained belief in the "attainment of truth, of beauty, of justice, of freedom" thanks to the possibility created by the subject's phantasy (Tomkins, 2008, p. 265), or imagery to use Tomkins's term.

Klein's reparation recalls Tomkins's consideration of joy as a reducer of negative affects. During the phase of ekphrastic fear, the subaltern subject is indeed in their deepest moment of fragmentation. Their ego is weakened to the point of strong paranoia: every split part of their traumatic self is considered an enemy to their mental safety. Nonetheless, the subaltern subject also experiences brief moments of reparation by overcoming the paranoid position. As introduced above, a depressive position enables the self to repair different parts of their split ego into a new whole (Garvey, 2023, p. 54; Klein, 1946, p. 105). Reparation is rooted in this position, but it is foremost rooted in love for the object (Sedgwick, 2003, p. 128). The self perceives, thus, the other, the resident alien, no longer as a threat, but as something they need to restore their mental well-being. This process can have different outcomes, both of which are relevant in subaltern ekphrasis. Either the subject realises with "sad recognition" that the object represents a traumatised part of the psyche "that cannot be repaired" (Spillius & Hinshelwood, 2011, p. 471), or the reparation of the ekphrastic objects provides the I with "a way out of despair" (Spillius & Hinshelwood, 2011, p. 470).

Both results improve the subaltern subject's mental well-being. In fact, both the recognition of damage and the reparation of a love object engender awareness of trauma and subalternity and have the power to heal an unconsciously open wound. It is noteworthy that, as for Tomkins, imagination is strictly linked with the affect of joy, so for Klein, all creative practice happens during the act of reparation in the realm of phantasy (Sedgwick, 2011, p. 126). Taking this a step further: during ekphrastic joy, the subaltern subject recognises in the gazed other a beloved ekphrastic object, an ally made up by a collection of split parts of the self. The subject can now repair their traumatised ego through the description of the images produced by their depressive phantasy. It is through this joyous articulation that the subaltern can finally speak.[19]

For this final ekphrastic moment, I will consider two ekphrases from the last chapters of *Troubling Love*. Each of these instances of ekphrastic writing articulates Delia's newly gained awareness of her subaltern condition and the effects this awareness has on her mental well-being. The first ekphrasis takes place in the ruin of the café in which Delia was abused as a child. Here, the first-person narrator encounters an old dress of her mother. Delia's ekphrasis evokes a moment of healing between fragmented parts of her ego. Until this moment, the main character had been unable to recognise these parts as constituents of her traumatised self. The narrative she imposed on the ekphrastic object-Amalia was indeed a patriarchal one. Instead of recognising the traumatic and subaltern nature of the object, in whose condition she partakes, Delia continued to regard the object as a reflection of Amalia's betrayal of normative gender roles, such as her affair, her divorce, and her way of dressing. The ekphrasis eventually induces a realisation of the transgenerational nature of the violence the two women have to endure (see Wehling-Giorgi, 2023, p. 258). "I felt that that old garment was the final narrative that my mother had left me, and that now, with all the necessary adjustments, it fit me like a glove." (Ferrante, 2006, p. 134).[20] The inherited dress-ekphrastic object-narrative brings about a realisation and thus, an articulation of both the shared subaltern condition and the irreparable damage that hegemonic power structures have inflicted on them.

The novel ends with a last moment of ekphrastic joy. Delia is on the shore where Amalia was found dead, and begins to alter her own identity card photo. In opposition to the moment of ekphrastic fear, Delia does not need to erase the other in the object to confront it. The last ekphrasis of the first-person narrator ratifies Delia's acceptance of the other as split parts of her ego, the acceptance of Amalia within herself, and the awareness of a transgenerational subaltern status, of a communal story of violence and trauma. Describing the altered picture, she comments, "I looked at myself, smiled at myself. That old-fashioned hairstyle, popular in the forties but already rare at the end of the fifties, suited me. *Amalia had been. I was Amalia* [emphasis added]." (Ferrante, 2006, p. 139).[21] Delia's subaltern ekphrastic experience concludes with the novel's final sentence. Ferrante manages to demonstrate that ekphrastic writing can enable subaltern subjects to articulate their experiences, gain awareness of their subaltern status and traumata, and, as such, work towards mental well-being.

FINAL REMARKS

The journey through classical theories of ekphrasis culminates here, in a repaired approach that gives voice to the subaltern subject. During their encounter with the ekphrastic object, subaltern viewers discover, through three moments of fascination, the true nature of their object of relation. Initially, the subaltern subject regards the object with excitement, then with fear, and ultimately, in a joyful moment, they recognise the true nature of the ekphrastic other. The fragmented, weakened, and subaltern I can now repair the object—composed of various split parts of the self—into a new whole. The articulation of this reparation within ekphrastic writings marks the beginning of a path towards mental well-being.

This chapter does not investigate the role of an important character in the dynamics of ekphrastic writings, that of the reader. Indeed, only the relationship between subaltern subjects and objects in the realm of fiction is analysed. The potential effects and affects a subaltern reader might have in response to subaltern ekphrasis require further examination. This chapter hopes to have contributed with its reasoning to the field of medical humanities. It wishes to promote, with the support of psychology and neuroscience, additional questioning regarding the potential of ekphrasis and of rhetorical devices in general for humans' mental health.

Delia's ekphrastic relationship with Amalia's imagery provides a fitting final reflection for this chapter. Delia's novel-length ekphrastic experience has unfolded in several glances at the image of her mother over the three moments of the ekphrastic encounter. Amalia was initially a ghost, whose description sparked excitement and hope within a religion of the subaltern. A religion that had the imperative to contain the negative effects and affect that confronting the split parts of the self could engender. However, the true nature of said religion lies in the failure of its intentions. A failure that brings about fear and extreme paranoia. Consequently, Delia had to erase Amalia's identity, as further investigation into the mother's nature could have endangered the stability of the protagonist's fragmented I. Finally, Delia has been repaired through and with Amalia. The main character has accepted the traumata she endured and, consequently, can now joyously face and repair her beloved ekphrastic object. From the construction of a religion of the subaltern to the destruction of the other's identity, and ultimately to the acceptance of the other as a collection of split parts of one's fragmented self, Ferrante demonstrates how the subaltern I can acquire awareness of their status through the articulation of their affect, imagery, and consciousness, towards a repaired and regained mental well-being.

REFERENCES

Ahern, S. (2024). Affect Theory and Literary Criticism. *Emotion Review*, *16*(2), 96–106.

Ahmed, S. (2020). Happy Objects. In Gregg, M., & Seigworth, G. J. (Eds.), *The Affect Theory Reader* (pp. 29–51). Duke University Press.

Atkinson, M. (2017). *The Poetics of Transgenerational Trauma*. Bloomsbury Academic & Professional.

Bisceglia, A. (2023, March 15). *Pittura e Poesia | Opere | Le Gallerie degli Uffizi*. Le Gallerie degli Uffizi. https://www.uffizi.it/opere/pittura-e-poesia

Clough, P. T. (Ed.). (2007). *The Affective Turn*. Duke University Press.

Clüver, C. (2018). On Gazers' Encounters with Visual Art: Ekphrasis, Readers, 'Iconotexts'. In Kennedy, D., & Meek, R. (Eds.), *Ekphrastic Encounters: New Interdisciplinary Essays on Literature and the Visual Arts* (pp. 237–256).

Cometa, M. (2024). *The Literary Life of Pictures: A Theory of Description* (1st ed. 2024). Springer Nature Switzerland. DOI: 10.1007/978-3-031-52897-2

De Rogatis, T. (2018). *Elena Ferrante: Parole chiave*. Edizioni e/o.

Demos, E. V. (2019). *The Affect Theory of Silvan Tomkins for Psychoanalysis and Psychotherapy: Recasting the Essentials*. Routledge.

Ferrante, E. (1992). *L'amore molesto*. Edizionie/o.

Ferrante, E. (2006). *Troubling Love* (1st ed.). (Goldstein, A., Trans.). Europa Editions.

Ferrante, E. (2016a). *Frantumaglia: A Writer's Journey* (A. Goldstein, Trans.; Unabridged and updated edition). Europa Editions.

Ferrante, E. (2016b). *La frantumaglia: Carte (1991-2003), Tessere (2003-2007), Lettere (2011-2016)*. Edizioni e/o.

Ferrante, E. (2021). *I margini e il dettato*. Edizioni e/o.

Frank, A. J., & Wilson, E. A. (2020). *A Silvan Tomkins Handbook: Foundations for Affect Theory*. University of Minnesota Press. DOI: 10.5749/j.ctv182jthz

Furini, F. (1626). *Pittura e Poesia* (Palazzo Pitti, Galleria Palatina, Sala di Berenice) [Oil painting on canvas]. https://www.uffizi.it/opere/pittura-e-poesia

Garvey, P. (2023). *Melanie Klein: A Contemporary Introduction* (1st ed.). Routledge. DOI: 10.4324/9781003215714

Gramsci, A. (1992). *Selections from the prison notebooks of Antonio Gramsci* (Hoare, Q., & Nowell Smith, G., Eds.). International Publishers.

Heffernan, J. A. W. (1993). *Museum of words: The poetics of ekphrasis from Homer to Ashbery*. University of Chicago Press.

Heffernan, J. A. W. (2015). Ekphrasis: Theory. In Rippl, G. (Ed.), *Handbook of Intermediality: Literature—Image—Sound—Music* (pp. 35–49). De Gruyter.

Jansson, M. (2018). Ekphrasis and Digital Media. *Poetics Today, 39*(2), 299–318. DOI: 10.1215/03335372-4324468

Kennedy, D. (2016). *The Ekphrastic Encounter in Contemporary British Poetry and Elsewhere*. Routledge.

Kennedy, D., & Meek, R. (2018). Introduction: From paragone to encounter. In Kennedy, D., & Meek, R. (Eds.), *Ekphrastic encounters: New interdisciplinary essays on literature and the visual arts* (pp. 1–24). Manchester University Press.

Klein, M. (1946). Notes on Some Schizoid Mechanisms. *The International Journal of Psycho-Analysis, XXVII*(3 & 4), 99–110. PMID: 20261821

Klein, M. (1984). *Envy and gratitude, and other works, 1946-1963* (Free Press ed, Vol. 3). Free Press.

Lessing, G. E. (2012). *Laokoon, oder, Über die Grenzen der Malerei und Poesie: Studienausgabe* (Vollhardt, F., Ed.). Reclam.

Lindhé, C. (2013). "A Visual Sense is Born in the Fingertips": Towards a Digital Ekphrasis. *Digital Humanities Quarterly*, 7(1).

Louvel, L. (2018). Types of Ekphrasis. *Poetics Today, 39*(2), 245–263. DOI: 10.1215/03335372-4324432

Maturana, H. R. (1970). *Biology of Cognition. Biological Computer Laboratory Research Report BCL 9.0*. University of Illinois.

Maturana, H. R., & Varela, F. J. (with Beer, S.). (1980). *Autopoiesis and Cognition: The Realization of the Living*. D. Reidel Publishing Company.

Milkova, S. (2016). Elena Ferrante's Visual Poetics: Ekphrasis in Troubling Love, My Brilliant Friend, and The Story of a New Name. In G. Russo Bullaro & S. V. Love (Eds.), *The Works of Elena Ferrante. Reconfiguring the Margins* (pp. 159–182). Palgrave Macmillan US.

Milkova, S. (2021). *Elena Ferrante as world literature*. Bloomsbury Academic.

Mitchell, W. J. T. (1986). *Iconology: Image, text, ideology*. University of Chicago Press.

Mitchell, W. J. T. (1994). *Picture Theory*. University of Chicago Press.

Morante, E. (1990). *Alibi* (1. ed). Garzanti.

Muñoz, J. E. (2006). Feeling Brown, Feeling Down: Latina Affect, the Performativity of Race, and the Depressive Position. *Signs (Chicago, Ill.)*, *31*(3), 675–688. DOI: 10.1086/499080

Schwab, G. (2010). *Haunting legacies: Violent histories and transgenerational trauma*. Columbia University Press.

Sedgwick, E. K. (with Frank, A.). (2003). *Touching Feeling: Affect, Pedagogy, Performativity*. Duke University Press.

Sedgwick, E. K. (2011). *The weather in Proust* (Goldberg, J., Ed.). Duke University Press.

Sedgwick, E. K., & Frank, A. (1995). Shame in the Cybernetic Fold: Reading Silvan Tomkins. *Critical Inquiry*, *21*(2), 496–522. DOI: 10.1086/448761

Spillius, E. B., & Hinshelwood, R. D. (2011). *The new dictionary of Kleinian thought*. Routledge.

Spivak, G. C. (2007). Can the Subaltern Speak? In C. Nelson & L. Grossberg (Eds.), *Marxism and the interpretation of culture* (pp. 271–313). University of Illinois Press.

Tomkins, S. S. (1995). *Shame and its sisters: A Silvan Tomkins reader* (Sedgwick, E. K., Ed.). Duke University Press.

Tomkins, S. S. (2008). *Affect Imagery Consciousness*. Springer Pub.

Webb, R. (2009). *Ekphrasis, imagination and persuasion in ancient rhetorical theory and practice*. Ashgate.

Wehling-Giorgi, K. (2016). 'Ero separata da me': Memory, Selfhood and Mother-Tongue in Goliarda Sapienza and Elena Ferrante. In Bazzoni, A., Fortini, L., Bond, E., & Wehling-Giorgi, K. (Eds.), *Goliarda Sapienza in Context: Intertextual Relationships with Italian and European Culture* (pp. 288–311). Fairleigh Dickinson University Press.

Wehling-Giorgi, K. (2023). Unspeakable Things Spoken: Transgenerational Trauma, Fractured Bodies and Visual Tropes in Toni Morrison, Elsa Morante and Elena Ferrante's Works. *Romance Studies*, *41*(4), 248–266.

ENDNOTES

1 "Only to those who love the Other lights its splendour." (Morante, 1990, p. 73; my translation).

2 As far as the interdisciplinary aspect of affect theory is concerned, two streams of thought dominate the present academic discourse. On the one hand, Silvan Tomkins's system is used as an instrument to overcome "ideological … binary opposites" (Ahern, 2024, p. 96), and on the other hand, the reading by Brian Massumi of philosopher Gilles Deleuze's work is considered as a fruitful tool to depart "from abstract conceptions of 'The Body' and to think instead about actual bodies embedded in and affected by networks of relation." (Ahern, 2024, p. 97).

3 "Ho letto con molta passione Melanie Klein." (Ferrante, 2016b, p. 116).

4 For literature as a medium expressing affectively transmitted trauma across generations, see Atkinson (2017) and Schwab (2010).

5 Heffernan is aware "that his early definition of ekphrasis may have its limitations" (Kennedy & Meek, 2018, p. 18), nevertheless he has not changed his maxim yet. As a consequence, I will still refer to the definition given above as the one considered most appropriate by the scholar.

6 The competition or comparison between various art forms, especially painting and poetry, is referred to as 'paragone' in Renaissance Italy. Artists and theorists often argued over the superiority of one art form over another during this period.

7 Horace's *Ars Poetica* is the source of the expression 'ut pictura poësis', which means 'as is painting, so is poetry'. This idea emphasises how the two disciplines can enhance rather than simply compete with one another.

8 This gender/genre dichotomy and its patriarchal structure pervade *Laokoon* in almost every page, but some sections could be considered particularly exemplary of this conception of the artistic world (see Lessing, 2012, Chapter I; II; III; IV; XVIII).

9 "Ho messo a punto una narratrice in prima persona che, sovraeccitata dagli spintoni casuali tra lei e il mondo, deformava la forma che si era faticosamente attribuita e da quelle ammaccature e distorsioni e lesioni spremeva fuori altre possibilità insospettate." (Ferrante, 2021, p. 60).

10 As far as Klein's system is concerned, the methods outlined in this chapter apply the psychoanalyst's theories on the development of the infant's mind to the growth of the subaltern's psyche during the ekphrastic encounter with an object.

11 "Qui per capirsi dobbiamo parlare di come il dolore modifica l'immagine del tempo. L'insorgere della sofferenza nulla il tempo lineare, lo spezza, ne fa vorticosi scarabocchi. La notte dei tempi si raccoglie ai bordi dell'aurora d'oggi e di domani. Il dolore ci sprofonda tra le antenate unicellulari, tra i borbottii rissosi o terrorizzati dentro le caverne, tra le divinità femminili ricacciate nel buio della terra, pur tenendoci ancorate ... al computer su cui stiamo scrivendo. I sentimenti forti sono così: stanno saltare la cronologia. Un'emozione è un salto mortale, una capriola, una piroetta vorticosa." (Ferrante, 2016b, p. 102).

12 "La sorveglianza invece, sebbene intesa, è piuttosto una disposizione affettiva di tutto il corpo, un suo distendersi e germogliare sopra e intorno." (Ferrante, 2016b, p. 98).

13 "Non avevo dubbi che gli schizzi col pastello riproducevano il corpo di mia madre. ... Ciò che gli veniva meglio erano i capelli. Lasciava quelle donne senza volto ma sul l'ovale vuoto del viso tratteggiava con efficacia una costruzione maestosa, inequivocabilmente simile alla bella pettinatura che Amalia sapeva realizzare coi suoi lunghi capelli." (Ferrante, 1992, pp. 141–142)

14 In the introduction to his volume, Maturana and Varela also recount the origin of the neologism "autopoiesis". The term derives from the ancient Greek philosophical opposition between the concepts of "*praxis*", action and "*poiesis*", creation, construct with the addition of the prefix "*auto-*". The authors stress also how the use of a neologism freed them from the bonds with earlier research and engendered the potentiality for a novel approach, thus stressing the relevance of language in his theory from the very beginning (Maturana & Varela, 1980, p. xvii).

15 "'Sei un fantasma' dissi alla donna nello specchio. Aveva la faccia di una persona intorno ai quaranta, chiudeva prima un occhio, poi l'altro, e su ciascuno passava una matita nera. Era scarna, aguzza, con zigomi marcati, miracolosamente senza rughe. Portava capelli tagliati cortissimi per ostentarne il meno possibile il colore corvino, che del resto con sollievo andava finalmente

sbiadendo e si preparava a sparire per sempre. Passai il mascara." (Ferrante, 1992, pp. 48–49).

16 "'Non ti assomiglio' le sussurrai mentre mi davo un po' di fard. E per non essere smentita, cercai di non guardarla." (Ferrante, 1992, p. 49).

17 "Non avevo dimenticato niente ma non volevo ricordare. All'occorrenza, avrei potuto raccontarmi tutto, per filo e per segno; ma perché farlo? Mi raccontavo solo quello che serviva, a seconda dei casi, decidendo di volta in volta sull'onda della necessita." (Ferrante, 1992, p. 57).

18 "I lunghi capelli baroccamente architettati sulla fronte e intorno al viso erano stati accuratamente raschiati via. Il bianco emerso intorno alla testa era stato mutato con una matita in un grigio nebuloso. Con la stessa matita qualcuno aveva lievemente indurito i lineamenti del viso. La donna della foto non era Amalia: ero io." (Ferrante, 1992, p. 73).

19 José E. Muñoz demonstrates that the arts through their affective power give the subaltern a tool to speak (see Muñoz, 2006, p. 677). Muñoz directly challenges with his concept Gayatri C. Spivak's famous essay on the subaltern's impossibility to articulate their status (see Spivak, 2007, pp. 271–313).

20 "Sentii quell'abito vecchio come la narrazione estrema che mia madre mi aveva lasciato e che ora con tutti gli artifici necessari mi calzava a pennello." (Ferrante, 1992, p. 171).

21 "Mi guardai, mi sorrisi. Quell'acconciatura antiquata, in uso negli anni Quaranta ma già rara alla fine degli anni Cinquanta, mi donava. Amalia c'era stata. Io ero Amalia." (Ferrante, 1992, p. 178).

Chapter 6
The Socratic Dialogue That Restores the Enchantment of the World:
A Study on the Methodology of the MemoGen Project

Patrizia Piredda
http://orcid.org/0000-0003-4510-4498
MemoGen Project - Centro Studi Sereno Regis, Italy

ABSTRACT

This chapter investigates the method applied in the project "The Legacy of the Second World War in the Memory of the Third Generation," which collects a corpus of video interviews with Italian people born between the 1960s and the 1980s. The interviews are dialogues developed according to the Socratic dialeghestai, which is based on listening and understanding and is aimed at developing a critical reflection that starts with the recollections of the past to reach our contemporaneity. This chapter investigates how this methodology produces well-being in the witnesses in connection with the pleasure of remembering their childhood and grandparents. Eventually, it is claimed that the interviewees' well-being partially derives from aesthetic pleasure and, by referring to Fischer-Lichte's aesthetics, the interviewer is defined as a maieutic director.

DOI: 10.4018/979-8-3373-3521-6.ch006

INTRODUCTION

Over the last twenty years, scholarship has investigated the long-term impact of the Second World War and its legacy on people, families, and communities in European countries, especially in terms of psychological effects, for example, in Germany concerning the legacy of the Holocaust on the second and third generation (Hirsch, 2012; Kundnani, 2011; Fossion, 2014). Such a legacy has been recently investigated in Eastern countries too, for example in Japan, where the long-term traumatic effects of the war have haunted thousands of families for generations (Tsutsui, 2009; Allen & Sakamoto, 2013; Hashimoto, 2015; Saito, 2017). In Italy, oral historians started to consider the impact of the war on people in the 1960s (Revelli, 1966; Revelli, 1977), and continued to investigate the legacy of the conflict in recent years (Portelli, 1999; Gribaudi, 2005). However, researchers have mainly focused on living witnesses of the war still in the early 2000s, neglecting to investigate how the legacy of the Second World War evolved among the following generations.

To fill this gap, the MemoGen project was launched in early 2024 in Italy to understand the relevance of the Second World War for Italians born between the 1960s and 1980s.[1] These people constitute the last generation that could hear the stories of direct witnesses of the war in their families, first and foremost grandparents or sometimes parents. This "emotional imprinting" shaped the legacy of the war in the minds and language of this group that today must deal with challenges other than those the previous generations were confronted with. Unlike the works by Hirsch and Fossion, which are mainly hinged on the concept of trauma, the MemoGen project aims to assess the extent to which people consider the Second World War a historical event capable of affecting their lives, ideas, ethical views and even well-being after eighty years.[2] Several interviewees recall the harshest episodes of their ancestors' experiences with emotional participation, showing feelings of sympathy and compassion; however, those events rarely affect them post-traumatically.

There is no selection process beforehand for the group. The interviewees are invited either personally or through intermediaries, who may be former interviewees or other people. The methodology used is modeled on the example provided by Italian oral historian Nuto Revelli, whose interviewees were people he had got acquainted with in the first place. The interview, therefore, is not conceived as an abstract task but as a particular form of social interaction that takes place within a broader framework of sociability that includes dialogue as a fundamental form of cultural and ethical interaction. Finally, a small number of interviewees have contacted us through the MemoGen website and mailing lists: in those cases, the interview was not prepared by any preparatory form of social interaction. The project involves people from all cultural and social backgrounds, many of whom have no scholarly involvement in the study of the Second World War. Therefore, as the interviewees are asked to recall their grandparents' experiences, they report things they heard of in the form of storytelling. Their relationship with the war is indirect and mediated by stories, both heard within the family and learned from books, movies, and other media over the years. This makes the Second World War a layered object, the knowledge of which may be blurred; nonetheless, its legacy still affects ethics, identity, political ideas, and even daily habits. In Italy, where historical consciousness of the Second World War has been divisive, most people still perceive Fascism as a "stain" on the history of the nation and are aware that the Italian Republic was born out of civil war, which makes the legacy of the Second World War complex and emotionally entangled.

Thus, speaking about the Second World War engages the interviewees intellectually, ethically, and emotionally. Then, soon after the project started, I began to notice the interviews unexpectedly produced a state of well-being in the interviewees that became manifest both in verbal and non-verbal terms, viz. as the explicit statement of pleasure and satisfaction and the implicit physical display of relaxation. In my article, I will claim that the project's methodology based on the principle of dialogue produces well-being in the interviewees along with the aesthetic pleasure of performing the interview as a process aimed at restoring the enchantment of the world.

WELL-BEING RESULTING FROM THE EXPERIENCE OF SHARING MEMORIES AND FEELINGS

In Western philosophy, well-being is connected to moral philosophy, is opposed to the deontological conception of the categorical imperative of Kantian tradition and is a constituent part of eudemonism. In Greek philosophy, *eudemonia* means the condition of human flourishing or living well (Shiner & Jost, 2003) and, according to Plato's testimony, it means to have a good *daimon*, which in the case of Socrates "accompanies him till the end of his life-giving benefits on him and, through him, also on his interlocutors" (Stavru, 2021, p. 363)[3] and prevents him from doing the wrong thing. *Eudemonia* can be reached by leading a good and virtuous life characterised by the two maxims carved in the *pronaos* of the temple of Apollo at Delphi, "know yourself" (*γνῶθι σαυτόν*) and "nothing in excess" (*μηδὲν ἄγαν*).[4] Well-being is therefore connected to self-awareness and awareness of the world around us, to knowing how to well evaluate every situation, and finally, to the ideas of balance and proportionality, that is, living well without ever falling into excess or defect.

In the Italian language, well-being is literally translated with the word *benessere* (*bene* [well] and *essere* [being]) and has two meanings, one negative and one positive. In the corpus of over 180 interviews collected so far by the MemoGen project, the word *benessere* is mentioned in terms of wealth, which is positive, but also more than

57 times in terms of consumerism and the tendency to waste things and resources. Well-being, understood in the second way, is a degeneration of the original Greek meaning: such an interpretation of well-being as material and transitory satisfaction is often nuanced as the cause of environmental damage (global warming, pollution, etc.) (MEMO01, 02, 27, 68, 83, 87, 140, 141), loss of critical thought (MEMO15, 19, 38, 64, 65, 74, 88, 90, 97, 109, 117, 125), and overconsumption of industrial low-quality food (MEMO15, 104, 142, 149). One interviewee spoke of material well-being as a "bubble" and a "taming narcotic" (MEMO97).

Still, another type of well-being also emerges from the interviews more inherent to the original meaning of *eudemonia* as a state of happiness and psychophysical relaxedness. Since it is difficult, if not impossible, to exhaustively define the meaning of this type of well-being, I quote some of the interviewees' comments published on the project's website (*italics* added):[5]

1) The interview was a *pleasant experience* that took me back to a time I did not experience directly but made me understand or even strengthened the idea that we ought not to lose our historical memory (*M. M*);
2) My interview was a *pleasant surprise*. I did not know what to expect, nor did I know what questions I would be asked, but *I am glad* I remained open to the experience. *I immediately felt at ease* in what turned out to be *an enriching exchange that pleasantly permitted* me to focus on several aspects of my family and my own life, which I treasure (*I.C.*);
3) Taking part in the MemoGen project was one of the most *touching and engaging experiences* I ever had the *pleasure* to have (*V.P.*);
4) Talking about my late grandparents was like opening a box full of memories whose key I thought I had lost. I personally felt that it was *like family therapy* because the war and the post-war left a scar not only on the generation who lived those events but also on us. And seeing how those scars affected my life and choices was *a real revelation*. Thank you very much (*Giuli*);
5) The interview I recorded with Gianluca Cinelli unfolded as *a maieutic process* that facilitates sharing personal memories of the Second World War (*Saverio*);
6) Speaking with you about my family and their war memories *stirred many emotions* (*C.C.*);
7) A return, a connection, an introspection into the inheritance of my DNA... Thank you for reminding me that there are *emotions that resurface thanks to sharing "words"* (*M.C.*);
8) The interview was very interesting and *a compelling opportunity to revisit in-depth, almost like meditation*, tales and memories of the past. You also allowed me to reflect more thoroughly on aspects related to freedom and ethics that are mostly neglected in everyday life (*S*);

9) An *almost thaumaturgical experience*. There is *something miraculous*, nowadays, in having the possibility to talk about one's life and the memories that we carry with us. Thank you! (*L*).

These comments highlight the perception of the interview as "pleasant," "emotionally stirring," "profound," "unexpected," "mind-soothing," and even "therapeutic". Each interview includes a valedictory moment in the end, before the recording is interrupted or immediately afterwards, when the interviewees share their impressions on the experience:

I never imagined I would share these things with someone outside my family. I am happy about that because now these stories will be collected in an archive that speaks about us all, which is precious. (MEMO70)

It was a gift, thank you. (MEMO53)

I said things I didn't think I knew. (MEMO127)

It was a beautiful experience because things surfaced, and that made me glad. You asked questions that helped those things to come out. I think we should do that more often, to focus on our memories and permit them to grow. That would help us today face this time that is neither happy nor quiet. (MEMO145)

I am glad because we don't have many opportunities to talk about such things in our daily lives. I am very happy and sincerely satisfied ... the project is really good, for it permits us to reconnect with our past and find meaning. (MEMO130)

Look, if we ever meet I want you to know I will hug you in silence. And in that silence, I will make you feel all the good I felt tonight. Thank you, heartily. I have a lump in my throat. Believe me, I am feeling emotional. (MEMO44)

Notably, the pleasure of sharing private memories also depends on the cultural turn of the last decades that has urged people to seek in the private sphere of memory and experience those cultural roots and ethical values that traditional ideologies and political institutions no longer provide (Macioti, 1995, pp. 6–7). The encounter between private and public spheres is largely facilitated by the presence of intermediaries who involve the interviewee in the project. The intermediaries are often former interviewees, and their role is crucial to building a relationship of trust between the participants and the researchers.[6] Trust is established through the provision of legal guarantees regarding data protection, privacy, rights, and mutual obligations (basically based on the GDPR). Trust is then reinforced during the interview through a non-judgmental approach of the interviewers, who interact dialogically, sometimes sharing their own personal views and memories, enhancing mutual understanding. Furthermore, the first contact with new interviewees occurs via email or WhatsApp, generally followed by an informal phone call, during which the researchers explain the method and purposes of the project and illustrate how the interview unfolds, thus laying the groundwork for dialogue.

In summary, the interview is built on trust and reciprocal acceptance, which is a contributing factor to triggering a feeling of relaxation and confidence. Therefore, the interview is often perceived as a pleasant and surprising experience, an enriching exchange, a revelation, a maieutic process, or even like some sort of meditation or therapy.[7] On the whole, the comments speak for an experience that stirs emotions and feelings of happiness, satisfaction, amity, and compassion. In the next paragraph, I would like to explore how pleasure connects to the aesthetic pleasure of surprise and active participation in the creation of a performance.

WELL-BEING AND PERFORMANCE: THE RE-ENCHANTMENT OF THE WORLD

What is the connection between well-being, oral sources and performance? According to Walter Ong, oral history produces performances, not written texts (1982), and that also applies to video interviews. A written text profoundly differs from oral dialogue: Italian oral historian Sandro Portelli writes that

the difference between written and oral sources is that the former are mostly documents, the latter are always acts; they should not be conceived in terms of substantives and things but of verbs and processes; not memoires and tales, but remembering and storytelling.[8] (Portelli, 1999, p. 15)

The act of storytelling, Portelli goes on,

depends on the existence of someone who listens. One of the things that makes oral sources different is precisely that they are the result of a joint effort between the narrators and the researcher, who goes looking for narrators, listens to them, and questions them.[9] (p. 16)

The video interview is therefore not mere communication, but the establishment of a relationship on a "common ground" that "does not necessarily … consist of a common identity (of class, gender, ideology...) but can be delimited, or better must be delimited mainly by the willingness to listen to each other, and to accept each other" (Portelli, 2014, p. 2).[10]

The witnesses' well-being partially derives from playing an active role in this performance and can be described as a declination of Erika Fischer-Lichte's notion of "re-enchantment of the world". Fischer-Lichte uses this expression to define a new aesthetic conception of performance in the theatrical field, in which the fourth wall disappears in favour of a free and bi-directional exchange of experience between actors and audience. In the case of video interviews, the free exchange of experience does not occur between the witnesses and the audience because the latter are absent. Instead, the free exchange of experience occurs between the witnesses and the interviewer. However, even if the audience are absent, all the witnesses act as if *someone else* was listening and watching: they are aware of the public dimension of their verbal and non-verbal acts. Some address directly the future watchers: for example, the interviewees of MEMO94 and 107 apologize for having used bad words; in MEMO24, 99, and 144, the interviewees ask for permission to smoke even though they are at home, connected on Zoom; in MEMO68 the interviewee greets the audience at the beginning of the recording. As for that, in the video interviews recorded in person (not on Zoom), it is noticeable how every interviewee thanks and says goodbye staring at the camera rather than at the interviewer, who is sitting next to them in the same room.[11]

The interviews unfold not by adhering to an inflexible format: they are designed, by contrast, to develop according to an open pattern. The interviewer leads the conversation, acting as a director/actor who guides the interviewee as a narrator/actor towards the realization of an aesthetic experience of pleasure, discovery, well-being and enrichment, both cultural and human: in other words, to experiencing the re-enchantment of the world. What does this expression mean? Re-enchantment implies that any phenomenon we previously looked at in amazement has become something trivial that no longer arouses interest and curiosity, and towards which we therefore experience a feeling of disenchantment. The term was first used by Max Weber[12] in the 1917 conference *Science as Vocation* (*Wissenschaft als Beruf*), where he identifies the cause of the *Entzauberung der Welt* [disenchantment of the world] through the technicalisation of knowledge: in short, for Weber, "the disenchantment of the world lay right at the heart of Modernity" (Jenkins, 2000, p. 12). Disenchantment is the result of the process of secularization and rationalization of existence in all its spheres, which causes every mysterious and wonderful aspect to be eliminated by the faith in objective knowledge, founded on logical principles (such as cause and effect and the *tertium non datur*); Weber writes that the disenchantment of the world "means first and foremost that our relationship to the world is reduced to causality. But … causality is a mechanical and external relation. Magical and poetic relationships to the world rest on a deep *sympathy* that connects humans and things" (Han, 2024, p. x).

Therefore, placing one's trust in the idea of being able to logically and technically dominate all aspects of reality through reason and logical thought and provide an exhaustive explanation of all physical phenomena, means ruling out the possibility that something imponderable and mysterious may exist or happen:

> *Thus the growing process of intellectualization and rationalization does not imply a growing understanding of the conditions under which we live. It means something quite different. It is the knowledge or conviction that if only we wished to understand them we could do so at any time. It means in principle, then, we are ruled by mysterious, unpredictable forces, but that, on the contrary, we can in principle control everything by means of calculation. This in turn means the*

disenchantment of the world … let us consider this process of disenchantment that has been at work in Western culture for thousands of years and, in general, let us consider "progress," to which science belongs both as an integral part and a driving force. Can we say that it has any meaning over and above its practical and technical implications? … how should we respond to this? Does "progress" as such possess a recognizable meaning that goes beyond the technical so that devotion to progress can become a meaningful vocation? (Weber, 2004, p. 13)

The disenchantment of the world begins with the belief that the world can be known and modelled rationally in an exhaustive way but also with the belief that the existing cannot be other than what it is: we are disenchanted with reality, with the hope that we can change erroneous social habits, as well as nefarious visions of the world that seem to repeat themselves over and over. The disenchantment of the world is counterbalanced by every experience that reactivates the enchantment, that is, every experience that reaches beyond schemata and habituation, both practical and linguistic, that leads us to act and think always in the same way. Consequently, we are enchanted again when we manage to see beyond what has already been determined, when we experience something new or when we succeed in gaining new knowledge not in a logical way but in a connective way, that is, by seeing new connections amongst things, which leads us to feel dormant emotions. The re-enchantment of the world is thus an experience that involves the mind, the body and the emotions: it is therefore, in short, an aesthetic experience.

In philosophy, the expression "aesthetic experience" can mean different things. A declination of aesthetic experience that aptly describes what happens during the video interview is given by John Dewey in his *Art as Experience*. For Dewey, the aesthetic experience not only concerns art but is broader and concerns the relationship between the human being and the environment in which he lives: he writes that the aesthetic experience "is also something exceptional … for it forms, within the general experiential flow of human life, a particularly heightened and complex experiential condensation" (Puolakka, 2014, p. 4). Dewey distinguishes between ordinary experiences and aesthetic experiences and defines the latter as a subset of experience *toutcourt*. Many daily experiences can be aesthetic, not only the enjoyment of a work of art. Dewey provides no exhaustive definition of the aesthetic experience, but he defines its fundamental traits. First, he states that human beings constantly make experiences as they live in connection with their environment. However, these experiences are often "inchoated" because, rather than focusing on the experience, we are distracted by many factors so that "we start and then we stop, not because the experience has reached the end for the sake of which it was initiated but because of extraneous interruptions or of inner lethargy" (Dewey, 1980, p. 35). Thus, mere experience is often characterized by a lack of attention and superficiality and is mainly limited to the thing experienced here and now. In that case, we also see only given phenomena, but not the connections between them and other ones: for this reason, such an experience is just like a determined point in the Cartesian space-time system, as it were. Dewey defines such experiences as anaesthetic, which have "beginnings and cessations, but no genuine initiations and concluding. One thing replaces another, but does not absorb it and carry it on" (p. 40). This experience has not a particular beginning, a coherent development and a significant end since this experience ceases with an "arrest, constriction, proceeding from parts having only a mechanical connection with one another" (p. 40). Its opposite is the aesthetic experience, which is "vital" and has a completion and an evolution in time during which all its elements relate to each other and evolve together:

In such experiences, every successive part flows freely, without seam and without unfilled banks, into what ensues ... because of continuous merging, there are no holes, mechanical junctions, and dead centers when we have an experience. There are pauses, places of rest, but they punctuate and define the quality of movement. They sum up what has been undergone and prevent its dissipation and idle evaporation. (p. 36)

Aesthetic experiences, being concluded, orderly move towards a direction so that their conclusions are never random but the fruit of a fertile path. In short, the aesthetic experience for Dewey has a beginning that can be triggered by different phenomena, including the start of a dialogue; it then has a duration and evolves through integrated phases until it reaches its conclusion, which is ultimately what makes the experience a significant unit: "When these different parts form a distinctive kind of orderly developing unity that stands out from the general experiential stream of our lives, the experience in question is aesthetic" (Leddy & Puolakka, 2023). A fundamental element that constitutes the aesthetic experience is emotion. Dewey underlines that emotions are not autonomous elements concerning the experience. It is the experience itself that is emotional: emotion is therefore "the moving and cementing force" (Dewey, 1980, p. 42) that makes the aesthetic experience particularly significant. In the case of a conversation, emotionality is present when the dialogue does not occur mechanically. Dewey gives the example of two people with different positions who meet and writes:

The interview may be mechanical, consisting of set questions, the replies to which perfunctorily settle the matter. There is no experience in which the two men meet, nothing that is not a repetition, by way of acceptance or dismissal, of something which has happened a score of times. The situation is disposed of as if it were an exercise in bookkeeping. But an interplay may take place in which a new experience develops. (p. 43)

Following Dewey's example, we can say that an interview is an aesthetic, ergo emotional, experience when it unfolds in a non-mechanical way, that is, when the questions and answers are not parts of a pre-established conversational pattern (for example, a questionnaire), but when are connected in a continuous harmonic flow which, starting from a point, ends in a synthesis or a significant reflection.[13] This flow forms what we call a dialogue, during which reflection and rational evaluation are accompanied by an emotional state that varies in intensity depending on the context.

Such a process of re-enchantment of the world occurs during the interviews in the form of storytelling and dialogue, which together constitute the performance and inspire feelings of satisfaction, accomplishment, and relief. The interview can be described as an aesthetic experience because it begins with amazement, unfolds by blending storytelling, critical thinking and dialogue, and ends with the attainment of closure and catharsis.

AMAZEMENT

Amazement is produced by the fact that the interviewees, not knowing in advance how the video interview will unfold, are amazed at having an unexpected experience of dialogue, sharing critical introspection, which is rare in daily-life communication (MEMO26, 66, 115, 70). Some interviewees admitted that the interview led them to reflect for the first time on aspects of their lives to which they never gave any thought before (MEMO60, 86, 89, 98), while others were happy to remember and honour their ancestors in the context of public discourse (MEMO02, 53, 72, 85, 90, 91, 99, 146). This exploration of private memories conducts many interviewees to rediscover and reassess things they remember of their families in a new light from a fresh perspective, especially those connected with powerful emotions such as, for example, visiting the Nazi extermination camps (MEMO24, 47, 49, 72). Notably, a remarkable number of interviewees react to the interviewers' questions by saying "I had never thought about that…" or "now that you make me think of that…," thus signalling that memories re-emerge in response to the stimuli of the dialogue. Finally, it happens sometimes that such a sudden return of memories and related emotions move the interviewees to tears (MEMO32, 34, 44, 56, 101, 113, 128, 144, 146, 148, 152).

STORYTELLING, CRITICAL THINKING AND PERFORMATIVITY

The trust established between the witnesses and the interviewer makes the interviewees take the interview very seriously: many anticipate the event by doing research, asking questions among their parents and relatives, and searching for any written sources (postcards, letters and diaries) their grandparents left. The awareness of the public dimension of the interview contributes to perceiving it as a sort of performance based on oral storytelling. First of all, a stage is set for the interview, which is generally a quiet and familiar space at home or in an office, where the interviewee takes place comfortably seated, allowing oneself to smoke or sip from a beverage, and leaving out stressful interactions with telephones and other external sources of distraction. At times the background is blurred, but in most of the cases the interviewees include the background of their domestic space in the interview, which contributes to creating an atmosphere of intimacy and relaxation. Throughout the interview, both the interviewer and interviewees stay focused on the dialogue, without distractions, and keep high levels of concentration. However, the tension is occasionally diffused by a joke or wit, or by interventions of the interviewer who reports personal episodes comparable with those the witnesses talk about, thus sharing experiences.

Invited to speak about their grandparents' war experiences, the interviewees dive into their memories and start recounting without being bound to any given pattern, be it chronological or thematic. They may unfold articulate biographical sketches, as well as they may prefer to browse memories randomly, moving forward and backward along the timeline of events. They often justify that approach by explaining that they ignore the precise temporal setting of the mentioned anecdotes, nor do they possess the contextual details of the stories (for example, concerning their grandfathers' military career, place and time of deployment, the identity of other military units mentioned). From storytelling emerges that most of the interviewees draw pleasure from mentioning places, people, and events involved in their stories locally, viz. in the environment of their family. By contrast, they do not seem to pay too much attention to broader historical events and contexts such as, for example, military campaigns. That is partially due to the fact that the grandparents did not expound on these aspects in the first place; and partially to the focalisation of the interview on an individual, i.e. microhistorical and anecdotal perspective. After all, the dialogue is not aimed at determining the truth of singular facts or opinions, because what lingers in the memory of the interviewees is often impressions and emotions that permitted them to "grasp the human (and inhuman) side of the war in a more universal way" (Portelli, 1999, pp. 375–376), reaching far beyond the historical information learned at school or absorbed as adults in the course of their lives. As Paul Ricoeur observed, when one looks a reality by changing the scale, one stops seeing the same things differently and begins noting different things (2000, p. 270).

Since the interview's starting point consists of recounting someone else's story, the core of the storytelling is not fully autobiographical but hybrid: along as the autobiographical "I" unfolds the narration, other characters emerge as the protagonists of tales, who are the real owners of the war experiences. This structure coincides with Dewey's definition of the aesthetic experience and with Aristotle's well-known description of *mythos* [story] as a discourse that begins, unfolds, and reaches its conclusions.[14] The attainment of such a goal is a source of pleasure for many an interviewee, and I will quote two examples starting with a man from the city of Civitavecchia (60 km north of Rome), which the Americans bombed for the first time on 14 May 1943:

My father always told me this beautiful story. Until the day of the bombing, my grandfather was employed at the port, a job he was proud of. In a few minutes, his life was turned upside down ... they quickly fled to Vetralla [near Viterbo] with nothing. But the story is beautiful because to make ends meet, my grandfather rode his bicycle every day from Vetralla to the port of Civitavecchia, a very tiring journey to get the salt that he resold in the village, something that my father always told me with emotion ... this story has always fascinated me. It taught me a precious lesson. He got back on his feet despite having lost everything in an instant ... it was also a tragedy because, in that same bombing, my father lost an eye. He was only seven ... I liked this idea of transforming a tragedy into an opportunity. Even today, when something bad happens, I try to see something positive. (MEMO70)[15]

The second example was narrated by a man from Tuscany, whose great-uncle was murdered by the Germans on the Greek island of Rhodes:

One source was my grandmother Armida, also because the war deeply affected her family. She had a photo on her bedside table. I remember it well, for it had always struck me. It portrayed her younger brother Bruno, shot by the Germans on the Greek island of Rhodes in February 1945. It was a traumatic experience for her ... her brother had not ended up in Rhodes by chance, and not even during the war. Someone had sent him there, and this is the story: I come from a poor peasant family, and Uncle Bruno had fallen in love with the daughter of the local fascist boss. As soon as this thing reached his ears, he immediately rushed to my grandmother's house saying, "this story must end here". But not content, when Bruno was drafted, he had him sent as far away as possible, to Rhodes. ... It was 1939 and he never returned ... in 1946, my grandmother met someone who was with Bruno in Rhodes and learned that her brother had been shot ... She told me then: "The pain was so strong that I felt like I was being lifted into the air and cast to the ground." I made myself an idea of the impact.

The interviewee then recalled that during a trip to Rhodes in the early 2000s, he looked for the cemetery where his uncle was buried:

The night before leaving, I was in a tavern whose owner spoke good Italian. I told him my uncle's story and asked about the cemetery, and he said: "Yes, I know it, but it's not a real cemetery. It's a place behind the old city where the Germans used to shoot the Greeks and the Italians." ... The next day I bought some flowers and went there. I found a small monument. I still remember the gale, and as I put the flowers down, the wind would blow them away. I came back to Italy quite happy with my discovery." (MEMO135)

These examples show how the experiences handed down within the family have transmitted to the children and grandchildren the pleasure of storytelling as a form of reconnection with the "mythical" roots of the family. Moreover, the oral nature of storytelling includes a physical component of non-verbal language and imitation of idioms (often in dialect), gestures and voices of grandparents or other people (MEMO 15, 64, 82, 93, 101, and 102). Finally, the interviewees interact with the interviewer who steers the conversation, playing both the roles of actor and director in the performance. This aspect is fundamental because it permits the interviewees to reach beyond the boundaries of mere storytelling and move to the higher ground of meta-narration, that is, critical thinking. Questions like "what did it feel like, listening to the stories?", "can you remember what emotions your grandparents' displayed while telling their stories?", "have you ever crosschecked the anecdotes for historical consistency?", or "did the storytelling occur randomly or on special occasions?" divert the interviewees' attention from storytelling to its multifaceted and temporally layered contexts.

This process of blending storytelling with critical thinking imprints the performance as an open-ended dialogue, for the interviewee cannot know in advance what questions will be asked, while the interviewer cannot foresee what stories is bound to listen to. This question-and-answer structure stimulates the interviewees to scan their memories in search for novel meanings or different interpretations, and to reassess previous points of view, especially when they are asked about the value their grandparents' stories have today in their lives. Starting mainly by saying "that's a good question" they ask themselves—often for the first time—about the legacy of the Second World War in their families, interviewees realise that it is a remarkable heritage of ethical teachings, habits, values, and examples:

I must say that although these events remained in the background, they have always aroused great emotion ... perhaps it was the first time I heard about the imprisonment of human beings or the fact that people could somehow lock up other people in fences or houses—I imagined these places to be very uncomfortable—just because they didn't share their thoughts and beliefs. My attention to the dynamics of marginalization stemmed from there since I was a boy. (MEMO33)

I certainly learned to help others in hardship, not as a dogma but as an almost natural urge, and not to gain visibility. So I still feel this sense of community, maybe because I live in a small village or maybe—I am just thinking out loud ... although I didn't talk much with my grandparents or uncles, I have learned something from the stories I heard as a child. (MEMO141)

I am grateful to my grandfather. I am lucky to have received such first-hand accounts that influenced my way of thinking. Those things he told me still have an influence on me today. (MEMO85)

I believe they taught me to reject war and verbal violence, too. That is something I cannot stand. (MEMO74)

The pleasure of performing is therefore enhanced by the experience of dialogue, which connects the tales of the past to present storytelling through an experience of sharing and meaning-building.

THE PLEASURE OF DIALOGUE: MAIEUTICS, THERAPY AND INTROSPECTION

Now, I would like to analyse the dialogue as a source of well-being in video interviews, which from Hans-Georg Gadamer's perspective is based on listening on context and the willingness to change one's prejudiced perspectives through the encounter with others and their unexpected answers (2006, pp. 352–361). The dialogue established in the video interviews is similar to the Socratic dialogue because it allows the interviewer and the interviewee to pave the way towards introspection and a shared reflection on history, society, family bonds, and nature.

The Socratic dialogue, like the interviews, is based on the interaction between the two interlocutors through questions and answers, and is opposed to the technique of making long speeches that characterizes sophistic arguments. This latter type of argumentation is aimed at persuading an audience, like in propaganda speeches (Garth & O'Donnell, 2015), while Socratic dialogue can "establish an adequate plan of interaction, … control the effects of the speech, … calibrate the communication methods from time to time, … verify mutual understanding" (Ferrari, 2007, p. 31). Like in the Socratic dialogue, the interviewee and the interviewer reach a mutual understanding and a point of agreement, which in Socratic dialogue is called *homologia*: this is a very important point because "the *homologia* reached between Socrates and his interlocutors is not yet an episteme" (Ferber, 2007, p. 266), i.e. scientific knowledge. Therefore, knowledge attained through dialogue is not definitive and irrefutable objectivity, but a good steppingstone on which to place one's foot to continue the research journey.

Another point that the interviews and the Socratic dialogue have in common is the maieutics. The interviewer is directly involved in the investigation and research process, and not only learns new historical facts but receives new stimuli, which permits him or her to see new connections, from which further questions and reflections derive. This virtuous process offers the interviewee the possibility to reflect on topics from a different perspective, to question beliefs and find new answers.

This methodology is very close to Socratic maieutics. This concept comes from the Greek *μαιευτική* [midwife] (*τέχνη* [art] and *μαῖα* [mother]), and as we read in Plato's *Theaetetus*, the word is used by Socrates to explain that he does not proceed from pre-established truths like a sophist, but acts like a midwife, helping others to "give birth" to their truth: through dialogue, Socrates urges his interlocutors to search for their own truths in the most autonomous way possible. For Socrates, the method of the true philosopher (not the sophist) is not to hand down his knowledge as if it were some liquid to pour from one vessel into another: the philosopher's ability is to allow knowledge to bloom in the interlocutor's mind through dialogue at different interconnected levels, such as "learning about one's own assumptions through critically examining and interrogating them with another; learning about a particular topic through definition and induction; and learning about the process of creating knowledge through participating in the dialogue" (Rule, 2015, p. 8). The description that Socrates gives of this method is not logical-rational but analogical-metaphorical and can be found in the *Theaetetus*:

> *All that is true of their art of midwifery is true also of mine, but mine differs from theirs in being practised upon men, not women, and in tending their souls in labour, not their bodies. But the greatest thing about my art is this, that it can test in every way whether the mind of the young man is bringing forth a mere image, an imposture, or a real and genuine offspring. … I am, then, not at all a wise person myself, nor have I any wise invention, the offspring born of my own soul; but those who associate with me, although at first some of them seem very ignorant, yet, as our acquaintance advances, all of them to whom the god is gracious make wonderful progress, not only in their own opinion, but in that of others as well. And it is clear that they do this, not because they have ever learned anything from me, but because they have found in themselves many fair things and have brought them forth. (Plato, 1921, 150b–d)*

There are also some differences between the Socratic maieutics and that of the MemoGen project. First of all, the interviews are not tailored to a specific group (while in Greek culture at Socrates' time, education mainly addressed men): every Italian-born person aged between 40 and 60 is welcome to join as an interviewee regardless of gender, level of education, geographical origin or social level. Furthermore, methodologically speaking, Socrates seeks out people who claim to be expert in a certain field because he wants to learn from them, until he finds out that they are actually ignorant and that their statements are contradictory and false. Socrates, therefore, ironically places himself below his interlocutor by claiming he is aware of his own ignorance, but in the end, he unquestionably demonstrates that he is actually the wiser man (Vlastos, 1991). Instead, the interviewer and the interviewee of the MemoGen project meet each other on the same level. This creates a relationship of trust that puts the two interlocutors at ease. The questioning is not aimed at refuting others' opinions but evaluating them from the dialogic perspective of collaboration, so as to arrive at producing non-obvious reflections on the historical reality we dwell. Thus, the dialogue reactivates memories with a strong emotional imprinting. That is the glue that permits one to absorb the content of the stories as ethical teachings. Such teachings concern solidarity, sharing, courage, dignity, the feeling of gratitude, the value of frugality and recycling, as well as emancipation, the sense of justice, generosity, fraternity, the value of choice and respect. That is why the objective account of what happened is not the most important goal: the facts narrated may be imprecise, inexact or blurry but this is not necessarily a drawback because, as Portelli says,

> *The lack of memory involves a loss of meaning and knowledge, but also opens up spaces for imagination and re-elaboration. To the extent that they are less informed, [the interviewees] are sometimes induced to try and reconstruct interpretation and meaning by themselves, starting with the little data available.*[16] *(1999, p. 373)*

What is important in the performative dialogue is the act of remembering childhood, sharing memories, critically evaluating opinions, and finally, the teachings learned from the elders and the pleasure of seeing that those teachings and memories can be an important perspective from which to look at reality.

CLOSURE AND CATHARSIS

Grandparents' stories and examples planted seeds in their descendants' minds that later mature through experience, eventually growing to fundamental factors in the formation of the younger generations' ethical conscience and self-knowledge. This purpose was expressed in the Greek world through the phrase *gnōthi seauton* (*γνῶθι σεαυτόν*), translated in English as "know thyself".[17] Self-knowledge in the Greek world was thought of as the *telos* [purpose] of the human being, meaning that everyone should first of all devote one's life to self-understanding. Such an endeavour was connected to the *epimèleia heautoù* (*ἐπιμέλεια ἑαυτου*), translated in English as "self-care," consisting of a series of practices, techniques, and spiritual and physical exercises to perform at different times of the day (Foucault, 1984; Hadot, 1987).[18] The Greeks considered this aim so important that they engraved it above the gate of Apollo's temple in Delphi: to lead a good life, human beings ought to constantly question themselves throughout their lives about who they are, and understand their inclinations, desires and passions in such a way as to develop virtues and keep vices under control. Such self-knowledge reaches beyond the apprehension of superficial evidence about oneself and gives access to a more thorough understanding of what one does and why.

By revisiting one's family roots and reconfiguring memories in a new context, the dialogue functions during the interview as a kind of exercise that helps the interviewees to refocus on themselves, their lives and habits, their views of the world and social interactions in a non-judgemental way. Most of the time, the interviewees show compassion for their grandparents and express profound gratitude for their surviving the war, permitting their families to thrive (MEMO02, 53, 129). In some cases, such reconnection also includes healing and reconciliation (MEMO50, 83, 84), or the pleasure of transmitting the family heritage to the following generations (MEMO39, 50, 128, 142, 148, 152).

In the case of one interviewee from Genoa, whose paternal grand-uncle fought as a partisan and was murdered in 1944, the interview interprets an event that profoundly imprinted her family:

That certainly created trauma in the family. For example, he was shot on Easter Sunday, so Easter was not celebrated in my father's family. My father never received an Easter egg. That may seem no big deal, but for a child, it was ... I remember him saying our surname weighed as a burden, though I didn't understand why ... nonetheless, I received their stories with pride. I felt the strength of these people who stood up following their ethics and were not crushed ... all that accompanied me into my adulthood. (MEMO88)

During the interview, she explained how she attempted to build the "energetic genealogical tree" of her family to understand how that event had affected her family for decades:

From the point of view of the family tree, I can feel this depth: what my ancestor did not resolve, I might have taken on. So, those who work on their family tree can attain liberation on a personal level, freeing their families from ties, too. It is a mutual liberation that brings lightness where there is none. (MEMO88)

Eventually, the interviewees experience catharsis, when the last words are spent talking about their feelings and impressions. All the interviewees are thankful for having been involved in the project and say, smiling, they are happy to have had this experience.

CONCLUSION

The methodology used for the interviews of the MemoGen project allows for the development of a dialogue that produces well-being both on an emotional and intellectual level in the interviewees, as well as in the interviewers, at multiple levels: the first concerns the enthusiasm of being involved in scientific research as active actors. The second consists of revisiting an emotionally engaging past within the framework of a dialogue based on trust and listening. The third depends on the aesthetic nature of the interview, which activates the re-enchantment of the world as the past is revived in the present conversation. The fourth factor contributing to producing well-being is the fact that the maieutic dialogue helps the interviewees to focus on the present moment.

The kind of pleasure produced by the interview can be compared with that in Eastern forms of meditation based on "practice without practicing" (Watts, 1989, p. 108) or "doing by not doing" (Suzuki, 1993, p. 111). The interviewees and the interviewer unfold their conversation in a state of full immersion, leaving the dialogue flow. Staying so focused on the play, they perform the interview as an event using their bodies (voice, facial expressions, emotions, posture, and gestures) as well as their minds to produce an "oral text," that is, a discourse in which the non-verbal component contributes to the process of meaning-building. As Mihaly Csikszentmihalyi states in his 1990 book *Flow*, complete immersion in an experience permits one to enjoy it profoundly and optimally, even though that may require great cost in terms of time and effort. Such an experience of "flow" described "as the pleasure, delight, creativity, and process when we are completely immersed in life" (García & Miralles, 2017, p. 40) is also enacted during the interview as an aesthetic experience.

In an "enchanted world," people perceive themselves in relation to the whole and not detached from others: their understanding of the world does not consist in the egotistic attempt to subjugate it to reason and logic, but rather in the pursuit of a broaden insight into reality as a dynamic and layered network of experiences. As Csikszentmihalyi reminds us,

> *Having a record of the past can make a great contribution to the quality of life. It frees us from the tyranny of the present, and makes it possible for consciousness to revisit former times. It makes it possible to select and preserve in memory events that are especially pleasant and meaningful, and so to "create" a past that will help us deal with the future. Of course such a past might not be literally true. But then the past can never be literally true in memory: it must be continuously edited, and the question is only whether we take creative control of the editing or not (1990, p. 133)*

The maieutic dialogue does not aim to assess the validity of the interviewees' statements about past events: by contrast, it invites the interviewees to tell the story of their ancestors and families during the war by participating in that legacy as an active part of its memory through time.

REFERENCES

Allen, M., & Sakamoto, R. (2013). War and peace: War memories and museums in Japan. *History Compass*, *11*(12), 1047–1058.

Aristotle. (1932). *Poetics*. In *Aristotle in 23 volumes* (Vol. 23). Harvard University Press. http://data.perseus.org/texts/urn:cts:greekLit:tlg0086.tlg034.perseus-eng1

Csikszentmihalyi, M. (1990). *Flow: The psychology of optimal experience*. HarperCollins.

Dewey, J. (1980). *Art as experience*. Perigee Books.

Ferber, R. (2007). What did Socrates know and how did he know it? In L. Brisson & M. Erler (Eds.), *Gorgias, Meno: Selected papers from the Seventh Symposium Platonicum* (pp. 263–267). Academia Verlag.

Ferrari, F. (2007). Socrate e la filosofia. In Ferrari, F. (Ed.), *Socrate tra personaggio e mito* (pp. 11–86). Rizzoli.

Fischer-Lichte, E. (2008). *The transformative power of performance: A new aesthetics*. Routledge.

Fossion, P., Rejas, M. C., Servais, L., Pelc, I., & Hirsch, S. (2014). Transgenerational transmission of trauma in families of Holocaust survivors. *Journal of Affective Disorders*, *171*, 48–53. PMID: 25285898

Foucault, M. (1984). *Le souci de soi*. Gallimard.

Gadamer, H.-G. (2006). *Truth and method*. Continuum.

García, H., & Miralles, F. (2017). *Ikigai: The Japanese secret to a long and happy life*. Penguin.

Garth, S. J., & O'Donnell, V. (2015). *Propaganda and persuasion*. SAGE Publications.

Gorelick, K. (1987). Greek tragedy and ancient healing. *Journal of Poetry Therapy*, *1*(1), 38–43.

Gottschall, J. (2012). *The storytelling animal: How stories make us human*. Houghton Mifflin Harcourt.

Gribaudi, G. (2005). *Guerra totale. Tra bombe alleate e violenze naziste. Napoli e il fronte meridionale 1940-1944*. Bollati Boringhieri.

Hadot, P. (1987). *Spiritual exercises and ancient philosophy*. Études Augustiniennes.

Han, B-C. (2024, March 20). The disenchantment of the world. *The Paris Review*. https://www.theparisreview.org/blog/2024/03/20/the-disenchantment-of-the-world/

Hashimoto, A. (2015). *The long defeat: Cultural trauma, memory, and identity in Japan*. Oxford University Press.

Heraclitus, . (1987). *Fragments*. University of Toronto Press.

Hirsch, M. (1997). *Family frames: Photography, narrative, and postmemory*. Harvard University Press.

Hirsch, M. (2012). *The generation of postmemory: Writing and visual culture after the Holocaust*. Columbia University Press.

Ingemark, C. A. (Ed.). (2013). *Therapeutic uses of storytelling: An interdisciplinary approach*. Nordic Academic Press.

Jenkins, R. (2000). Disenchantment, enchantment and re-enchantment. *Max Weber Studies*, *1*(1), 11–32.

Kundnani, H. (2011). Perpetrators and victims. *German Life and Letters*, *64*(2), 272–282.

LaCapra, D. (1994). *Representing the Holocaust: History, theory, trauma*. Cornell University Press.

Leddy, T., & Puolakka, K. (2023). Dewey's aesthetics. In Zalta, E. N., & Nodelman, U. (Eds.), *The Stanford Encyclopedia of Philosophy* (Winter 2023 ed.). https://plato.stanford.edu/archives/win2023/entries/dewey-aesthetics/

Macioti, M. (1995). *Oralità e vissuto. L'uso delle storie di vita nelle scienze sociali* (2nd ed.). Liguori.

Marcus Aurelius. (1906). *Meditations*. Dent.

Napolitano Valditara, L. (2003). Alle origini del "gnōthi sautòn". Da Delfi al sapere socratico di non sapere. *Esercizi Filosofici*, *2*, 110–125.

Ong, W. J. (1982). *Orality and literacy: The technologizing of the word*. Routledge.

Plato. (1921). *Theaetetus*. In *Plato in twelve volumes* (Vol. 12). Harvard University Press. https://www.perseus.tufts.edu/hopper/text?doc=Perseus%3Atext%3A1999.01.0172

Plato. (1955). *Alcibiades I*. In *Plato in twelve volumes* (Vol. 8). Harvard University Press.

Plato. (1967a). *Meno*. In *Plato in twelve volumes* (Vol. 3). Harvard University Press.

Plato. (1967b). *Protagoras*. In *Plato in twelve volumes* (Vol. 3). Harvard University Press.

Portelli, A. (2014). Un lavoro di relazione. Osservazioni sulla storia orale. https://www.aisoitalia.org/wp-content/uploads/2014/04/Alessandro-Portelli-Storia-orale-un-lavoro-di-relazione.pdf

Portelli, A. (2019). *L'ordine è già stato eseguito. Roma, le Fosse Ardeatine, la memoria*. Donzelli.

Puolakka, K. (2014). Dewey and everyday aesthetics. *Contemporary Aesthetics*, *12*, 1–15.

Revelli, N. (1966). *La strada del davai*. Einaudi.

Revelli, N. (1977). *Il mondo dei vinti. Storie di vita contadina* (Vol. 1–2). Einaudi.

Ricoeur, P. (2000). *La mémoire, l'histoire, l'oubli*. Seuil.

Rojcewicz, S. (2004). Poetry therapy in ancient Greek literature. *Journal of Poetry Therapy*, *17*(4), 209–213.

Rule, P. (2015). *Dialogue and boundary learning*. Sense Publishers.

Saito, H. (2017). *The history problem*. University of Hawai'i Press.

Shiner, R. A., & Jost, L. (2003). *Eudaimonia and well-being*. Academic Printing and Publishing.

Slivinske, J., & Slivinske, L. (2013). *Therapeutic storytelling for adolescents and young adults*. Oxford University Press.

Stavru, A. (2021). Eudaimonia e protrettica socratica in Platone, Senofonte ed Eschine: Rendere migliori gli altri per essere felici? *Thaumàzein, 9*(1), 363–367. https://rivista.thaumazein.it/index.php/thaum/article/view/170

Suzuki, D. T. (1993). *Zen and Japanese culture*. Charles E. Tuttle. (Original work published 1959)

Thompson, P. (1984). Historians and oral history. In Puissant, J. (Ed.), *Collective memories* (pp. 281–295). Éditions de l'Université de Bruxelles.

Tsutsui, K. (2009). The trajectory of perpetrators' trauma. *Social Forces*, *87*(3), 1389–1422.

van Alphen, E. (1997). *Caught by history*. Stanford University Press.

Vlastos, G. (1991). *Socrates: Ironist and moral philosopher*. Cornell University Press.

Watts, A. (1989). *The way of Zen*. Vintage Books. (Original work published 1957)

Weber, M. (2004). Science as a vocation. In Owen, D., & Strong, T. (Eds.), *The vocation lectures* (pp. 1–33). Hackett.

Wilkins, E. G. (1927). ΕΓΓΥΑ, ΠΑΡΑ ΔΑΤΗ. *Classical Philology*, *22*(2), 121–135.

Young, J. E. (2000). *At memory's edge*. Yale University Press.

ENDNOTES

1 The MemoGen Project, founded in 2024 by Patrizia Piredda and Gianluca Cinelli, is implemented in collaboration with the Archivio Ligure della Scrittura Popolare (University of Genoa) and the Centro Studi "Sereno Regis" (Turin), with the support of "La Mola ltd" and "Bylogix ltd". To learn more, see the project website at www.memogenenglish.wordpress.com.

2 One question to ask about the MemoGen project's methodology is whether and how it aligns with other studies that collect oral histories of the Second World War. Many of these research projects focus on memory and representation of the Holocaust, including texts like LaCapra (1994), van Alphen (1997), Hirsch (1997), and Young (2000). Apel's study, *Memory Effects: The Holocaust and the Art of Secondary Witnessing*, is among these. Like MemoGen, Apel's project involves artists who could not directly witness the Holocaust, having not experienced it. Instead, they analyze the effects of the memory of the event, along with existing material traces, seeing what implications they have for the present. However, in my opinion, these studies, including Apel's, cannot be applied to the MemoGen project because while the latter concerns the study of second-generation art and artists, MemoGen concerns the third generation, i.e. a group that has a completely different relationship with the stories of those who fought in the war. Moreover, the MemoGen project does not address artists specifically. The focus shifts from the father-son (second generation) to the grandfather-grandson relationship, and none of the interviewees has intergenerational trauma, not even in the cases in which the interviewees are Jewish and have relatives who were persecuted and died in concentration camps. The MemoGen interviewees generally report a peaceful relationship with the past. At any rate, that relationship is not traumatic, even in the cases where grandparents suffered war trauma, which has not affected the third generation.

3 “Che lo accompagna per tutta la vita fino in punto di morte, elargendo benefici a lui e, per suo tramite, anche ai suoi interlocutori.”

4 The third maxim of wisdom is “Certainty brings ruins” (Wilkins, 1927 p. 121).

5 https://memogenenglish.wordpress.com/the-interviewees-said/. The Italian original version can be found here: https://memogen3.wordpress.com/dicono-i-testimoni/.

6 Equality between interviewees and interviewers is assumed. Education, social position, gender, religious and political orientation, or ethnicity do not interfere with the social interaction or with the methodological approach to interviewing: the same questions are asked, every answer is listened to, no statement is criticised or censured, mistakes may be corrected by both interviewees and interviewer if that is relevant to the conversation.

7 The therapeutic function of storytelling does not concern only recounting one's memories but belongs to the act of telling stories itself. Storytelling is one of the fundamental characteristics of the human species (Gottschall, 2012). All Greek poetic and dramatic production highlights the therapeutic and ethical power of storytelling (Gorelick, 1987; Rojcewicz, 2004). Today, this power is studied in depth not only from an aesthetic-literary perspective but also from a psychological and cognitive one, and is used as a practical therapeutic methodology (Slivinske & Slivinske, 2013; Ingemark, 2013).

8 “La differenza fra le fonti scritte e le fonti orali è che le prime sono per lo più documenti, le seconde sono sempre atti; non vanno pensate in termini sostantivi e di cose ma di verbi e di processi; non la memoria e il racconto, ma ricordare, raccontare”.

9 “Dipende dall'esistenza di qualcuno che ascolti. Una delle cose che rendono differenti le fonti orali è appunto che sono l'esito di un lavoro comune fra le narratrici e il ricercatore, che le va a cercare, le ascolta, le interroga.”

10 “Terreno comune” che “non deve necessariamente consistere in una comune identità (di classe, di genere, di ideologia…) ma può essere delimitato, anzi deve, principalmente dalla disponibilità all'ascolto reciproco, alla reciproca accettazione.”

11 The interviewers are aware that the practice itself of the interview is distortive and therefore potentially manipulative. Some interviewers may be reticent or willing to provide well-told stories, but in general they approach the interview in a relaxed mindset, and do not worry if they remember too little or too blurrily. Moreover, the interviewers strive to reduce the distortive potential to

a minimum. The dialogue plays a major role in that: the interviewer guides the interview while engaging in dialogue. Interviewees are free to express themselves, reason why questions are formulated in such a way as to avoid piloting the answer in a predetermined direction.

12 Weber borrowed the term from Schiller, who had used it in the poem *Die Götter Griechenlandes* [*The Gods of Greece*], 1788.

13 "La qualité de la témoignage dépend aussi essentiellement du style de l'interview. L'historien doit apprendre à encourager un témoin, à l'écouter, et par-dessus tout à jamais l'interrompre ; mais il doit également venir avec des questions bien préparées, avec dans sa tête une suite de sujets, de telle manière que le témoin puisse être encouragé et gentiment aiguillé, à travers la discussion. Ceci amène de résultats plus riches qu'un questionnaire d'interview structuré de manière rigide" (Thompson, 1984, p. 287).

14 "A whole is what has a beginning and middle and end. A beginning is that which is not a necessary consequent of anything else but after which something else exists or happens as a natural result. An end on the contrary is that which is inevitably or, as a rule, the natural result of something else but from which nothing else follows; a middle follows something else and something follows from it. Well constructed plots must not therefore begin and end at random" (Aristotle, 1932, 1450b).

15 All the translations of the interviews are mine.

16 "La mancanza di memoria infatti comporta una perdita di senso e di conoscenza, ma apre anche degli spazi di immaginazione e di rielaborazione. Nella misura in cui sono meno informati, [gli intervistati] sono a volte indotti a cercare di ricostruirsi interpretazione e senso da soli, a partire dai pochi dati a disposizione."

17 Traces of this "know thyself" culture can be found already in fragments 93, 101, and 116 by Heraclitus (1987); in verse 311 of Aeschylus' *Prometheus Bound*, Ocean commands Prometheus to "know himself" (1926); in Plato's *Protagoras*, the three engravings of Apollo's shrine are quoted, "those maxims which are on every tongue— 'Know thyself' and 'Nothing overmuch'" (1967b, 343b); and finally, in Plato's *Alcibiades I* (1955, 133 B 2–10), *Meno* (1967a, 84 A 3–C 6), *Theaetetus* (1921, 189 E 6–7) and above all *Socrates' Apology*. For further reading about classical sources of the "know thyself," see Napolitano Valditara (2003).

18 The stoic philosophy, which was imported into the Latin world and became the dominant philosophical current during the imperial age, changed the Western approach to the body-mind interaction. Roman emperor Marcus Aurelius was well-versed in philosophical meditation which included rules such as contenting oneself with a spare diet, letting go of negative emotions, pursuing sexual continence, and keeping one's body fit and steady (1906). All in all, however, the stoic doctrine tended to hold the soul in higher consideration than the body, thus imprinting the following Western conception of the body-mind interaction. The practice of exercising the mind over the body passed into Christianity, where the practices of self-inflicted bodily pain through flagellation, sexual abstinence, or severe fasting were diffused among the monastic orders. The acme of this tradition was reached with the formulation of Ignatius de Loyola's "spiritual exercises" in 1548. This manifesto of the Jesuitical religiousness calls spiritual exercise "any method of examining one's own conscience; also of meditating, contemplating, praying mentally and vocally, and, finally, of performing any other spiritual operations" (1847, p. 1). As one can see, the body is utterly expelled from the scope of the exercises.

Chapter 7
Manic Hand and Mobile Self:
Ghérasim Luca's Transformative Aesthetics, From Fragment to Healing Flow

Charlène Clonts
http://orcid.org/0000-0003-4228-4868
Kyushu University, Japan

ABSTRACT

The chapter studies the transformative aesthetics of Ghérasim Luca, a Francophone poet and visual artist, whose practice, allegedly obsessive, mobilizes the body as both medium and site of metamorphosis. His "manic hand" enacts a performative gesture that disrupts normative structures, reconfiguring materiality, imagination, and affect. Through close readings of his cubomanies, Objectively Offered Objects, and handmade albums, the chapter examines how they foster emotional resilience, sensory awareness, and epistemic dissent. Luca's art resists fixed representation, instead cultivating liminal spaces where identity, perception, and relationality are continuously renegotiated. The chapter argues that his poetics constitute a participatory model of care – not through normative restoration, but through the affirmation of multiplicity, ambiguity, and imaginative freedom. In this context, well-being is redefined as a dynamic and relational state, emerging from creative engagement and the continual reconfiguration of the self in relation to others and to the environment.

DOI: 10.4018/979-8-3373-3521-6.ch007

INTRODUCTION

Central to the work of Ghérasim Luca—a French–speaking poet and visual artist (Bucharest 1913–Paris 1994)—is the act of "making oneself," conceived as a legitimate creative process in which the craftsman's hand at work becomes especially prominent. It is rooted in the etymology of the word "poetry," originally associated with craftsmanship and praxis. The ancient Greek verb ποιέω [*poieo*] first meant "to do," later acquiring the sense of "to make, to execute, to produce," particularly in relation to manual labor and artistic creation, especially statuary. Over time, it came to evoke creation and generation, and more specifically poetic composition and imagination. It also conveys ideas of action and efficiency, and ultimately "to do for oneself" and "to do by oneself" (*Bailly* Ancient Greek Dictionary). From this perspective, Luca emphasizes the manual dimension of poetic and plastic creation through an etymological redundancy: in his own word, he seeks to affirm a "practical poetry" (Clonts, 2021) whose dynamic and active forms resist normative petrification.

More broadly, Luca's engagement with reality often involves a process of manipulation that treats language and images as materials. The French term *manipulation* derives from medieval Latin *manipulare*, meaning "to lead by the hand" (*TLFi* Dictionary). In Latin, the word *manus* [the hand] carries numerous figurative implications that enrich the idea of artistic manipulation: action, violence, artistic handling, scribe writing, throwing the dice, power, and might (*Gaffiot* Dictionary). Similar associations appear throughout Luca's work. One technique he invented combines the roll of the dice with the hand: the *cubomanies*—collages of squares cut from reproductions of famous paintings—are rearranged, allegedly according to the laws of chance. This recalls the medieval meaning of the French word *chance*, understood as a roll of the dice, and further evokes Stéphane Mallarmé's *Un Coup de dés jamais n'abolira le hasard*, along with Luca's own spatialization of poetic writing.

Luca's deconstruction–construction 'mania,' however, stems from a feigned and humorous obsession that desacralizes the distinctions between behavioral disorder—monomania—and the alleged 'noble' making of art, leaving room for a hovering in–between. Luca's 'manic hand' appears in both his poetry and visual art as a means of highlighting figural renewals through mobile combinations, as seen in his *Objets Objectivement Offerts* [Objectively Offered Objects] (O.O.O.), *cubomanies*[1], homemade editions and postcards, scrapbooking albums, *écriture aux points* [dot writing], and photocopied ready–made. Based on a series of gestures performed in his studio during the creative process, this chapter explores how Luca's composition, practice, and thought exploit relationships that generate shifts or displacements from fixed and petrified cultural forms to fluid, dynamic and mobile forms of life. According to Dick Hebdige, such shifts mark a subculture—distinguished from classical and conservative culture as a standard of excellence—and are perceived as an integral way of life (Hebdige, p. 7). By questioning the study of his own work by a PhD. student in the early 1990's (personal notes in his archives), Luca had already grasped this cultural duality, linked to the patrimonialization process. Therefore, this chapter examines Luca's poetic and visual practices as a singular form of body–mind engagement that challenges normative structures, focusing particularly on perception, identity, and mental health care. While Luca is not typically associated with discourses of well–being in a conventional or therapeutic sense, his work offers a radically different approach to emotional resilience and healing. His poetic and performative gestures were deeply infused with existential urgency and ontological instability, reflecting his lifelong engagement with the limits of perception, identity, and language. His work does not promise comfort or resolution, but instead proposes a healing flow through the destabilization of fixed identities and the creation of transitional spaces—what Dominique Rabaté describes as "seeking to exit from within" [chercher à sortir par le dedans] (Rabaté p. 236). In this sense, Luca's aesthetics are profoundly transformative: they enact a movement from fragmentation toward relationality, from anxiety toward a form of poetic survival. Whether through his texts, vocal performances, or visual assemblages, Luca's work proposes a transformative aesthetics where the manic hand and mobile self converge—not to resolve anxiety, but to inhabit it creatively and relationally.

Through deliberately obsessive manual techniques, Luca constructs a poetics of fragmentation and recomposition of the self, mobilizing the body as both a site and a medium of transformation. His 'manic hand' enacts a performative gesture that disrupts established forms and reconfigures the relationship among materiality, imagination, and affect. By disrupting hegemonic visual and textual codes, Luca's work opens space for alternative forms of life and knowledge, offering a model for how artistic practices can support emotional resilience, sensory awareness, and the reconditioning of everyday experience. Situated within the context of 20th–century French–speaking East European experimentation and diasporic marginality, Luca's work resists fixed representation and instead fosters a dynamic interplay between sensory experience and cognitive reorientation. His artistic strategies—cutting, assembling, collaging—function as embodied acts of resistance and renewal, producing liminal spaces where the boundaries between self and other, subject and object, are continuously renegotiated. I argue that Luca's practice constitutes a participatory aesthetic of self–care, associated with an epistemic dissent, wherein the act of making becomes a means of healing. Through close reading of Luca's visual and poetic assemblages, and by offering in conclusion a precise definition of well–being in the context of his work, this study demonstrates how artistic creation can cultivate well–being—not through normative healing, but through the affirmation of difference, mobility, and imaginative freedom. By foregrounding the tactile, the rhythmic, and the relational, Luca's work proposes a noninstitutional model of a holistic and transformative body–mind practice, while embracing multiplicity, dissonance, and the irreducible complexity of lived experience. This chapter contributes to the volume's holistic perspective on well–being by examining Luca's artistic gestures as body–mind practices that foster emotional resilience, sensory awareness, and creative transformation. His work offers an alternative model of healing—one rooted in poetic disruption and relational aesthetics.

EMBODIED RECONFIGURATIONS: HANDS–ON POETICS FOR AN "OBJECTIVE" REALITY

Sensory Awareness and Tactile Imagination

In Luca's cubomanies, the motif of the hand appears recurrently. It functions as a reflexive *mise en abyme* of the artist—supposedly obsessive cutter—who repeatedly extracts squares of identical format from reproductions of artworks originally representing or commissioned by influential figures such as popes, aristocrats, wealthy merchants, and ambassadors. At the same time, it evokes the poet's hand that writes: although eventually circumstantial, the cubomanies often depict, through their poetic titles and selected images, thinkers and writers such as Erasmus and Antonin Artaud. In addition, motifs featuring letters of the alphabet and signs of writing—such as signatures and phylacteries—signal a persistent questioning of the hand that traces. Luca's own signature, sometimes superimposed on that of well–known painters, also appears as a visual motif, indicating a shift in the value attributed to the artist's signature in favor of an inquiry about the commodification of art from a postmodern perspective. The *detournement* and extraction of these signs from their original context foster new readings of the artwork, momentarily freed from the economic, temporal, and spatial circumstances of its original production. The evocation of the hand—that makes and traces—underscores the processes of figural construction. It highlights the materiality and artisanal dimension of artistic creation while introducing divergence at the core of a system to which it simultaneously belongs—economy and contingencies. Cubomania infiltrates the capitalist organization of art—for example, the signature certifying the origin of a piece or reproductions of famous merchants' portraits—to create space for alternative representations of individuals and their social status, thereby raising questions about labelling. For Luca, existence cannot be reduced to a word or formula, that is, to a fixed form. His self–generating work, whose deep structure operates as a continuous variation (Clonts, 2020), thus moves toward a broader organic art that seeks to produce corporeality. This is why Luca offers the following definition in his first exhibition of cubomanies: "Cubomania is the instantaneous ocular correspondent of our behavior toward the outside world, a behavior that consists in the refusal to consider the axiomatic human condition as an objective reality, even in its apparently immutable aspects[2]" (Luca & Trost, n.p.). This definition implies a vision of the world that turns away from the representationist system by avoiding the drawback of an otherness and exteriority that would exist only outside of oneself in a fixed state, absorbed by the senses during perception or objectified in a subject–object relationship. Cubomania focuses on interactional processes—including transactional and transitional—where interiority/exteriority and otherness/identity sustain circulation and constant transformation. This practice seeks to escape unilateral representation. Luca considers the cubomanies "objective"—impartial objects—because their processes diverge from unilateral representation, offering a more comprehensive scope of the world. In this context, the cubomaniac practice interrogates the human relationship to the otherness.

The question first arises through the viewer–object bond. From the perspective of the reception, the cubomanies initially appear as flat works. However, when collected and glued on various supports, the squares create a subtle relief. Their handmade cuts reveal both regularities and irregularities, reinforcing a non–machinic, human presence, and evoking a gesture that is also lyrical—one that surfaces in both the poet's texts and the titles of the cubomanies. The processes of representation are reframed by combining the regularity of the alleged monomania, the rhythm of repeated cuts from reproductions of artworks, and the contingent trembling contour of handmade production. This rhythmic gesture, obsessive yet lyrical, resonates with Henri Meschonnic's conception of rhythm as a mode of subjectivation and meaning–making that exceeds metric regularity and engages the body, language, and affect in continuous transformation (Meschonnic, 1982). Luca's gesture oscillates between the cutting hand and the technical reproducibility, a dynamic in which the artist plays with repetition and variation. The combination of squares produces something close to what François Lyotard calls the "figures–images," which "deconstruct the percept" and "are accomplished in a space of difference[3]" (Lyotard, 1971 p. 277), accumulating multiple layers of interpretation. In this sense, duplicating a canonical work is not merely copying but rather bestowing a form of thickness. The restless manic hand thus disrupts the established order and transforms the viewer–object relationship by introducing unpredictability.

The cubomaniac space may as well be related to Gilles Deleuze's *diagram*: a "zone of indistinguishability or objective indeterminacy, which opposes and imposes on the sight an unbridled manual power[4]" (p. 88). The maker's gesture and the metamorphoses imposed on the original figures reach the viewer through propelling, sensitive perceptions. The space of the cubomanies is crossed by visual effects of sliding, translation, whirling, and reversal. In this "tactile–optical space[5]" (Deleuze,

p. 81), the viewer's eye acts like a hand, aspiring to motion and creating an imaginary movement. Psychology and neuroscience studies show that motor imagery profoundly impacts the body, for example in mental training or in the rehabilitation of injured athlete (Bonnechère, 2017; Herrera & Vargas, 2019; Chacon, 2020). Through this cognitive and emotional relationship to imagery, a "haptic" function (Deleuze, p. 79) emerges. It enables a mobile life that no longer belongs entirely to the artist but becomes an appropriation of the body–mind movement. Consequently, the cubomanies should not appear as petrified works of art. They constitute an integral process, comparable to a relentless image recycling—human–powered by an alternative body–mind.

Recycled Knowledge: Crafting New Epistemes Through Body–Mind Engagement

Luca practiced a recycling form of art as a mode of circulation and transformation of consumer goods. He searched for vintage objects, albums, and photographs at the Saint–Ouen flea market. The collection of heterogeneous elements is at the origin of many works. For instance, the artist found a box of multicolored glassware that he used to create the poetry collection *Le Sorcier noir* [The Dark Wizard] (1962), accompanied by an etching by Jacques Hérold. Similarly, he repurposed a 19th-century photography album for the handmade book *Le Tangage de ma langue* [The Pitching of My Tongue] (n.d.), created with paintings by Micheline Catti. The same approach applies to colonial images, almanacs, and old dictionaries that enabled him to produce the plates of the *Série Brésil* [Brazil Series] (1960–1970, 1988–1989[6]). These plates consist of photographs onto which words taken from dictionaries—often illustrated—were pasted. The knowledge conveyed by these photographs and encyclopaedic drawings is old–fashioned. Similar to scrapbooking, the boards of the *Série Brésil* compel the viewer to constantly adjust the gaze, shifting between holistic and detailed perception. In addition, the photographic reading is disrupted by collaged elements that conceal some parts while revealing others. As in a scrapbook album, the association of apparently heterogeneous elements alters the original reading of the pasted documents: texts lose their primary informative purpose and acquire new value through collage and juxtaposition. In the scrapbooking, these elements often take on memorial significance, seeking to suspend a moment in the time–space of the album. The *Série Brésil*, however, reverses this process. Luca does not aim to preserve the memory conveyed by the images—at least not in the way colonial photography originally represented it from the sole perspective of the colonizer. In contrast to the initial objective of the photograph, the plates of the *Série Brésil* do not fix meaning, they set it in motion.

Oscillating between widely distributed ethnographic photographs, almanac rebuses, and encyclopaedic illustrations, the viewer's gaze gradually adjusts through the recognition of sound and graphic repetitions of shapes and letters in the collages. This perception of a rhythm becomes the transmission belt that links heterogeneous elements and generates relationships. Despite the sociohistorical context of the original photographs—and their biased anthropological aims within a colonial context—Luca's processes create a humorous and playful atmosphere. Puns and rebuses appear throughout. The viewer still perceives the colonial perspective of the initial photographs, even though the photographer's name has been removed. From one glued word or drawing to another, satiric and rhythmic progressions produce contrasts with the original images. This unexpected contiguity of heterogeneous elements introduces a strangeness that makes sense: Luca sheds new light on photography. He short–circuits the initial meanings of colonial photographs of Afro–Brazilians and Native Americans in the Amazon. His goal is not to erase their historical weight but to underline forms of life that were unnoticed and made minor in the colonial context. Over a period from 1960 to 1989, applying vignettes depicting handcuffs and shackles to colonial–era ethnographic photographs makes it an eminently political gesture. In the case of *Série Brésil*, this gesture condemns the appropriation of Amerindian lands and the enslavement of Afro-Brazilians—a practice not abolished until 1888. Abolition itself had been subjected to limitations, to which was opposed the nascent Black press of São Paulo and Rio in the 1930s and 1950s, later by the Black movement, and highlighted in a UNESCO report commissioned to sociologists in 1950 (Saillant & Araujo, p. 458).

Nonetheless, the *Série Brésil*, like the cubomanies, cannot be reduced to a dialectical synthesis that merely opposes criticism and the affirmation of viable solutions—settling only in difference by opposition. Luca's writing and visual works are not, strictly speaking, 'engaged works.' Nevertheless, they bear political features and reflect an ethic. Words taken from dictionaries and pasted onto old photographs mimic and divert the naturalistic classification of the colonizer found in old–fashioned anthropological photographs. This nomenclature implicitly comments on the relationship between colonial photography and the natural sciences. Beginning with the history of slavery, Luca's collages open onto a broader ethical–political function. They question the human impulse to catalogue and find typologies that belong to the representation of forms—a tendency that can lead to inhumanity, as in slavery and colonialism—while also pointing toward struggles for freedom, such as the Black movement and the abolitionist movement in Brazil. For Luca, handmade practice becomes a way to produce reality rather than merely oppose it. This construction of a reality to be invented relies on photographic reproductions as historical and socio-cultural documents. Such combination forms what Leibovici (2007, p. 24) names a "poetic document," in which one can read "the instituting stages, linguistic and visual, of the making of the world," simultaneously functioning as an "intellectual technology that produces reality.[7]" Crafting, therefore, is making reality. Despite its association with fixation, the verb "to paste" means "to join together," "to be in close contact," and "to stick as close as possible to reality" (*TLFi* Dictionary). Selecting, cutting, assembling, and gluing become the primary actions of a serial reprocessing of preexisting knowledge. The heterogeneity of these collages suspends documentary and stereotyped interpretation of ethnographic photographs, thereby transforms epistemes. Crafting becomes both an aesthetic paradigm for transforming the world through an impartial recasting of the referential function of texts and images, and a critique of discourses that present themselves as absolute truth.

SUBCULTURAL MEDIATIONS AS VERBAL AND NONVERBAL PATHWAYS TO EMOTIONAL EXPRESSION

Relationalities: Otherness, Emotional Resilience, and Creative Healing

Luca's poetic and artistic practice has often been described as radically disruptive, notably through Dominique Carlat's lens of an "intempestive poetics." This poetic is characterized by resistance to closure, an embrace of contradiction, and the disruption of linear meaning. According to Carlat, Luca's work systematically undermines binary oppositions and conventional narrative structures, producing a divided enunciation and a paradoxical rhythm that highlights internal tension—eminently visible in the *Objets Objectivement Offerts* [Objectively Offered Objects] (O.O.O.) [8] (Carlat, pp. 145–160). This framework also extends to Luca's vocal performances, which challenge the notion of orality as expressive unity. Instead, they present the voice as a site of semantic instability and theatrical distance. Building on this interpretation, the present analysis seeks to extend Carlat's framework by foregrounding the material, relational, and affective dimensions of the O.O.O.s. Luca did not radically consider the O.O.O.s as objects of art. Yet, with their explicit name, they correspond in every way to the criteria of DIY. They are made from found objects—sourced from flea markets or among personal belongings—and assembled by the artist. Close to a ready–made but bearing another meaning, each assemblage is given a title and generally self–gifted or offered to a third party (e.g., André Breton, Victor Brauner, Déline, Hélène, Satan). The objects used are varied: dolls' parts, figurines, mannequin heads, letters, ink pens, sieves, *Fantômas*' book covers, cut–out images, horns, and marbles. In this analysis, rather than treating these objects solely as poetic devices that embody internal tensions, I examine them as ephemeral acts of offering operating within a broader economy of emotional transmission. Their capacity to mediate unconscious expression, initiate peer–to–peer communication, and engage with mythical or nonhuman entities suggests a performative and transformative function that exceeds the bounds of textual contradiction. In this sense, the O.O.O.s not only reflect Luca's poetics of paradox but also enact a dynamic of relational projection and reception, where the object becomes a medium of connection, disruption, and reconfiguration—both of the self and of the other.

Till now, no physical traces of the O.O.O.s remain, except for photographs by Théodore Brauner included in *Le Vampire Passif* [The Passive Vampire] (1945), first published clandestinely in Bucharest. Their disappearance situates them among ephemeral acts of offering manufactured objects or homemade gifts. The poetic prose of *Le Vampire passif* provides insight into the power of these objects, which speak their own language. Luca deciphers the meaning of each handmade piece, crafted on a particular occasion to materialize the unconscious of the giver. For instance, *Le Bouquet tragique* [The Tragic Bouquet] was created from a cover of *Fantômas* depicting a frightened woman holding flowers. This object inspires an entire poetic reflection centered on love, physical intimacy, and the desire to offer flowers to a specific woman known to Luca, enriched with erotic metaphor. The poet records sensations experienced during creation, describing them as a meaningful form rooted in both dream and waking life. The object is perceived as a liberating experience of the "subject that exteriorizes itself[9]" (*Le Vampire passif*, p. 69). It stands in contrast with "I think therefore I am" and instead expresses "I create, therefore I move toward the other." Writing begins with attempts to fictionally capture the recipient's thoughts—Mrs. A.—as a peer–to–peer distance communication with the "receptive subject[10]" (*Le Vampire passif*, p. 69). Thus, an O.O.O. reveals the maker's unconscious while carrying seeds of a future response from its recipient. It acts as a medium, bridging people. Like a Voodoo doll, whether positive or negative, it can instantly act on and transmit a message to the recipient—even one unknown to its creator at the moment of the crafting. The accompanying poetic texts draw out the deeper meaning of these objects, which function not as isolated creations but as components of a larger machinery of human connection and emotional exchange.

Human beings are not the only recipients of O.O.O.s; they can also be offered to mythical figures or even to other objects, transforming them into *Objets Objectivement Offerts aux Objets* [Objectively Offered Objects to Objects]. This practice reflects the belief that the true power of these offerings lies in their ability to reveal hidden processes within the universe: "But the eyes alone are useless in a universe in which the moon is black, and the pretension of separating the perceptible from the imperceptible does not count on the secret mechanism of the retina[11]." (*Le Vampire passif*, p. 69) Echoing Gérard de Nerval's "soleil soir de la mélancolie" [black sun of melancholia], the black moon introduces a nocturnal and feminine counterpart to perception. The mention of flowers in Luca's text also evokes Nerval's poem "El Desdichado," where "the vine with the rose joins forces[12]" on the lovers' tomb (Nerval, 2005, p. 29). Still, Luca transforms the solitude through intricate networks of meaning and the distance communication of the O.O.O.s, which subvert the melancholic descent from the "desolate heart[13]" poet (Nerval, p. 29). The proliferation of vegetal images associated with lovers' union is no longer confined to the symbolic void of Nerval's tomb but expands into the universe's amorous potential, beyond dyadic interaction. The term "Objectively Offered Objects" reflects an effort to maintain impartiality and to facilitate the emergence of latent, subterranean processes into visible and interpretable forms. The repeated use of the letter "O" serves as a graphic symbol for the rupture of boundaries, suggesting openings, circulations, and transitional spaces that expose the elusive nature of human self–conception and the dynamics of interpersonal relationships. These objects challenge norms and assumptions surrounding their very existence: "Humanity in panic asked itself for the first time a question resembling a slip of the tongue: what is an ear? Is it a shell/a typo? A trap? A curl/loop? An echo? Anatomy leaves the old instruments that are out of use and seeks an equivalence in the shadows that it casts inside and outside human like a living mask[14]." (*Le Vampire passif*, p. 71) Much like Vincent van Gogh's symbolic gesture of offering his ear to his beloved, the artist who presents an O.O.O. engages with the projective force of art and the body–mind intensity of its reception. This act disrupts established social conventions, classifications, and functions, emphasizing on the paradoxical potential of both absolute impossibility and relative offering.

In sum, Luca's O.O.O.s emerge not only as poetic assemblages but as dynamic instruments of emotional and figurative exchange. Their ephemeral nature, capacity to channel unconscious impulses, and openness to multiple forms of relationality—human, mythical, and material—position them as key sites of transformative aesthetics. By highlighting the act of offering as a gesture of connection and disruption, these objects challenge fixed categories of art, identity, and perception. They invite to reconsider the boundaries between self and other, fragmentation and healing, and reveal in Luca's manic hand the generative force of a mobile, relational self.

Crafting Duets: Handmade Albums and the Fluidity of Identity

Luca's use of recycled objects from flea markets can be attributed to the material constraints he faced after moving to Paris. Similarly, his handmade books often stemmed from material difficulties, unfinished projects or the absence of plans for formal publication. But beyond these practical reasons, Luca's crafting reflects a deeper impulse: a continual reimagining of the self, others, and artistic creation itself.

Working with homemade or found materials offered creative freedom, even within the limits of availability. He produced artisanal editions of his works, including *Le Jour sans souvenir* [The Day Without Memory] (1954) with an ink drawing by Béatrice de la Sablière, *Souvenir de vacances* [Vacation Souvenir] (1961), *Mot–clef sur porte–parole* [Keyword/Word–Key on Spokesperson/Spoken Medium] (1962) with dot drawings, *POEMETTO (Ready-made)* (1965) and *Passionnément* [Passionately] (1992) with painted papers by Isabelle Vorle. These homemade works take the form of a collaborative dialogue book, artist's books, and ready-mades. They operate similarly to animated books or collages, yet often derived from preexisting, commercially circulated albums whose original functions have been subverted.

Dedicated to the painter Victor Brauner, the artist's book *Mot–clef sur porte–parole* features a poem and a series of dot–based drawings arranged within the window frames of an old photo album, emptied of its original contents. Luca's dot compositions evoke both images and words through a dense constellation of spots that become legible only when viewed from a distance. This pointillist technique—seemingly obsessive or at least executed with great patience—engages with Mallarmé's idea of the constellation, inviting the reader to mentally connect the dots to form images or words, or to trace intuitive, free–form associations. Luca further distances himself from conventional poetic lines and extends the constellation metaphor by using punctuation as a material for drawing. The trace of the pointillist gesture materializes the emergence of figures in place of the original album's photographs. Whereas photography once fixed individuals in posture, time, and place, the dot drawings introduce dynamic potential. Though permanently inscribed by the artist's hand, the dots suggest a multiplicity of connections and interpretations, inviting the viewer to fill the spaces between them. This multiplicity contrasts with the idea that identity—particularly represented through photography—could be definitely fixed. Instead, identity appears mobile, elusive, and ever–changing, metaphorically marked by gaps and absences like the spaces between the dots. It also echoes Arthur Rimbaud's adage "Je est un autre" [I is another]. The dedication of his handcrafted work to Brauner, Luca's lifelong friend, further underscores otherness as a reflection of the self—not a mirror–like self but a wider, communal self. The constellation of dots thus suggests the multiplicity of the self and the inherent instability and wavering of a subject that both reflects on oneself and contemplates the other—while the latter also penetrates the self in return.

The poetry collection *Le Tangage de ma langue* [The Pitching of My Tongue] (post–1953) reflects a dynamic relationship to otherness. Conceived as a *book of dialogue*[15] [un livre de dialogue] —a book created with four or more hands—it merges poetry and visual art in a way that resists hierarchical relations between the two. Rather than illustration or subordination, the interplay of media affirms mutual autonomy and a shared creative space. The collection was assembled using an old picture album originally designed to illustrate scenes from medieval life, reminiscent of Poulain chocolate albums but executed in a more luxurious format. In the slots intended for printed images, painter Micheline Catti—also Luca's long–time partner—inserted abstract tinted cardboard pieces, while Luca contributed the poetic text "Le Tangage de ma langue". This collaborative intervention transforms the album into a hybrid work where visual abstraction and poetic language coexist without subordinating one medium to the other. The word "pitching" in the title evokes instability—a liminal zone oscillating between anchoring and falling. It is mirrored in the physical structure of the work itself: the poetry cards and the painted inserts placed within the album's notches remain unfixed, consistent with the original format of image albums. The reader is implicitly invited to rearrange the cards, reinforcing internal mobility as a foundational principle of the work. This openness to reconfiguration partly explains the choice of a home–produced format. Traditional mainstream publishing, by contrast, typically necessitates the fixation of text, favoring editorial decisions that enhance readability for a targeted audience, simplify distribution, and control production costs. Moreover, the use of a pre–existing album disrupts the initial conception of the book through the serendipity of chance encounters—such as discoveries at the Saint–Ouen flea market or the availability of second-hand albums at a retailer's stall. Adapting original ideas to an object that once belonged to an unknown third party transforms *Le Tangage de ma langue* into a multi–handed collaboration, where several contributors remain anonymous. This layering of contributions recalls the cubomaniac technique; yet it contrasts with the possessive tone of the title, "my tongue", highlighting the impossibility of fully approaching the means of expression as a solitary individual. It underscores the collective nature of creation, rooted in the artist's relationship with otherness in its broadest sense.

The materiality of the image album as a medium directly shapes the segmentation and layout of the poem "Le Tangage de ma langue" across its pages. Unlike the standardized formatting found in the introductory booklet in the double CD *Gherasim Luca par Gherasim Luca* (2001), the poem's presentation within the medieval album is fragmented and recontextualized. As Catherine Perret argues in *Le Temps de l'œuvre* [The Time of Artwork], the artwork is not a static object but a temporal and relational process that unfolds through discontinuities, rhythms, and embodied perception. Artistic creation resists the homogenizing temporality of industrial production, embracing instead a time of experience, hesitation, and transformation (Perret, 2019 pp. 15–18). Luca's handmade albums[16] exemplify this counter–temporality, where instability of form and tactile engagement—of both the viewer and the producer—generate a dynamic and relational experience of time. In *Le Tangage de ma langue*, section titles from the original album interrupt the poetic flow, while the text itself is distributed across multiple cardboard inserts placed in the album's notches and vertically oriented within its structure. Micheline Catti's painted cardboards introduce further discontinuities, suspending the temporality of the written word with that of the image, and vice versa. This interaction between text and image underscores the work's resistance to fixed interpretation and its embrace of material and semantic instability. The album's material constraints, along with the limited space on the cards—where only a few words can be inscribed—introduce variations in the poem's syntactic structure. Additionally, the physical fragmentation of the text, its spatial arrangement within an album originally conceived for images, and the use of painted cards alter the sonorous legibility of the text and generate anticipation. The slowed pace of reading, combined with the distribution of text across multiple cardboards on a single page, enables broader visual engagement and simultaneous interpretation. The reader's gaze moves freely across the page, capturing isolated words, images, or titles, constructing meaning through a mobile and non–linear reading experience.

Luca's handmade process forms the basis of a poetics of recycling, partly grounded in the dual criteria of *bricolage* as articulated by Claude Lévi–Strauss regarding mythical thought: "they have served, as the words of a discourse that mythical reflection 'dismantles', in the manner of the handyman taking care of the gables of an old dismantled alarm clock; and they may also serve the same or a different use if they are diverted from their first function[17]." (Lévi–Strauss, p. 50) Myths possess an infinite capacity for expansion, as their constituent elements can be endlessly recombined to generate new narratives and produce meanings that are concretely applicable. In Luca's work, recycled elements—originally embedded within different symbolic systems—are recontextualized through new performative frameworks. This process profoundly transforms their legibility, visibility, meaning, and organization. Detached from their original contexts and integrated with new components, these elements undergo a radical shift in function and interpretation. However, Luca's visual practice diverges from the classificatory impulse and desire to order that characterizes myths, thus departing from Lévi–Strauss' *bricolage*. Metaphorically, recycling albums into duets with close friends and partners allows Luca to bring his poetics into contact with that of other artists, creating a relational and fictional space that sparks new meanings. In this sense, his work tests the ideological foundation of standardized forms, including those shaping the artist himself and the meanings assigned within a given symbolic system. Luca's practice interrogates established symbolic structures by multiplying associations and opening diverse interpretative pathways. For this reason, even opposition and revolt—conventional modes of symbolic resistance—are surpassed by the deliberately obsessive, almost maniacal, gestures of the artist's hand. This hand gives rise to a body of work that resists comparison with the so–called "real world," which is itself a curated selection of what is preserved and what is marginalized within a hegemonic system. The manic hand generates borderline experiences that destabilize conventional meanings given to life, resulting in patchworks of bodies, faces, words, and images—constantly shifting, perpetually in motion, and suspended in a state of (dis)equilibrium.

Patchworks in Continuous Becoming: Multiplicity, Disruption, and the Poetics of Well–Being

In both poetry and visual art, Luca employs sound and graphic patchwork to disrupt the fabric of everyday life—not out of contempt for the ordinary, but from a need to explore alternative modes of expressing the multiplicity of being. Patchwork, a craft of sewing that joins small textile pieces of varied origins and textures, illustrates this approach. Despite its heterogeneity, patchwork produces coherence and rhythm while creating jumps and connections between fragments. Similarly, Luca seeks to liberate the multiplicity of being from the rigid structures that typically define certain forms of expression. He frequently articulates his struggle to apprehend what is conventionally called "reality", suggesting that naming inherently causes the named to elude us. Consequently, his oeuvre abounds with poetic and visual techniques centered on fragmentation and void—manifested through holes and cuts—that reflect this epistemological tension. In a framework where the signifier might grant access to the real, Luca attempts to apprehend the elusive presence through the absence marked by cuts and voids, or interruptions in the chain of signifiers. Simultaneously, he manipulates this chain through intricate sound and graphic play that permeates his writing, generating multiple layers of understanding. His work does not aim to represent the real through symbolic mediation; rather, it resists such representation altogether. This poetic and aesthetic ambition—central to what he calls the work of the "manic hand"—seeks to evoke a different kind of real, or even an "unreal" as conceived in psychoanalytic terms. Yet, from the perspective of anti–psychiatry—which conceives itself as a form of psychiatry—this 'unreal' is simply another modality of being–in–the–world. The presence Luca strives to capture is unstable and polymorphic, resembling the fragmented unity of patchwork or even the playful circulation of the fifteen–puzzle game. His images hover at the edge of the representable, engaging the signifier as *another*, through relentless manipulation of the signified and its associative networks. This approach also underpins his collaborative, multi–handed practices with fellow artists—across poetry, visual art, performance, and multisensory exhibitions. Through these practices, patchwork in continuous becoming turns out to be a method for staging differential processes in artistic production. In this regard, Jean-Luc Nancy's reflections in *Corpus* offer a useful conceptual lens. Rather than conceiving the body as a unified or interiorized entity, Nancy describes it as a site of exposure and spacing—a "corpus" that exists only in its fragmentation and in its relation to others (Nancy, 2000, pp. 15–18, 83–85).

Luca's visual and poetic strategies, focusing on discontinuity, tactile rhythm, and relational assemblage, enact a similar displacement of the body from any essential form toward a condition of shared exteriority.

This dynamic is notably present in the book of poetry *Satyre et satrape—Rébus super 8* [Satyr and Satrap—Super 8 Rebus] (1987), created in collaboration with visual artist and performer Joël Hubaut. Although the book is not strictly self–published or artisanal—having been released by CREM (Conceptuelle Rapide Et Maximale) [Conceptual Fast And Maximal], a publishing house founded by Hubaut himself—it nonetheless adopts mobile patchwork methodologies that permeate its creative processes. The seven visual art boards of "Super 8 Rebuses" contributed by Hubaut are emblematic of this approach: conceived as societal 'residues', they echo the logic of patchwork, which traditionally assembles fragments of fabric left over from previous sewing projects. These rebuses function not only as visual puzzles but also as cultural remnants, reinforcing the book's engagement with fragmentation, reuse, and multiplicity as aesthetic strategies. The patchwork structure is also set in motion, as suggested by the cinematographic reference to the Super 8 motion–picture format, a technology first introduced in 1965.

In *Satyre et Satrape*, the rebuses are explicitly defined as "REBUS = (secretion → sparse hybrid signals)" and "Word-image energy (super 8)[18]" (n.p.), underscoring their conceptual hybridity and dynamic interplay between text and image. These rebuses consist of densely packed pen drawings that visually saturate the page, reproducing fragments of ordinary life—comparable to cinematographic stripes—through the juxtaposition of words, numbers, and images. Their aggregation within single pages or across double–page spreads transforms the perception of these elements, which, when isolated, would appear mundane or contextually inert. Through this recontextualization, his work generates both humor and provocation. Hubaut's "Épidémik" [Epidemik] (n.p.) experiment, embedded within this project, positions itself against normative structures and embraces an aesthetic of proliferation. The rebuses function as visual and semantic contagions, resisting containment and coherence, while promoting excess, multiplicity, and disruption. This approach resembles the broader patchwork logic of the material collection but insists that fragmentation and junction together become a method of critique and creative renewal—set in motion by the sprockets of the Super 8 metaphor.

In one of the rebuses, signed "Don Joël Hubaut de la Mancha" (n.p.), the artist adopts a quasi–fictional, autobiographical persona that playfully echoes Miguel de Cervantes's *Don Quixote*. This self–stylization not only reinforces the ludic and parodic dimensions of the work but simultaneously situates Hubaut within a lineage of errant creators—figures who challenge normative frameworks through absurdity, excess, and fictional reconfiguration, and to whom Luca also relates, particularly in his early works in Romania, both in French and in Romanian (Clonts, 2016, pp.

279–305; Clonts, 2020). By invoking this alter ego, Hubaut blurs the boundaries between author and character, autobiography and fiction. This gesture goes along with the broader ethos of *Satyre et Satrape*, where identity, language, and meaning are continually destabilized through hybrid forms and proliferating signs. In an autobiographical work, Hubaut writes: "Interdisciplinarity seems natural to me against this imposed formatting. In an attempt to react to the conditioning of daily bureaucracy, I transform the word epidemic with a K in reference to Kafka, Mr. K., The Metamorphosis[19]." (*Re-mix épidémik—Esthétique de la dispersion*, p. 41)

Facing the rebuses, Luca's poem is laid out with spacious restraint, offering a stark graphic contrast to the dense, image-saturated rebuses. Despite the sobriety of the text, Luca revisits the procedure he termed "apostroph'apocalypse"—based on the title of his book *Apostroph'Apocalypse* (1967) with fourteen etchings by Wifredo Lam[20]. Here, the apostrophe disrupts words, generating neologisms that functions as puns, such as "je t'ouche" [I t'ouch you] placed near "je t'aime" [I love you] (n.p.). The fragmentation and stitching of words materialize both the bodily dimension of love and the encounter with otherness. Through cutting and recombining language, Luca produces a semantic rupture that opens space for new meanings to emerge. Yet, the apparent contrast between the poet's restrained layout and the visual artist's exuberant rebuses is superficial. The apostrophe, as a poetic device, enacts a process of deconstruction and reconstruction that implicates both writing and reading. Like the rebus, it demands an active interpretative engagement, inviting the reader to navigate and to participate in the creation of drifting and mobile meanings.

François Lyotard studied the complex interactions between discourse and figure, challenging the primacy of linguistic structures in meaning production. In his view, discourse—understood as rational, sequential, and syntactically governed—tends to suppress the figural, which operates through visual, affective, and spatial modalities. The figure resists discursive containment, introducing ruptures, intensities, and ambiguities that cannot be fully articulated through language alone. This tension between the discursive and the figural opens up space for aesthetic experience, where meaning is not fixed but emerges through the intertwinement of signs, sensations, and forms:

> *We can follow the recessus of speech [...] because there is anti–speech in speech, seeing within saying, continuity within articulation, difference even within opposition. A regressive inflection rather reflection, the opposite of dialectics [...]. One can follow it, and one must follow it, because it is precisely this mobility, introduced into the order of invariant spacings, that can reveal them: the ironic contribution of dead Eros to Eros–Logos. How the two forms of negation intersect, how that of showing can enter into the act of discoursing, how the text can become figure[21] [...]. (Lyotard, p. 60).*

Echoing Lyotard's reflections on the tension between discourse and figure, Luca's "apostroph'apocalysed" text and Hubaut's daily rebuses transform the temporality of reading—and thus of meaning—into a process of ongoing deconstruction and reconstruction. The reader is invited to navigate fragments of text and image, assembling and reassembling them into a dynamic, open–ended whole. Meaning emerges not as fixed or linear, but as fragmentary, uncertain, and mobile. In becoming a kind of expansive, collaborative rebus, the work deliberately cultivates ambiguity and resists closure, privileging the indeterminate and the in–between. Both artists substitute conventional elements—whether linguistic, social or image—with material drawn from elsewhere, displacing normative structures and opening space for alternative modes of signification.

Unlike the conventional rebus, Luca and Hubaut's work resists the idea of a singular, 'correct' reading. Instead, it foregrounds the interpretative operations the reader might perform—homonymy, graphic equivalence, lexical displacement into graphic space, redivision of the sonorous chain, fragmentation, and collage. These techniques disrupt the automatic processes of recognition that typically facilitate rapid comprehension, deliberately slowing down the act of reading. In doing so, the artists shift the focus from communication to signification, emphasizing displacements and peripheric pathways within a space that remains fundamentally open and under construction. The rebus, in this context, becomes a site of semantic play and figural excess, where meaning is not delivered but continually deferred and reconfigured.

CONCLUSION: TOWARD A POETICS OF BODY–MIND INTERACTIONS

Ghérasim Luca's artistic praxis, centered on the obsessive gesture of the "manic hand," offers a compelling model for holistic body–mind engagement. Through his manipulation of language, images, and found objects, Luca constructs a poetics of transformation that resists fixed representation and hegemonic norms. His cubomanies, homemade albums, and Objectively Offered Objects (O.O.O.) do not merely reflect reality—they actively reconfigure it, inviting viewers and readers into a participatory space of affective and cognitive renewal. This reconfiguration moves beyond traditional artistic boundaries and enters the space of embodied practice. Luca's practices—cutting, assembling, collaging—are not only aesthetic but therapeutic, fostering emotional resilience, sensory awareness, and epistemic dissent. By highlighting fragmentation, rhythm, and relationality, his creations become sites of healing—not through normative restoration, but through the affirmation of multiplicity and imaginative freedom.

At the heart of this transformative process lies a profound inquiry into the nature of the self. Luca interrogates the idea of a fixed, stable identity by engaging the body as both a medium and a site of metamorphosis. His expression of the "manic hand"—a performative, obsessive gesture—embodies this dynamic. The hand becomes a symbolic extension of the self, enacting a continual process of making and remaking identity. This is illustrated in Luca's cubomanies, which disrupt visual order and challenge the idea of representation as a mirror of reality. Instead, they propose a fluid, tactile engagement with the world, where the self is shaped through interaction, rhythm, and variation. Similarly, in *Le Tangage de ma langue*, the collaborative and reconfigurable format of the handmade album reflects a self that is mobile, unstable, and relational. The poetic and visual fragments resist resolution, suggesting that identity is not a solitary construct but a constellation of connections—"oneself as another," in Paul Ricoeur's terms. Further extending this relational view of the self, Luca's O.O.O.s function as bridges between individuals, between humans and objects, and between humans, objects, and a wider environment. These assemblages are not merely expressions of the maker's unconscious; they are invitations to dialogue. The self here is externalized, projected, and received—always in flux, always in relation.

Through these artistic strategies, Luca cultivates emotional resilience not by resolving tension, but by embracing ambiguity and transformation. From flea market finds to outdated colonial photography, his use of fragmented and recycled materials recontextualizes silenced histories and 'minor' forms of life, that is, persecuted, traumatized, marginalized or understated forms of life. This act of re–seeing and re–making fosters emotional endurance, allowing the viewer to confront discomfort, contradiction, and complexity without retreating into fixed narratives. Equally important is the haptic dimension of Luca's work. Especially in cubomanies and dot drawings, the viewer's body engages in a sensory dialogue. The eye becomes a hand, tracing movement and rhythm, activating motor imagery and embodied perception. This tactile–optical interaction supports sensory awareness, encouraging deeper attunement to the nuances of experience. Moreover, Luca's emphasis on non–linear reading, semantic play—sometimes with figural excess—opens new paths of comprehension, slows automatic recognition, and invites introspection. This deliberate disruption cultivates a reflective space where emotional and cognitive responses are not dictated but discovered.

Considering these practices, this chapter—though framed within an academic format—seeks to honor Luca's ethos of non–hegemonic perceptions of creation. As his work enters institutional spaces—museums, textbooks, theatres—it faces canonization, a process that Luca did not especially praise. Yet, as Dick Hebdige reminds us, no form remains eternally normalized. Luca's legacy, rooted in subcultural mediation and poetic recycling, continues to offer fertile ground for new diversions, new meanings, and new forms of life. Luca's "manic hand" exemplifies a holistic practice where making becomes a mode of being. It challenges us to rethink the boundaries between art and life, self and other, perception and creation. In the context of Luca's work, well–being can be understood as a dynamic and relational state of being that is generated through creative engagement with the world—where the body and mind are not separate entities but co–constitutive forces. It is not defined by stability or harmony but by the capacity to navigate fragmentation, ambiguity, and transformation with imaginative freedom. This form of well–being privileges sensory awareness, emotional openness, and the continual reconfiguration of the self in relation to others and to the material world.

REFERENCES

Bonnechère, B. (2017). Revalidation physique, entraînez le cerveau. *Medecine Sciences*, *33*, 887–890. PMID: 28994385

Carlat, D. (1998). *Gherasim Luca l'intempestif.* José Corti.

Chacon, Q. (2020). *La Préparation mentale au service du sportif blessé.* Master thesis, STAPS, Université de Bretagne.

Clonts, C. (2016). L'Avant–garde bucarestoise: Alge, de la revue à l'affiche. In *LiVres de pOésie Jeux d'eSpace* (pp. 279–305). Honoré Champion.

Clonts, C. (2020). *Gherasim Luca: Texte, Image, Son.* Peter Lang. DOI: 10.3726/b17339

Clonts, C. (2021). La Poésie Pratique de Ghérasim Luca. *Études des Lettres Françaises*, 56, 15–32. DOI: 10.20767/ELFK.56.0_15

Deleuze, G. (1981). *Francis Bacon—Logic of Sensation* (Vol. 1). La Différence.

Hebdige, D. (1994). *Subculture, the meaning of style.* Routlege.

Herrera, B.M., & Vargas, P.C. (2019). Benefits of Mental Practice in Sport Practice. *Apunts. Educació Física i Esports*, 35 (135), 82–99. DOI: 10.5672/apunts.2014-0983.es

Hubaut, J. (2006). *Joël Hubaut, Re–mix épidémik—Esthétique de la dispersion.* Les Presses du Réel.

Leibovici, F. (2007). *Des Documents poétiques.* Al Dante / Questions théoriques.

Lévi–Strauss, C. (1962). *La Pensée sauvage.* Plon.

Luca, G. (1962). *Ghérasim Luca.* Ghérasim Luca Archives, Bibliothèque Littéraire Doucet.

Luca, G. (2001). Le Tangage de ma langue. In *Gherasim Luca by Gherasim Luca.* José Corti / Rien de Commun, 2 CDs.

Luca, G. (2001). *Le Vampire passif.* José Corti. (Original work published 1945)

Luca, G. (2008). *Série Brésil.* CipM, sixteen plates.

Luca, G., & Catti, M. (post–1953). *Le Tangage de ma langue.* Ghérasim Luca Archives, Bibliothèque Littéraire Doucet.

Luca, G., & Hérold, J. (1953). *Héros–limite.* Le Soleil Noir.

Luca, G., & Hubaut, J. (1987). *Satyr and Satrap—Rebus Super 8*. Éditions de la C.R.E.M.

Luca, G., & Lam, W. (1967). *Apostroph'apocalypse*. Giorgio Upiglio.

Luca, G., & Trost, D. (1945). *Présentation de Graphies Colorées, Cubomanies et Objets*. Brezoianu Hall Exhibition.

Lyotard, J.-F. (1971). *Discours, Figure*. Klincksieck.

Meschonnic, H. (1982). *Critique du rythme—Anthropologie historique du langage*. Verdier/poche.

Nancy, J.-L. (2000). *Corpus*. Métailié.

Nerval, G. (2005). *Les Chimères, La Bohème galante, Petits Châteaux de Bohème*. Poésie/Gallimard. (Original work published 1854)

Perret, C. (2019). *Le Temps de l'œuvre*. Éditions de la Sorbonne.

Saillant, F., & Araujo, A. L. (2007). Slavery in Brazil: The work of the black movement. *Ethnologie française. Presses Universitaires de France*, *37*(3), 457–466.

ENDNOTES

1 From now on, the French neologism *cubomanie* will be translated as "cubomanie" when referring to the object of art, and as "cubomania" when referring to the practice or the thought leading to the object of art. All the translations from French to English in this chapter are mine. For an example of cubomanie, see Wikiart, https://www.wikiart.org/en/gherasim-luca/cubomanie-24 [accessed June 19, 2025].

2 Translated from French: "la cubomanie est le correspondant oculaire instantané de notre comportement vis-à-vis du monde extérieur, comportement qui consiste dans le refus de regarder comme une réalité objective l'axiomatique condition humaine même sous ses aspects apparemment immuables."

3 Translated from French: les "figures-images" qui "déconstrui[sent] le percept" et "s'accompli[ssent] dans un espace de differénce".

4 Translated from French: "zone absolue d'indiscernabilité ou d'indétermination objective, qui oppose et impose à la vue une puissance manuelle déchaînée".

5 Translated from French: "l'espace tactile-optique".

[6] The exact dates still remain uncertain. For an example of a plate, see Centre Pompidou, https://www.centrepompidou.fr/fr/ressources/oeuvre/c79B4B [accessed June 24, 2025].

[7] Translated from French: "les documents poétiques" dans lesquels on peut lire "les étapes instituantes, linguistiques et visuelles, de fabrication du monde" qui sont simultanément une forme de "technologie intellectuelle productrice de réel".

[8] For an example of O.O.O., see Wikiart, https://www.wikiart.org/en/gherasim-luca/illustration-for-le-vampire-passif-1945 [accessed June 24, 2025].

[9] Translated from the French: "sujet qui s'extériorise".

[10] Translated from the French: "sujet réceptif".

[11] Translated from French: "Mais les yeux seuls sont inutiles dans un univers dans lequel la lune est noire, et la prétention de séparer le perceptible de l'imperceptible ne compte pas sur le mécanisme secret de la rétine."

[12] Translated from French: "le pampre à la rose s'allie".

[13] Translated from French: "cœur désolé".

[14] Translated from French: "L'humanité en panique se posait pour la première fois une question ressemblant à un lapsus: qu'est-ce qu'une oreille? Est-ce une coquille? un piège? une boucle? un écho? L'anatomie quitte les vieux instruments hors d'usage et recherche une équivalence dans les ombres qu'elle jette à l'intérieur et à l'extérieur de l'homme comme un masque vivant."

[15] I borrow this expression from Yves Peyré, *Peinture et Poésie*, 2001.

[16] See Clonts, 2020 for a developed analysis on the complete work of Luca, especially his collaborations with other artists and his handcrafted albums.

[17] Translated from the French: "ils ont servi, comme mots d'un discours que la réflexion mythique 'démonte', à la façon du bricoleur soignant les pignons d'un vieux réveil démonté; et ils peuvent encore servir au même usage ou à un usage différent pour peu qu'on les détourne de leur première fonction."

[18] Translated from French: "REBUS = (sécrétion → signaux hybrides épars)"; "énergie des mots-images (super 8)".

[19] Translated from French: "L'interdisciplinarité m'apparaît naturelle contre ces formatages imposés. Pour tenter de réagir au conditionnement de la bureaucratie

quotidienne, je transforme le mot épidémie par un K en référence à Kafka, monsieur K., La Métamorphose."

20 See Khalfa (ed.), *Wifredo Lam–Artist's Books*, 2025, Jean-Michel Place, for an extensive study on Luca's collaboration with the Cuban painter Wifredo Lam. See esp. Clonts, "Wifredo Lam et Ghérasim Luca: Apostroph'apocalypse / Wifredo Lam and Ghérasim Luca: Apostroph'Apocalypse", pp. 216-264.

21 Translated from French: "On peut suivre le recessus de la parole [...] parce qu'il y a de l'anti-parole dans la parole, du voir dans le dire, du continu dans l'articulé, de la différence jusque dans l'opposition. Flexion régressiste plutôt réflexion, le contraire de la dialectique [...]. On peut le suivre et on doit le suivre parce que c'est justement cette mobilité qui, introduite dans l'ordre des écartements invariants, peut les déceler: ironique contribution d'Éros mort à Éros-Logos. Comment les deux formes de la négation se recoupent, comment celle du montrer peut entrer dans celle du discourir, comment le texte peut se faire figure [...]."

Chapter 8
The Way of Sound:
Music as a Transformative Experience

Stefano Lombardi Vallauri
http://orcid.org/0000-0002-0253-6162
IULM University, Milan, Italy

ABSTRACT

The belief that music, both as a performing practice and as listening, can function as a way of physical-psycho-spiritual self-transformation crosses eras and cultures. From this perspective the chapter discusses the work of five contemporary classical Italian composers: Giacinto Scelsi, Luigi Nono, Domenico Guaccero, Salvatore Sciarrino, and Dario Buccino. All five organize a music-making and a musical form that urge the performer on one side and the listener on the other, each in their own way also physically involved, to open the perception to free configurations of sound, purified from the emotional and rational encrustations –often historical style elements– which hinder the full experience of the here and now. Consciousness opens to the liberated sound, immerses itself in the sound flow and, conforming to it, thus liberates itself in turn. The different conception of each composer, inherent to both vocal and instrumental performance (as well as possibly to improvisation and theatre), is examined in its technical specificity.

1. BRIEF EXPOSITION

The belief that music—both as a performing practice and as listening—can function as a way of physical-psycho-spiritual self-transformation spans eras and cultures, Western and Eastern alike, from the Pythagorean school (Guanti, 1999, pp. 11–23) and the Indian treatise *Nā yaśāstra* (Higgins, 2003; Magno, 2009) to today's

DOI: 10.4018/979-8-3373-3521-6.ch008

transcultural integrations. From this perspective, this study examines the work of five contemporary Italian composers active in so-called "classical experimental" music: Giacinto Scelsi, Luigi Nono, Domenico Guaccero, Salvatore Sciarrino, and Dario Buccino. Each of them articulates a musical practice and a formal conception that engage both performer and listener—each physically involved in their own way—in opening perception to free configurations of sound, purified from the emotional and rational encrustations (often elements of historical styles) that hinder the full experience of the here and now. In short, what occurs is that consciousness opens to liberated sound, immerses itself in the flow of sound, and, by conforming to it, liberates itself in turn. Each composer's individual conception, inherent in both vocal and instrumental performance (as well as in some cases improvisation and theatre), entails distinct stylistic and technical characteristics, that call for focused reflection.

2. TERMINOLOGICAL CLARIFICATION

I use the term *physical-psycho-spiritual* to indicate that the three levels of human experience—physical, psychological, and spiritual—while certainly distinct, also form a unified whole. In some circumstances, separating the bodily, the psychological, and the spiritual dimensions prevents a deep understanding of the experience itself. Using a now widespread term, one might say that the experience is *holistic*. But the term *holistic* lacks, by definition (or rather, by vocation), the capacity to articulate the distinct components that constitute the unity. Conversely, the compound terms *psychophysical* and *psychospiritual*, although also common, fail to fully convey the complete unity of certain experiences that involve body, mind (*psyché*), and spirit in an integrated way. By spirit, I refer to that aspect of mental experience that is distinct from the psychological, as it concerns conceptions that are also intellectual in nature, relating to the meaning of human existence and, more broadly, of the world.

3. MEANING AND VALUE OF MUSIC

The question of the physical-psycho-spiritual value of music is intertwined with the ancient aesthetic-semiotic question about the meaning of music. Value and meaning are not the same thing. We can define the value of something as the manner and measure in which that something is important to someone; and meaning as what something—through a process of semiotic transposition—represents, rather than simply being literally itself. For example, the meaning of a sentence is the concept it conveys, a concept that is ontologically distinct and different from the sentence itself, whether the sentence is a string of phonemes in spoken language, a string of graphemes in written language, or a string of dots and dashes in Morse code, and so on.

That music holds value for a great many human beings is not a controversial fact. Although some thinkers and philosophers—such as Kant (Guanti, 1999, pp. 242–248)—have questioned this, it does not change the reality that, in the lives of countless individuals and human groups, music plays an important and sometimes extremely important role. What is controversial, instead, is the question of the meaning of music. It is presumably the most debated issue in the millennia of reflection on music in the West, and no less persistently in recent decades.[1] In a very brief summary, the debate can be reduced to two positions. The formalist position maintains that music is the organization of pure sound forms, that it is not a sign of something else, and therefore does not have meaning. The most obvious reason for this view is that music does not function like language, which is the primary model for all human systems of signification; and the clearest clue supporting this view is that, indeed, if one tries to say what a segment of music means, one cannot do so—at least not in the way one can state the meaning of a linguistic utterance. The expressivist position holds that, although music does not function and signify in the same way as language, it nonetheless does generate in listeners certain psychological experiences and mental representations that are ontologically distinct and different from the music itself. In a broad sense, these experiences and representations could be understood as the meaning of music.

It is interesting that the most historically recurring argument used to deny that music has value is its (supposed) lack of meaning. Not that anyone confuses the two characteristics. But according to this view, the domain of meaning—the realm of conceptualizing and verbalizing reason—is where the humanity of human beings is expressed at the highest level. Therefore, music, although it belongs to the noble category of the fine arts, is not considered to have the same dignity as other arts, such as the linguistic or visual ones, since it is not, like them, capable of representing objects or concepts.

In any case, setting aside for a moment the question of whether and how music has meaning or not, music still has value precisely because and to the extent that human beings, rightly or wrongly, attribute meaning to it due to the experiences it evokes in them. One piece of music—for example, a Beethoven sonata—may have value because, by attentively following its formal development with rational focus, I form a mental representation of it (a meaning?), which I consider beautiful, and since beauty has value, music too has value (NB: personally, I find such a description of the experience of listening to a Beethoven sonata reductive, but I present it here to do justice to the formalists' position); another piece of music—for example, an improvisation by the Dagar Brothers—may have value because, by following and emotionally engaging with the gradual unfolding of the sound events over time, my consciousness attunes to their expressiveness (a meaning?), and I reach a desirable psychophysical state, and since a positive mood has value, music too has value (NB: I also find this description of a musical experience reductive); yet another piece of music—for example, a Stevie Wonder song—may have value because, while listening to it with my ears, through the decoding performed by the brain (a meaning?), yet my whole body feels invited to follow its rhythmic and phrasing patterns by dancing, and since dancing has value, music too has value (NB: I also find this description reductive). And so on.

Thus, even hypothetically admitting that music has no meaning, music still has value because of the value people attribute to the experiences it fosters. Regardless of whether music possesses spiritual meanings or not, if music itself fosters spiritual experiences, then music has spiritual value. I do not intend here to argue my position in the debate on the meaning of music in a detailed manner. I only assert, apodictically, that I consider music to be endowed with meaning, and that in the present reflection I will treat it accordingly. Therefore, without any difficulty, all the more so, I recognize spiritual value in it.

There are three distinct levels on which it happens that meaning is attributed to music, and consequently, value as well: (1) formal level; (2) content level; (3) pragmatic level.

1) On the formal level, meaning is found within the music itself—namely, in its aesthetic form, that is, in its perceived material structure.
2) On the content level, music is endowed with meaning by association; it is not the music itself that possesses meaning, but rather the meaning that is projected onto it, deriving from various external strata (language, video, etc.) associated with music in a multi-artistic work.
3) The pragmatic level concerns the way music is actually created and situated within real-world circumstances. On this level, meaning is attributed to music based on the way it is realized in specific contexts—interpersonal, social, economic, and so on.

That said, I am stating here what is only my belief: there exist certain types of music whose experience, when fully realized, can serve as a path toward physical-psycho-spiritual improvement for the individual, insofar as they influence both philosophical worldview and concrete daily behavior.

Let us now consider, one by one, the cases of the five composers listed.

3a. Giacinto Scelsi (1905–1988)

Scelsi was a practitioner. He was familiar with and engaged in Eastern physical-psycho-spiritual disciplines, such as yoga and meditation (Fondazione Isabella Scelsi, n.d.). He willingly involved the instrumentalists who performed his music in practice sessions aimed at achieving a physical-psycho-spiritual state that he deemed appropriate—not only in accordance with the ethical principles governing daily life, but also with those he believed governed the very nature of musical creation. Scelsi was convinced that music connects this world with an otherworldly plane from which it originates; as a composer, he did not see himself as a creator, but rather as a medium through which music could manifest itself. In order for both himself and the performers to serve as such a medium, he considered essential what we might call a form of personal attunement—something to be cultivated through the aforementioned practices.

But are we required to share Scelsi's metaphysical beliefs in order to attribute a physical-psycho-spiritual dimension to his music? Absolutely not. First and foremost, because in my view those beliefs are not at all credible (the burden of proof that an otherworldly plane exists—and that anything, including music, might descend from it into this world—lies entirely with those who make such claims, and such claims have never been substantiated). More importantly, however, these are meanings attached to the music from the outside; they are extrinsic, not inherent to the music itself. It is far more interesting when the physical-psycho-spiritual quality of music derives from its very mode of being and functioning, independently of any declarations by the composer or anyone else.

Scelsi's music, in its mature stylistic phase, consists in the magnification—even through large ensembles such as the orchestra—of the smallest salient sonic phenomenon. This phenomenon is smaller even than a single discrete sound; rather, it is a subtle difference emerging within the sound itself. Thus, for example, his music may present itself as the orchestral thickening of a single pitch—a solitary note—expanded into a vast bundle of sounds with varying timbres, dynamic intensities, temporal movements, and even slightly different pitch levels (through microtonal discrepancies). This technique endows the sound with an exceptional degree of presence, a kind of material and perceptual vividness. A human consciousness that focuses on such a sound, immersing itself in this flow of sonic energy, is called upon to respond with maximal sensitivity to minimal stimuli. This act of magnifying nuance—the microacoustic element—of emphasizing and solemnizing it to the point of transforming it into the eruption of an entire sonic cosmos, closely resembles the intensification of present experience characteristic of Tantric practice (Gnoli, 1994) (if one wishes to associate Scelsi's music with a specific tradition, although his spirituality was, in truth, eclectic).

3b. Luigi Nono (1924–1990)

Nono was a committed atheist communist. On paper, therefore, he would be considered an adversary of physical-psycho-spiritual practices, which are not necessarily—but often are—linked to religious, even metaphysical beliefs, and in any case are oriented toward individual self-work rather than the improvement of society on economic and material levels. However, his music, especially that of his late period (beginning in the late 1970s), takes a different turn. While the political motivation for societal improvement remains recognizable, it is pursued through the awakening of individual consciousness. According to Nono himself, the opening of consciousness is achieved through the opening of perception (Nono, 2001c). On the compositional level, this entails dwelling on nuance, on the smallest difference inherent in pitch intervals, timbre, and dynamics. As in Scelsi, albeit in a different manner, this means acknowledging the maximum importance of the minimum detail.

Moreover, in his late period, Nono also altered his typical compositional process by incorporating elements of improvisation. He often had his collaborating instrumentalists perform and improvise while being recorded, after which he would process the sonic material they produced into electroacoustic pieces. Above all, he specialized in live electronics, a form of extemporaneity in which sound direction is guided by the same perceptual openness and sensitivity to nuance previously discussed. The interaction between instrumentalists and sound direction takes place within a condition of heightened perceptual openness to the smallest sonic event, thereby fostering a comparable liminal sensitivity in the listener.

3c. Domenico Guaccero (1927–1984)

To the best of my knowledge, Guaccero was the first composer to conceive the idea of what is now known as *art as a vehicle*, even anticipating the famous formulations of Jerzy Grotowski—not by chance, like Grotowski, through an approach that combines music and theatre (Lombardi Vallauri, 2015). A particularly relevant example is his musical theatre work *Rappresentazione et Esercizio* (1968), written for twelve performers (including six singers), which he described as an *azione sacra* [sacred action]—where the term *sacred* must be understood in a "rigorosamente laico e profano" [strictly secular and profane] sense (Guaccero, 2005b, p. 162; see also Mastropietro, 2020, pp. 374–382). Beyond the subtitle, the two key terms that define the work are those contained in the title itself: *Rappresentazione* [representation] and *Esercizio* [exercise].

The essential distinction should be noted: *Rappresentazione* corresponds to the most common model of theatre in the Western tradition, especially in its modern form—as a spectacle, something performed by those who do it and, etymologically, something seen by those who do not, representing a fundamentally aesthetic experience. *Esercizio*, by contrast, revives a model of theatre typical of the pre-modern West as well as of extra-Western traditions: something to be done, and to be done not only by the actors but also by the spectators, who are invited to participate. The intention is not purely aesthetic, but one of self-transformative practice (Grotowski, 2007; De Marinis, 2000, pp. 246–251). What is of particular interest here is action rather than representation—specifically, action understood in terms of its potential for self-transformation on the part of the performer, even before considering its implications for the spectator.

Let us therefore examine the repertoire of actions performed by the performers in the work. Focusing first on vocal actions, we observe that the work explores a wide variety of vocal techniques, both singing and, above all, non-singing vocalizations. This requires the performers to become aware of the vast expressive range of the human voice—both artistic and *extra-daily*[2] as well as everyday—and in particular of their own individual and highly personal vocal apparatus. Moreover, another remarkable feature of this work is that each performer's repertoire of actions is broad not only in depth, but also across artistic genres. Thus, while Guaccero values the singularity of each interpreter, he simultaneously emphasizes their universality, asking each of them to transcend the limits of their own specialization (singer, actor, mime, dancer) in order to become total performers.

In *Rappresentazione et Esercizio*, across all layers of its musical-theatrical form, performers are called to a form of engagement that involves them comprehensively and holistically—as body, mind, and spirit, as individuals and as participants in a relational dynamic—toward a process of perceptual awakening and the refinement of cognitive and emotional faculties. This type of involvement is not unlike that promoted by various human traditions as tools for ethical self-development (such as meditation, yoga, and "internal" martial arts): music and theatre are conceived here essentially as *action*, as action undertaken by the performers upon themselves, aimed at transforming their way of being in the world (Lombardi Vallauri, 2017b).

3d. Salvatore Sciarrino (1947)

Salvatore Sciarrino is a master of liminality (Lombardi Vallauri, 2024). For him, the threshold between sound and silence constitutes an entirely natural habitat—somewhere to remain, to linger, without any concern that the sound might fail to be heard. In his poetics, there is no such risk. The risk that Sciarrino actively avoids, rather, is that of failing to contribute to the sharpening of the listener's perceptive faculties. Being in proximity to silence heightens perception, and thereby opens up consciousness (the self): I perceive the slightest hint of sound; I realize, at the same time, that what I hear is indeed a mere hint; I recognize that this hint—though minimal—is nonetheless a salient event (on a cognitive and emotional level as well as a perceptual one); I may even conclude that the hint, the slightest difference—not only in sound—is something that deserves to be understood and respected, something to *be*, and something to *love*. To linger on the threshold, at the passage between silence and sound, between nothingness and matter and form, thus becomes the foundation of what has been described as Sciarrino's "ecological" stance: an openness of consciousness to the world.

Such an orientation is also evident in his decision to embrace the elective presence of another, equally significant threshold: that between pitched sound and noise. Sciarrino is renowned for his musical recognition of sounds that had, for centuries, been excluded from Western musical culture: the anomalous, residual, noisy, and defective sounds produced by musical instruments—or even by non-musical objects. In this case, the recognition and simultaneous dismantling of the threshold—it is noise, yes, but it is also music—entails the acceptance of disorder, of the untamable, as a source of spiritual richness.

3e. Dario Buccino (1968)

Buccino has developed a composition system called the "HN system," that is, "*hic et nunc* (here and now) system" (Buccino, 2006), in which the physical-psycho-spiritual work primarily concerns the performer and subsequently the listener. Buccino's writing is a type of "action notation," rather than result notation; that is, it indicates to instrumentalists not—or not only—the desired sound outcomes, but the bodily actions necessary to achieve them. Furthermore, these actions are conceived to constitute a profound ignition of consciousness—consciousness in the body, specifically the body of the musician as a human being, even more than as an instrumentalist.

Buccino aims to transform musical action into sound, and to transform into musical action the bodily act of a person whose present psychophysical experience is at its most ignited, made incandescent by adherence to a flow that is at once free and open, because partly improvised (decided *hic et nunc*), and also perfect, because partly determined according to highly demanding compositional criteria. He seeks to combine the aesthetic merits of extemporaneity with those of thoughtful selectivity (Lombardi Vallauri, 2011). He goes beyond standard instrumentalism and calls on the musician to transcend themselves and to become—as one might say in yoga or Advaita terminology (though this is not Buccino's jargon)—a "living liberated": a being freed from the smallness of the ego and from the automatisms of the mind.

The composer's long-standing experimental work with performers on the variables of sound, performance, and experience fosters a process of global personal development—not only musical—for both him and the musicians. In turn, through participation in a total act rather than a form, the listener is invited to become a "testimone" [witness] to "un'esperienza vitale del tempo" [a vital experience of time] (Buccino, 2005, p. 4), and possibly to share in the transformation. In this sense, it is also relevant to invoke the category of embodied empathy, as we can assume that the spectator of a Buccino performance experiences a pre-rational understanding of the bodily actions performed by the musicians, through an identification with their movements made possible by the brain mechanism of mirror neurons. These, as is well known, are neurons that fire both when a person performs an action and when they merely observe or hear it—this latter point being especially significant in the case of musical actions (Lombardi Vallauri, 2012). The spectator's empathic adherence to bodily actions so dense with psychological and spiritual meaning is rare in the musical field, where actions—however refined—are for the most part strictly functional to the achievement of a sonic result, within an overall process in which the spiritual value lies more in the sonic outcome itself than in the means used to attain it (to return to the tripartition discussed in paragraph 3, it resides more on the level of form than on the pragmatic level).

4. ETHICAL MUSIC LISTENING

It may seem implausible that musical listening could be a practice conducive to psychospiritual self-transformation—that is to say, improvement. There are two main reasons for this skepticism. The first is that listening is commonly regarded as a passive activity: it requires no physical action, and the mind need only receive information coming from the outside. The second is that, even when directed toward spiritually elevated music, listening remains an essentially aesthetic activity—one that belongs to a domain of human experience considered superfluous by many, even frivolous, and therefore not suitable for positively influencing a person's practical ethos. (An extreme example sometimes cited to support this view is the notorious passion of Nazi officials for excellent music; but the counterproof is lacking: we do not know whether, had they not engaged in good musical listening, they might have been even more barbaric.)

1) On the first point, we may object that listening can be a practice that is anything but passive (Cavicchi, 2002). Who would call thinking passive? Listening is thinking—mental activity—as well as potentially bodily activity (the body may respond to music not only when dancing, but always, through virtual, embryonic, unexpressed movements that follow the rhythmic and phraseological flow, and the formal tensions unfolding in time). Listening is musical thought: musical, but thought; not linguistic, but still thought. Indeed, precisely because it is not linguistic—not tied to verbalization or conceptualization—musical listening is a kind of mental

(and bodily) activity particularly suited to engaging consciousness not at the level of explicit declarations of principle (which may be superficial or empty—the "preach" in "Practice what you preach"), but at the level of actual ethos: the level where reason, emotion, and motivation meet and converge in shaping action (the "practice" in that same phrase) (Lombardi Vallauri, 2016b).

2) On the second point, I would argue that although listening may indeed be entirely useless for a person's improvement, it is not impossible for it to be useful. Everything depends on the listener's willingness to be oriented—to allow their practical ethos to be influenced—by the teachings they derive from the listening experience. Like any other teaching, the teachings of music are seeds that can fall on rocky ground, or be cultivated with care and allowed to flourish. For example, it has been suggested that listening to opera may serve as a form of emotional education (Bianconi, 2008), since opera deals primarily with emotions—especially on the level of content (that is, the linguistic and representational meanings associated with music), but also on the level of musical form, which is capable of supporting and powerfully amplifying that content. The same could be said, for instance, of the song genre; or of cinema, which makes extensive and essential use of music. As for the music of the composers discussed here, in a similar vein, it is plausible to suggest that it may serve as a form of psychospiritual education. It constitutes what might be called an ethical invitation.

It is so in its very form, which, through the organization of sound, represents: the collapse of dogmatic certainties (musically, through the rejection of uncritically inherited elements of traditional compositional systems); the disposition to live the present moment intensely—the here and now—rather than to revisit the past pointlessly or project oneself anxiously into the future (through the abandonment of teleological form, as well as of tonal and modal melodic-harmonic tensions); the inclination to find value in the quality of infinitesimal events, seemingly insignificant but in fact forming the very fabric of the present (through the appreciation of the slightest perceptual differences—of pitch, timbre, dynamics); the affirmation that everything that exists is worthy of contemplation, simply because it exists (through the adoption of a universal listening attitude, open to all kinds of sound, not only those traditionally considered musical); the acceptance of reality, free from the individual's vain desire to control it—what Buddhism calls *choiceless awareness* (through allowing musical form to be determined by processes not governed by the composer); a prolonged and patient concentration on recurring events, such as breathing (through formal construction based on a dialectic between repetition and modular micro-variation); ultimately, freedom (through the sum of all these elements, which liberate composition from the constraints of convention). These are all psychospiritual principles akin to those encouraged and cultivated by traditional wisdom paths and by physical-psycho-spiritual practices from the East—as well as, increasingly, from the West.

In addition, in the work of these composers, any extramusical content associated with the musical form—whether found in linguistic texts, paratexts, or within a representational and/or narrative theatrical layer—also constitutes an ethical invitation. And so do pragmatic factors: for instance, the fact that, at times and in various ways or stages, the creative process includes a certain degree of improvisation—that is, the immersion of open consciousness in the unbiased flow of the present moment (in the cases of Scelsi, late Nono, some works by Guaccero, and Buccino); or the de-specialization of performers (in *Rappresentazione et Esercizio* by Guaccero, and in some works by Buccino), where the required actions are not solely musical, but also choreographic and theatrical—in short, fully human actions (Lombardi Vallauri, 2016a). Thus, in conclusion, this reveals that beyond what could be called a "vertical" holistic integration—of body, mind, and spirit—these musical works also promote a "horizontal" holistic integration across the various domains of human artistic (and even non-artistic) action.

5. CAGEAN LEGACY

> *Thus, the composers [...] on whom the culture industry has fixated, offering glossy and sweetened versions in order to weaken their historical significance, are precisely those who point toward the liberation of sound and, through it, the possibility of glimpsing the liberation of both the subject and the social sphere. In these musicians—such as Feldman, Scelsi, Nono, and Cage—the core of speculation is not technique or style, but rather the reflection on ethical form, on the persuasive power that the organization of sound exerts on society, on the listening subject, and on the composer's responsibility.*[3] *(Incardona, 2018, p. 124)*

John Cage (1912–1992) is the twentieth-century composer—and perhaps the composer of all time—whose influence has been most decisive specifically in the ethical domain, in addition to the musical and, more broadly, artistic spheres. From our perspective, what makes him truly central is that the ethical significance and value of his paradigm are entirely embedded within the music itself: in its form, in its pragmatic dimensions, as well as in the conceptual content he explicitly articulated (through writings, interviews, and so forth). All five of the composers we consider here work within a context in which Cagean conceptions are well present to all. And with the exception of Scelsi (due both to his age and to a certain distance from the mainstream circuits of contemporary music),[4] the other four composers may each be seen, in different ways, as heirs to Cage.

To assert this about Nono might seem fallacious and even irreverent, given that Nono's aversion to Cage's technical-stylistic positions—indeterminate and aleatory, and therefore, in Nono's view, absolving the composer of responsibility toward his societal commitment, which for him was non-negotiable—is well known (Nono, 2001b, 2001c)[5]. However, the truth is that over time Nono's attitude changed radically, and although belatedly and perhaps in an apocryphal form—in the sense that one could say Cagean ideas were circulating "in the air"—he nevertheless came to embrace Cage's teaching. In Nono's case, this teaching consists, at minimum, in a degree of spontaneity within the creative process, achieved through collaboration between the composer and performers, who are partially called upon to improvise (albeit within strict compositional guidelines); and in the dissolution of formal teleological tensions in favor of immersion in an extended, contemplative present time.

Unlike Nono, Guaccero instead embraces Cage's teachings extensively, frequently invoking him—indeed more than any other composer—even in his writings (Guaccero, 2005a). Presumably, Guaccero's approach to the despecialization of performers is also related to Cage's breaking down of boundaries between the arts (see his openness to gesture, dance, visual arts, sound poetry, up to the extreme case of happenings). Above all, the cluster of *alea*/indeterminacy/improvisation, along with the related issues concerning notation and graphic notation, constitutes a central set of compositional problems in Guaccero's reflection and work, always ideally referencing Cage and consistently oriented toward the liberation of musical practice.

Sciarrino, of a subsequent generation, is immersed in Cagean influence transmitted through his initial models Franco Evangelisti and Sylvano Bussotti (Lombardi Vallauri, 2017a), who, despite being diametrically opposed to each other, both deeply embrace Cage—particularly regarding the indeterminacy of the work, the inclination toward residual sounds (extra-instrumental, especially Evangelisti), the form achieved through repetition (especially Evangelisti), the ateleological present, and the inventiveness of graphic notation (especially Bussotti). Except for indeterminacy—since the form of his pieces is always determined—Sciarrino incorporates all these Cagean elements: he composes through graphic processes, emphasizes residual sounds, and creates temporal form through varied repetition that produces an extended, elegantly unsentimental present.

Buccino also derives fundamental elements of his compositional conception from Cage (Lombardi Vallauri, 2013). First and foremost, partial indeterminacy at all structural levels, and the consequent amount of improvisation, which he organizes through the "HN System" and which, as noted above, aims not only to open musical form but also to generate elevated physical-psycho-spiritual experiences. Another Cagean element is the integration of noise—or rather, any kind of sound, including extra-musical sounds—into music. This openness carries not only aesthetic implications, as it expands the boundaries of what can be considered artistic material, but also ethical ones, because it abolishes the hierarchy of values represented by the traditional classification of artistic materials. Such classification regards noise—which actually is nothing but unpitched sound—as something insufficiently noble to constitute the foundational material of a piece, whereas it is simply acoustically complex sound, thus not reducible to scales, exceeding the cultural systems of rationalizing material, and therefore, in a certain sense, wild, untamable (Arbo, 2004). In Buccino's output—particularly during a period when he himself often performed as a percussionist—there is an abundance of pieces for ensembles that include a type of steel sheet capable of responding to the impulses of the entire human body, from head to toe, across a range spanning from maximum violence to maximum subtlety, with timbral-articulative possibilities that are highly varied. This very total bodily involvement serves as a means to work on the performer's entire physical-psycho-spiritual wholeness. Finally, Buccino attributes to Cage a formal conception—which he adopts alongside others (including the opposing one)—that constructs musical form as a proposal rather than a constraint: that is, events are not made to follow one another according to criteria of an (alleged) necessity, logical and coercive, which would also be constraining for the listener, who, in order to respond appropriately, *must*—so to speak—continuously conform their consciousness to that same logic; instead, events are allowed to follow one another in absolute freedom, so the listener can attend to the constructive logic but also disregard it, simply dwelling in the flow of sounds with a freely contemplative attitude.

REFERENCES

Arbo, A. (2004). Breve storia del rumore, da Rousseau a Grisey. *Musicalia. Annuario internazionale di studi musicologici, 1*, 29–51. http://www.libraweb.net/riviste.php?chiave=52&h=432&w=300

Barba, E., & Savarese, N. (1996). *L'arte segreta dell'attore: Un dizionario di antropologia teatrale*. Argo.

Bianconi, L. (2008). La forma musicale come scuola dei sentimenti. In La Face Bianconi, G., & Frabboni, F. (Eds.), *Educazione musicale e formazione* (pp. 85–120). FrancoAngeli.

Buccino, D. (2005). *Ma vero* [Unpublished dossier]. Retrieved from http://www.dariobuccino.com

Buccino, D. (2006). *Sistema HN* [Online article]. Retrieved from http://www.dariobuccino.com

Cavicchi, D. (2002). From the bottom up: Thinking about Tia DeNora's Music in Everyday Life. *Action, Criticism, and Theory for Music Education, 1*(2). https://act.maydaygroup.org/volume-1-issue-2

De Marinis, M. (2000). *In cerca dell'attore. Un bilancio del Novecento teatrale*. Bulzoni.

Fondazione Isabella Scelsi. (n.d.). *Biography of Giacinto Scelsi*. Fondazione Isabella Scelsi. Retrieved from https://www.scelsi.it/en/biography/

Gnoli, R. (1994). *Iniziazione= Kālacakra*. Adelphi.

Grotowski, J. (2007). Dalla compagnia teatrale a L'arte come veicolo (1993). In Attisani, A., & Biagini, M. (Eds.), *J. Grotowski, Testi 1968-1998* (pp. 89–113). Bulzoni.

Guaccero, D. (2005a). *"Un iter segnato". Scritti e interviste* (Mastropietro, A., Ed.). Ricordi-LIM.

Guaccero, D. (2005b). Postilla sul teatro musicale (1966). In Mastropietro, A. (Ed.), *D. Guaccero, "Un iter segnato". Scritti e interviste* (pp. 161–171). Ricordi-LIM.

Guanti, G. (1999). *Estetica musicale. La storia e le fonti*. La Nuova Italia.

Higgins, K. (2003). Comparative aesthetics. In Levinson, J. (Ed.), *The Oxford handbook of aesthetics* (pp. 679–692). Oxford University Press. DOI: 10.1093/oxfordhb/9780199279456.003.0040

Incardona, F. (2018). Presentazione (1989). In F. Incardona, *Scritti critici e di poetica* (S. Lombardi Vallauri, Ed.; with the collaboration of M. Crescimanno & M. Spagnolo; pp. 119–125). Aracne.

Lombardi Vallauri, S. (2011). Perfetta effimera accensione di vita: Formalizzazione sonora, performativa ed esperienziale nella musica di Dario Buccino. *Poli-Femo: Nuova serie di Lingua e Letteratura, 2*, 123–140.

Lombardi Vallauri, S. (2012). Azione fisica ed empatia nell'opera musicale-performativa di Dario Buccino. In C. Falletti & G. Sofia (Eds.), *Prospettive su teatro e neuroscienze: Dialoghi e sperimentazioni* (pp. 205–209). Bulzoni.

Lombardi Vallauri, S. (2013). Fedeli tradimenti: la ricezione cageana di tre compositori italiani nel Duemila. In Cuomo, V., & Distaso, L. V. (Eds.), *Il caso, il silenzio, la natura. La ricerca di John Cage* (pp. 41–59). Mimesis.

Lombardi Vallauri, S. (2015). L'*anti-opera* come veicolo: il teatro musicale come pratica autotrasformativa per il *performer*. In Ramerino, A. (Ed.), *Teatro e musica* (pp. 131–146). Bulzoni.

Lombardi Vallauri, S. (2016a). The composition of experience in the musical-holistic art of Dario Buccino. In A. Bratus & M. Lutzu (Eds.), *Dossier: "Analysis beyond notation in XXth and XXIst century music"* [Special issue]. *El Oído Pensante, 4*(1), 1–27. https://revistascientificas.filo.uba.ar/index.php/oidopensante/article/view/7531/6740

Lombardi Vallauri, S. (2016b). Sull'accompagnamento musicale del discorso filosofico. Sull'ascolto musicale come pratica sapienziale. In Bianchi, A. (Eds.), *Scritti per Luigi Lombardi Vallauri* (Vol. 1, pp. 793–807). Wolters Kluwer – CEDAM.

Lombardi Vallauri, S. (2017a). Interaction between noisy instrumental timbre and traditional intervallic systems in composers from Sicily, 1960–1985. In *Proceedings of the 9th European Music Analysis Conference*. In *EuroMAC 2017*. Université de Strasbourg., Retrieved from http://euromac2017.unistra.fr/wp-content/uploads/2017/05/Ext-lombardi-vallauri-stefano.pdf

Lombardi Vallauri, S. (2017b). Lo spazio teatrale-musicale come ambito di azione etica: *Rappresentazione et Esercizio* di Domenico Guaccero e *La Passion selon Sade* di Sylvano Bussotti. In G. Borio, G. Ferrari, & D. Tortora (a cura di), *Teatro di avanguardia e composizione sperimentale per la scena in Italia: 1950–1975* (pp. 187–209). Fondazione Giorgio Cini Onlus. https://www.cini.it/publications/teatro-avanguardia-composizione-sperimentale-la-scena-italia-1950-1975

Lombardi Vallauri, S. (2024). Liminal music: Sciarrino, Mundry, Momi. In Bossini, O. (Ed.), *Absolute music* [Program booklet of the Venice Biennale Musica 2024]. (pp. 103–111). La Biennale di Venezia.

Magno, E. (2009). Introduzione all'estetica indiana. Arte e liberazione del sé. *Mimesis.*

Marconi, L. (2001). *Musica espressione emozione*. Clueb.

Mastropietro, A. (2020). *Nuovo teatro musicale fra Roma e Palermo, 1961–1973.* Libreria Musicale Italiana (LIM).

Nono, L. (2001b). *Il potere musicale* (1969). In De Benedictis, A. I., & Rizzardi, V. (Eds.), *L. Nono, Scritti e colloqui* (Vol. 1, pp. 261–271). Ricordi-LIM.

Nono, L. (2001c). L'errore come necessità (1983). In De Benedictis, A. I., & Rizzardi, V. (Eds.), *L. Nono, Scritti e colloqui* (Vol. 2, pp. 522–524). Ricordi-LIM.

Scelsi, G. (2010). *Il sogno 101* (Martinis, L., & Pellegrini, A. C., Eds.). Quodlibet.

ENDNOTES

1 On this topic, innumerable studies could be cited. I will allow myself the luxury of mentioning just one—Marconi's (2001) compendium, which I consider particularly valuable—notwithstanding its only flaw: it is not written in English. However, it takes into account the literature on the subject in all major Western languages, and even today, it would still deserve to be translated into English.

2 I derive the definition from Barba and Savarese (1996).

3 The English translation is mine. The original reads: "Così gli autori [...] sui quali l'industria culturale si è accanita per fornire versioni patinate, edulcorate, al fine di debilitarne la portata storica, sono quelli che guidano alla liberazione del suono e attraverso questo, a intravedere la liberazione del soggetto e del sociale. In questi musicisti, come Feldman, Scelsi, Nono e Cage il centro della speculazione non è la tecnica o lo stile, ma la riflessione sulla forma etica, sul potere suasivo che l'organizzazione del suono ha sul sociale, sul soggetto ascoltante, sulla responsabilità del compositore."

4 It was, however, Scelsi who hosted Cage in his home during the period of Cage's famous participation in the television quiz show *Lascia o raddoppia?* in 1958 (Scelsi, 2010, pp. 314–315).

5 Reviewing all of his interviews (in the second volume of his writings), it is evident that as late as 1972 Nono still associated Cage with the issue of power in music and U.S. colonialism, whereas starting from 1980 he began to acknowledge Cage's importance in positive terms. This is a conjecture, but we might even interpret this eight-year silence as the time Nono needed to process a reconsideration that surely was not an easy one.

Chapter 9

Questioning the Meliorative Agency of Art and Fiction in Relation to Family Memory Through Embodied Inquiry

Julie-Marie Duro Sasaki
http://orcid.org/0009-0002-1068-5405
University of Liège, Belgium

ABSTRACT

This chapter is grounded on feminist epistemology (Despret, Haraway), memory studies (Muxel, Hirsch) and literary theory (Viart, Demanze). It explores how verbal and visual narratives that include fiction challenge family memory in both its collective and individual dimensions by putting it in motion and stirring it. Such narrative practices are shown to contribute to well-being by fostering dialogue and improve family relations. These narratives operate not only as responses to generational silences, but also as tools for situated knowledge production. Anchored in somaesthetic philosophy and Deweyan pragmatism, this chapter examines how embodied artistic practices—such as walking, photography, and storytelling—can function as epistemic methods. The embodied research presented in this chapter demonstrates a methodology in which practice and theory are entangled. Rather than separating artistic creation, daily life, and scientific inquiry, this chapter advances an integrated mode of embodied research in which the human being as a whole is situated at the center of epistemic practices.

DOI: 10.4018/979-8-3373-3521-6.ch009

INTRODUCTION

"Tu m'as toujours dit de ne pas ouvrir la boîte de Pandore. Moi, je la remplis."[1]
Lou Dimay

This chapter dives into the theoretical and the narrative from the art project *Looking for my Japanese Family* centered on family memory that I conducted from 2014 to 2019. This artistic project led to several exhibitions (Musée de la Photographie, Galerie Satellite, Youkobo Art Space, among others) and resulted in 2019 in the publication of the photography book *Looking for my Japanese Family* (Duro, 2019).

Initially, the project began as a private quest for my unknown Japanese uncle, the son of my grandfather, whom I have still never met to this day. This search soon unfolded into a broader investigation of my grandfather's life in Japan. It also became a way of engaging with the silence that surrounded him in the family narrative. As a photographer, I started documenting my quest, but the narratives multiplied. Some narratives remained close to the facts, others became more fictional. These narratives disrupted and set in motion not only the discourses on family memory but also family relationships themselves. Gradually, the search transformed into research. What had started as an attempt to retrace an opaque family history evolved into a critical inquiry into how narratives and artistic practice itself could act as an agent to generate knowledges. The very processes of walking, photographing, and narrating revealed their epistemic potential, shifting my focus from the pursuit of biographical facts to the investigation of how narratives, especially fictional ones, act upon memory. Engaging in research, in this sense, was not an external addition but a necessity that arose from the project itself: the demand to create meaning and to understand was embedded in the artistic process, and it resonated with broader contemporary concerns about memory, transmission, and the epistemic role of art. It is from this transition that my doctoral research emerged. Rather than treating the artistic work as a preliminary stage followed by academic analysis, I conceive artistic practice as research in itself, simultaneously the method and the object of inquiry. In this sense, *Looking for my Japanese Family* did not simply precede the research but constitutes its first movement, from which the present chapter develops part of its theoretical and methodological scope.

This chapter interrogates how embodied artistic practice can serve not only as a method of inquiry but also as a space of repair and improved well-being within the family circle. Research has shown how narratives in the form of storytelling can be linked to individual and collective well-being and healing (Elias & Brown, 2022; Michell, 2015). According to these studies, telling stories about oneself and one's family may be beneficial to developing one's sense of self, and cultivating better relationships with others and the world one lives in. Narratives offer a framework in which past events are organized not only to facilitate the transmission of information, but mainly to continuously create new meanings and understandings (Fivush, 2008). The ability to talk about one's family history and the knowledge of it can even be correlated to well-being in the sense of self-esteem, family cohesiveness and intergenerational sense of self (Duke et al., 2008). In this chapter, I describe how verbal and/or visual narratives that include fiction challenge family memory in its collective and individual aspect, by putting it in motion and stirring it, resulting in improved well-being. I also argue that such narrative practices contribute to a form of well-being by engaging the body as a heuristic tool to explore inherited and unspoken memories and by activating the healing potential of fictional artistic gestures.

EMBODIED SENSITIVE ENQUIRY: PHILOSOPHY, ART AND LIFE

The use of the body as a heuristic tool of inquiry in this research is grounded in *somaesthetics,* the pragmatic philosophy theory developed by Richard Shusterman that is deeply rooted in the philosophy of John Dewey. Richard Shusterman (2008) defines somaesthetics "as concerned with the critical study and meliorative cultivation of how we experience and use the living body (or soma) as a site of sensory appreciation (aesthesis) and creative self-fashioning" (p. 1). His preference for the term *soma(*esthetics*)* instead of *body(*esthetics*)* is rich in implications and highlights how the *body* is not considered outside of the *body-mind.* As he clarifies in *Body Consciousness*, *soma* designates "the living, feeling, sentient body rather than a mere physical body" (Shusterman, 2008, p. 1) leaving behind the idea of the Cartesian dualism of body and mind. In the *Meditations on First Philosophy*, René Descartes explicitly insists on their "real distinction" (*Sixth Meditation*, 1641/1996, p. 72). Against this background, Richard Shusterman emphasizes the body as lived and felt, foregrounding embodiment as an active site of experience, knowledge, and aesthetic cultivation. Richard Shusterman integrates the idea of the human as a living creature, where the mind is always rooted in the organism and where the body is always accompanied with thoughts and feelings, and therefore deeply connected to aesthetics (Shusterman, 2012). This holistic view on the body-mind is also evident in the way somaesthetics engages epistemic issues through embodied research. According to Ben Spatz, embodied research cannot be reduced to forms of research in which the body functions only as a transparent tool. Of course, the biologist whose hands acquire technical dexterity in the lab, or the archaeologist whose body endures the physical demands of the dig are done with the body. In both cases, the body supports research but remains conceptually invisible. By contrast, embodied research foregrounds the body itself as one of its site and object of inquiry. It requires the researcher to ask: "what can bodies do?" (Spatz, 2017, p. 5). This reframing shifts the focus from the body as an auxiliary means to the body as a locus of epistemic potential, where meaning can be generated through practices. In the case of this research, it translates into asking: what can we learn with the body about family narratives ?

While Ben Spatz formulates embodied research as a methodological field that takes the body itself as a site of epistemic inquiry, Richard Shusterman defines its philosophical approach as an embodied philosophy, meaning a philosophy that gives "real body to thought through somatic style and behavior, demonstrating one's philosophy through one's own bodily example, expressing it through one's manner of living" (Shusterman, 2012, p. 4). Richard Shusterman (2008) develops somaesthetics into three branches or approaches to philosophy: an analytical approach, a pragmatic approach and a practical approach. Each unveils its own semantic regime, its own production of knowledge. Although they can be distinguished, Shusterman warns against treating them as isolated domains. Their interaction is what allows somaesthetics to act as an embodied transformative philosophy of life. The analytical approach aims at theoretical clarification and critical reflection. It examines the cultural, conceptual, and normative frameworks that shape our practices (and especially our bodily practices) and representations. Though often dominant in academic philosophy, this analytical work is not just an abstraction: it unveils the structures that underlie embodied experience[2]. As Shusterman (2008) writes, it is "an essential descriptive and theoretical enterprise devoted to explaining the nature of our bodily perceptions and practices and their function in our knowledge and construction of the world" (p. 23). The analytical approach sharpens our attention: it names, questions, reframes. It teaches us how we walk, and what walks through us-concepts, histories, norms.

However, the aim of somaesthetics is not only descriptive but also prescriptive, which is why its pragmatic branch develops concrete methods for improving embodied experience and our ways of knowing through embodied experiences. This improvement concerns, for example, the refinement of our habits, postures, and perceptions, not in order to standardize them, but to cultivate awareness and expand the range of possibilities for richer, more diverse, and more meaningful experiences. The goal is never to increase knowledge for itself, but to understand how knowledge can help us enrich our lives. Richard Shusterman is influenced by John Dewey, particularly by his theories of experience and inquiry. For John Dewey, inquiry is not a detached intellectual operation but a process of knowledge production that arises from, unfolds through, and returns to experience. As he explains in *Logic: The Theory of Inquiry*, "inquiry is the controlled or directed transformation of an indeterminate situation into one that is so determinate in its constituent distinctions and relations as to convert the elements of the original situation into a unified whole." (Dewey, 1938, p.108). The seeds of this conception were already present in *How We Think*, where Dewey identifies the first logical step of reflective thought as "a felt difficulty" (Dewey, 1997, p. 72), a formulation he later developed into the notion of the "indeterminate situation" or the "problematic situation" (Dewey, 1938, p.111). In both works, the need for inquiry arises from the very disruption of experience, when a situation becomes uncertain, unsettled, problematic. In other words, the need for inquiry arises exactly when a problematic, indeterminate situation disrupts the flow of experience: when a resistance in the environment is encountered. These resistances that give rise to inquiry function as catalysts for a process of active engagement with the environment, a process that transforms both the situation, and the agents involved. In Deweyan terms, this transformation is not a one-way adaptation, but a *transaction*: a mutual restructuring in which both the subject and the environment co-evolve through inquiry. In this sense, the original problem, the resisting experience, is not merely solved; the whole situation is reframed in a way that allows better quality experiences. To inquire, to think, implies to "bridge a gap in experience, to bind together facts or deeds otherwise isolated" (Dewey, 1997, p. 80). Thus, inquiry can be seen as a practice of reconciliation, of recomposing relations where discontinuity prevailed. It is through this effort to reconnect what has become disjointed that knowledge takes shape, not as abstract principle, but as a means for a life filled with continuity and richer experiences. This restored sense of coherence must however never be mistaken for a stable or final truth, but rather as a temporary equilibrium, always open to being shaken again. Improving one's experience is central to the entire work of John Dewey, as it allows the human being, as a living and embodied creature, to live more fully.

I suggest that inquiry-related experiences are no different than other experiences, and that to reach their full potential, they need to acquire aesthetic qualities. In *Art as Experience* (1934/2005), John Dewey analyzes, in a spiral logic of back-and-forth movement, how out of the ongoing flow of ordinary experiences there occasionally emerge certain experiences that are more "complete", which he calls *an experience*, and whose culmination is to be found in the aesthetic experience. Ordinary experiences are those that constitute the continuous, scattered, non-reflective flow of daily life, the threshold of everyday routine, the "commute-work-sleep" of experience. Pushed to the extreme, it is like finding one's glass of beer empty without even remembering having ordered it. Yet, amid these routine experiences, some stand out. They are memorable: *that meal, that bicycle ride along the Sumida River, that photograph*. They are no longer just one experience among others; they become *an experience*, something that can be named and situated. Such an experience is perceived as a whole, felt as complete, unfolding with a certain grace. But it also possesses a transformative value: after it, one is no longer quite the same, and the world to which one returns is itself altered. When an experience reaches its culmination, when its sensible, emotional, formal, and rhythmic elements interact in an organic and intense manner, experience acquires, for John Dewey, aesthetic qualities. (Dewey, 1934/2005).[3] In this perspective, the pragmatic approach of somaesthetics is not merely a process of knowledge production, but a way to cultivate richer, more meaningful, and more embodied and aesthetic experiences across all dimensions of life.

The analytical and the pragmatic approach would not be complete if they were not put through concrete action though practices; Shusterman writes that embodied philosophy "means putting one's body where one's mouth is: to really walk the walk, not just talk the talk" (2012, p. 4). Therefore, for Richard Shusterman philosophy is not just "a matter of producing text (...) it is instead about actually pursuing such care through intelligently disciplined practice aimed at somatic self-improvement" (2008, p.29). The practical approach is not simply an embodied application of given theoretical knowledge but is a way to inquire into the somatic space where one meets the world with one's body, where one listens, where experience insists, where one feels resistances. It is through one's bodily engagement that knowledge takes shape. Practice is a generative ground for inquiry.[4]

In this chapter, I will apply the aesthetic philosophical theories of Richard Shusterman and John Dewey to analyze family memory in relation to an experiential inquiry that involves the human being in his entirety, where thinking emerges from embodied practices, and where theory and practice are not dissociated. According to Richard Shusterman (2012b), "by integrating theory and practice through disciplined somatic training, it takes philosophy in a pragmatic, meliorist direction, reviving the ancient idea of philosophy as an embodied way of life rather than a mere discursive field of abstract theory" (p. 3). With this in mind, the analytical approach adopted in this research serves to examine how family memory operates in relation to fiction. The pragmatic dimension explores the conditions under which family storytelling can contribute to improved well-being. The practical dimension, finally, is grounded in embodied art practices (photography and storytelling) that do not illustrate the theoretical framework but actively participate in its construction. Since these three approaches of somaesthetics are not separated in the process of research, they are likewise intertwined in the outcome.

Accordingly, the narrative and artistic practices discussed in this chapter are not treated as secondary or decorative, but as an integral part of its epistemological development. From this perspective, artistic practice is neither an illustration of theory nor a passive object of analysis. It is itself a form of research. In *The Production of Knowledge in Artistic Research* (2012), Henk Borgdorff refers to Christopher Frayling's influential essay *Research in Art and Design* (1993), which introduced the now classic distinction between research *on* the arts (where art is treated as an object of study), research *for* the arts (where artistic practice is used instrumentally to serve external purposes), and research *in* the arts (where artistic practices are themselves recognized as forms of research that generate knowledge). My project aligns with this third perspective, which Henk Borgdorff designates as artistic research. Henk Borgdorff clarifies this position when he writes:

> *Art practice qualifies as research when its purpose is to broaden our knowledge and understanding through an original investigation. It begins with questions that are pertinent to the research context and the art world, and employs methods that are appropriate to the study. The process and outcomes of the research are appropriately documented and disseminated to the research community and to the wider public. (Borgdorff, 2012, p.43)*

This aligns with the notion of *recherche-compagne* (Havelange, 2014), a companion inquiry that Carl Havelange introduced precisely to move beyond the reductive diptych that opposes theory and practice, favoring instead a model of research *with* art. A companion inquiry "expresses 'the porosity of boundaries' and seeks to recognize and name zones of intersection where art and science can come together in the service of a shared project of expression or intelligibility" (Havelange, 2022). Far from conceiving art and science as separate territories, Carl Havelange calls for a form of inquiry attentive to their overlapping zones, where sensibility and intelligibility are continuously reconfigured. In this sense, the idea of a companion research resonates with this chapter, which does not aim at merging artistic and academic languages into one indistinct discourse, but at exploring their interstices as fertile grounds for knowledge. My aim is neither restricted to commenting on pre-existing artworks, nor to using art as a sole vehicle for philosophical content. Rather, art practice is conceived as co-agent of inquiry and a condition for its emergence. This model of inquiry implies that artistic practice actively contributes to the production of knowledge but also to its dissemination. The aim is to produce not only a form of rigorous knowledge but also a sensitive one that addresses the human being holistically, and that places aesthetic experience at the very heart of research.

The interrelation of experience, art, and inquiry resonates with a broader epistemological commitment towards a requalified conception of the research process and of *knowledge production*, not as opinion, but also in the scientific domain. In line with feminist epistemology, Sandra Harding (1986, 1991, 2015) critiques the pretense of scientific knowledge and production to *neutrality* and *objectivity*, where *neutrality* and *objectivity* are often assimilated with the standpoint of those in dominant positions hence rendered invisible, unmarked, through methodological conventions. According to Sandra Harding, "it is their economic, political, and cultural assumptions, intended or not, that tend to shape results of research" (Harding, 2015, p. 34). Sandra Harding refers to this type of objectivity as *weak objectivity* and proposes instead a *strong objectivity* that reflects critically on itself and takes into consideration the voices of the marginalized. She explains further that "The strong objectivity program argues that starting research from "outside" a discipline can enable the detection of the dominant values, interests, and assumptions that may or may not be widely prevalent, but which tend to serve primarily the most powerful social groups" (Harding, 2015, p. 34).

The famous example of Robert Rosenthal's rat experiments (Rosenthal et al., 2009)[5]—as revisited by Vinciane Despret (2009)—serves here as a powerful illustration of how experimenters' expectancy can influence the outcomes of their experiments. Robert Rosenthal arbitrarily divided laboratory rats into two groups, designating one as descending from "bright" ancestors and the other from less favorable lineages. The students conducting the experiments were explicitly informed not only of the supposed differences between the groups, but also of the expected results they might confirm through their own experiments. And indeed, the experimenters obtained results that confirmed the superior abilities attributed to the "bright" rats. However, in reality, all the rats came from the same animal supplier and were therefore probably all related. Robert Rosenthal acknowledged the small possibility that the animals labeled "bright" might by chance have been brighter than those labeled "dull", which is why some attempts were made to match the rats in order to reduce this bias. But he explained that the difference in results was due to artifacts, defined as "influences that are not of direct interest to the investigator" (Rosenthal et al., 2009, p. v). According to Robert Rosenthal's own observations, the students who believed they were working with "bright" rats expected better results and, without realizing it, treated their animals more kindly than those who had been told their rats came from "dull" lineages. As a result, "those initial differences in the treatments accorded the animals might have led to different performances by subjects which could, in turn, reinforce experimenters' expectations about their animals and maintain the subtle differences in the treatment of the 'bright' and 'dull' rats" (Rosenthal et al., 2009, p. 438).

Robert Rosenthal's experiment demonstrated that experimenters' expectancy and beliefs affected the rats' behavior. Vinciane Despret (2009) reads these results as revealing how such expectations shaped not only the interpretation of the data but also the very performance of the research subjects. According to Robert Rosenthal, such artifacts should be identified and strictly controlled in order to produce scientific knowledge that can be generalized. Vinciane Despret agrees that they must be taken into account, but she refuses to treat them as biases to be neutralized. Instead, she proposes to situate the researcher and to acknowledge these variations as meaningful responses that reveal the animals' active participation in the experimental setting. Vinciane Despret regrets that Robert Rosenthal did not use these findings

> *to open the door to the idea that animals collaborate in research, and that they are not indifferent to the way they are addressed. But the psychologist's aim was not to open the door, but rather to close it—and if possible, to throw away the key. Rosenthal's real concern was the problem of generalization in science. What holds as a hypothesis for one rat must hold for all rats; to achieve this,*

absolute similarity of circumstances must be guaranteed. He therefore set out to eliminate the sources of variation. Rosenthal wanted to standardize experimenters by demanding greater neutrality, or greater indifference.(Despret, 2009, p. 16)

According to Vinciane Despret, Rosenthal's experiments revealed that the rats, and by extrapolation, the research subjects, are affected by the situation. Rats actively participate in the relational setup proposed to them, and that they become agents of a response, not mere reactions. Yet for such a response to be heard, scientists must consider their research objects as having a voice, and be willing to listen to what *they*, the rats, have to teach *them*, the scientists. This implies allowing oneself to be vulnerable and affected, or in Vinciane Despret's (2025) terms, "to allow ourselves to be instructed" (p. 17) by the field, that is, the situated web of relationships, affects, and resistances through which knowledge can emerge.

According to this, the present research proceeds from the premise that the field and the inquirer are interconnected, and that *I*, the researcher hidden behind this chapter, am not *neutral*, but *situated*.

Also drawing on Luigi Gariglio's proposal to rethink the field through the lens of the *hybrid field* (Gariglio, 2024), I treat the *field* not as a single, external location but as a heterogeneous and porous configuration. In my case, *hybridity* refers less to digital/physical settings than to the way domestic spaces, embodied routines, artistic devices, and theoretical reflection mutually shape one another and affect the inquiry. The *hybrid field* is a methodologically constructed, one where the researcher explicitly evaluates and selects the dimensions that matter, including those usually set aside in conventional inquiry, so that the field reflects the hybrid textures of life. This is even more evident as this research takes place within my own family and daily life, making it a form of indigenous research. Malika Gouirir defined it as a research done by a researcher "born and raised within the group" she researches (1998, p. 110) and by Florence Thiault as a research grounded in familiarity with the field and an emic position within the intimate terrain of lived experience (2009).

As it is the case with the art practice involved, my personal story is not anecdotal to the research; it is constitutive of it. In agreement with Joëlle Bahloul (1992) and Anne Muxel's (2007) work on family memory, I argue that the researcher's personal involvement plays a crucial role in clarifying the often complex and opaque processes through which family histories are constructed, transmitted, and interpreted. The epistemological commitment here is not to the neutrality of an outsider, but to the attention, response, and care of an insider of the family.

To this end, I frame my research, and this chapter, within the autoethnographic method. As Tony Adams, Stacy Holman Jones, and Carolyn Ellis define it, autoethnography is "a research method that uses a researcher's personal experience to describe and critique cultural beliefs, practices, and experiences" (2015, p. 1). Autoethnography relies on reflexivity to interrogate the intersections between self and society, balances the rigor of critical reflexion with emotion and creativity, and seeks to make life more just and meaningful. In this perspective, the form of this chapter, combining narrative, reflexive, and analytical sections[6], follows the very logic of autoethnography which joins "artistic and analytic demonstrations of how we come to know, name, and interpret personal and cultural experience" (Adams, Holman Jones & Ellis, 2015, p. 1). Performing autoethnographic research implies situated autoethnographic narratives where the researcher is aware and critical of their own position as privileged and/or as biased. Autoethnographic writing "resists (…) the façade of objective research that decontextualizes subjects and searches for singular truths" (Spry, 2001, p. 710). It also recognizes the researcher as a living person with a body and with a subjectivity that is central to an embodied methodological praxis. Spry (2001) goes further by asserting that "self-reflective critique upon one's positionality as researcher inspires readers to reflect critically upon their own life experience" (p. 711). Therefore, this chapter does not simply use narrative as illustration, but treats writing itself as a method of inquiry that entangles theory, emotion, and embodied experience (Richardson, 2000). Following Laurel Richardson's proposal to consider writing as a way of knowing rather than a mere vehicle for reporting results, I situate this work within what she named creative analytic practices (CAP ethnography). In this framework, form and content are co-constitutive, and evocative texts are understood as analytic in their own right rather than as secondary to "theory". Creative analytic practices explore *evocative representations* that use "literary devices to re-create lived experience and evoke emotional responses" (Richardson, 2005, p. 931) as a methodological choice that foregrounds the situated, partial, and affective dimensions of inquiry. This view has led me to shift my philosophical inquiries away from abstraction and toward the textures of ordinary life and embodied sensible experiences. It is thus from the intersection of daily life, artistic practice, and theoretical inquiry into family heritages that the question at the heart of this chapter emerged, not as a preformulated problem, but as a response shaped by the practice of writing itself. In accord with autoethnographical standard, rather than separating theory and storytelling, this chapter seeks to include narrative form within scholarly inquiry as both method and expression according to the imaginative-creative style defined by Heewon Chang (2008, p. 148). Storytelling is not simply a narrative technique, but a heuristic and methodological tool. This research engages with the idea that research itself is a way of living and relating to others, as an embodied emotional practice that is not a separate intellectual act. In what follows, I unfold this inquiry not only through theoretical analysis, but also through situated narratives where embodied experience, artistic practices, and fictional storytelling operate together as epistemic tools.

NOVELISTIC FICTION: OPENING A SPACE FOR SENSITIVE NARRATIVES

Before turning to theoretical developments on fiction, I would like to ground this inquiry in a moment that shaped it: a photograph I took nearly a decade ago.

Figure 1. Looking for my Japanese Family

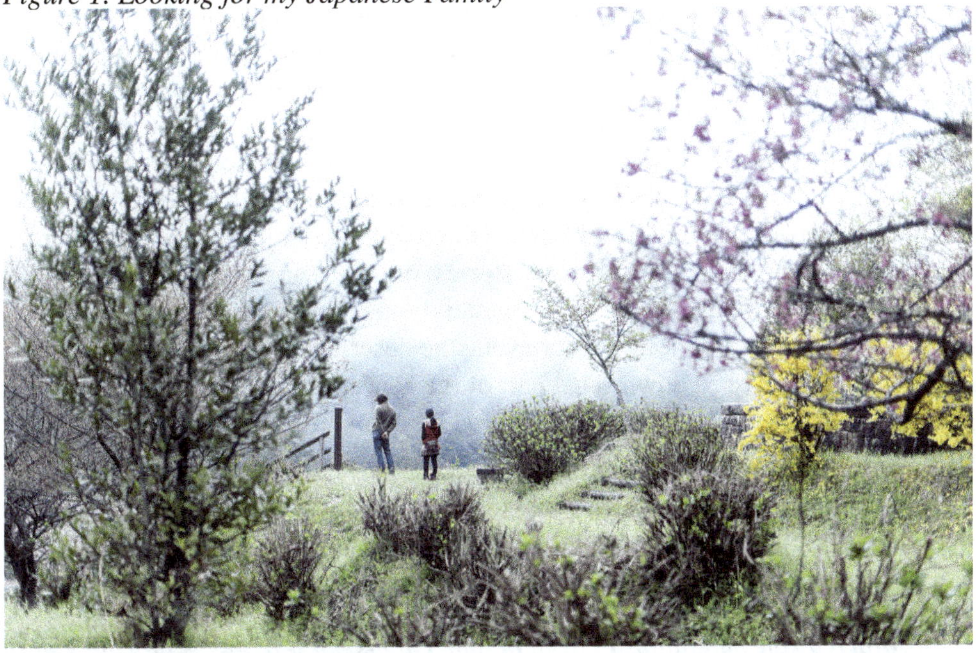

photograph by the author (Julie-Marie Duro, 2019)

You might have seen a man and a woman.
They are facing a chain of mountains that is kept hidden by a sea of clouds. Even if the cherry trees and shrubs were not in bloom, you could tell by the vivid light green of the newly sprouted leaves that it was spring. The woman is three steps back of the man. The place women were supposed to occupy according to Japanese tradition. Yet no shadow is there to be seen. He is looking down. Relaxed. She's looking straight in front of her, her legs in waiting position.
Had you met them, you would know that those were Yuki and Akiko. And that they were waiting for me.
Akiko ran a small café close by. They organized music events and organic fairs. I do not remember much about Yuki's life. He did not live there most of the time. And it does not really matter to our story.

Because when I looked at them on that day, my gaze slipped. And in that shift, sudden, somatic, involuntary, the figures before me became other. Onto their bodies, I projected the image of my grandfather and the woman who, decades ago, had loved him in Japan. A perceptual and affective superimposition took place. She, in my mind, was no longer Akiko.

And she, she was waiting for him.

In the moment I took the photograph, I no longer felt my act of seeing with detachment. It became inhabited by memory, by longing, by something lived through the body. This photograph became the emblem of the whole project, both my art book titled *Looking for my Japanese Family* (Duro, 2019) and the present research. Both started with the story of a man who remained a mystery, an absent grandfather, an absent presence in the family narratives, almost like the missing character of a novel. All that was known about him is that during the 1970s, he had lived and worked between Belgium and Japan. He brought back gifts. He sent postcards. Upon returning home, he shared many stories, most of which revolved around the city of Kyoto. Yet, while Kyoto was frequently mentioned, the actual content of those stories, the facts, anecdotes, or events he described, was never remembered and therefore not passed down. That part of the conversation remained untold. The photograph of Yuki and Akiko was captured not long after the discovery of an old postcard at an antique dealer in the suburbs of Kyoto: a postcard onto which I had also decided to project the image of my grandfather, this man who had remained almost unknown to me until then.

On the postcard, a man beside a temple on a clear day.

A few scattered clouds soften the blue sky, perfecting the composition. He appears absorbed by the mountains in front of him. On his back, a bag. A pilgrim's staff in one hand. Everything seems to whisper ready to depart. So, I departed too. I set out to walk the mountains that encircle Kyoto, the mountains of the postcard, the mountains of my grandfather.

Step by step.

I tried to trace his invisible footsteps.

Were his feet and mine following the same paths? I wondered. Could our bodies, through this landscape, become momentarily connected? Through my own bodily presence, could I feel what he once felt, see what he once saw, nourish myself with what had once sustained him?

I had arrived in Japan with no intention of turning this quest into an embodied experience, or of using my own body as a tool for intelligibility.

Once it became clear that the information collected simply did not exist, walking gradually appeared as the only meaningful response.

One pace at the time.

Ethnographers are said to produce two books.

One of facts, the other of presence.
Only the latter seemed within my reach.
Thinking through the body.
Not because I had planned to, but because the quest itself demanded it.
The silence I encountered, the opacity of the traces left behind, the absence of archival material, all of these became invitations to shift register.
The quest called for another kind of engagement.
To pursue my quest, I had to let myself be instructed by the situation.
And so, I walked.

In Dewey's terms, an experience arises when the ordinary flow of life is interrupted by a rupture or a resistance that calls for resolution. The missing stories about my grandfather, the discovery of the postcard, and the impossibility of accessing factual information were all such interruptions that acted as *impulsion* and became the very condition for the inquiries to begin and to continue with. As John Dewey writes, "impulsions are the beginnings of complete experience because they proceed from need; from a hunger and demand that belongs to the organism as a whole and that can be supplied only by instituting definite relations (active relations, interactions) with the environment" (Dewey, 2005, p.61). However, this impulse cannot be reduced to a hunger to understand. If the postcard I found in the antique shop put me in motion, it is because that postcard had affected me, had touched me. And, as Vinciane Despret so beautifully writes in a remarkable book that deals, among other things, with the ways in which the dead set us in motion:

> *What touches, I learned, and it is an important dimension of the ecology of feelings, demands relays, reprisals: "Pass what touches, touch others in your turn." What touches us relates to viral ecology; without hosts, what touches withers, and can no longer touch anyone. What touches needs us.*[7] *(Despret, 2021, p. 56)*

The postcard had touched me, requiring me to begin inquiring through the walk in ways that, at the time, were beyond my understanding.

> *Those put in a position of being obliged are in that position, most of the time, without knowing exactly what is obliging them: "I had to do it, period." What people are trying for, when they respond to what is asked of them, is being up to the task. This experience has to be honored, not explained (Despret, 2025, p. 26).*

Now that the walk has been walked, new understandings emerge about how this postcard could have affected me. This image, being the only one at my disposal and, even though not a representation of my actual grandfather, called for intimacy and for what Carl Havelange (2016, p. 48) calls a "sensible intelligence".[8]

Another dimension had to be honored: the fact that each step of the quest left behind a residue, whether an unresolved grey area that kept the hunger for inquiry alive, or another event or object that touched me and required me to continue walking. These residues sustained relations both with myself and with the environment, whether through family members or through the field itself. How these relations unfold, how they foster greater awareness, and how they contribute to the growth of understanding is what this chapter will now explore. Because it was not just about walking, but *footstepping*.

THE BODY AS A SITE OF INQUIRY: FOOTSTEPPING AND EMBODIED EPISTEMIC INTIMACY

The performances of *footstepping*, walking in the traces of another's life, rarely leads to verifiable data or factual confirmation and does not necessarily bring the researcher closer to the empirical object of the inquiry. However, this method opens up another epistemological regime, one grounded in embodied intimate experience rather than in demonstration. It reconfigures the field of knowledge from that of proof to that of embodied attunement and affective proximity. Footstepping requires to live from inside, to feel with the body-mind, "to walk the talk" (Spry, 2001, p. 725). Footstepping can be closely linked to autoethnographic performance practices, where the body serves as a tool to acquire another form of knowledge, which is both sensible and intelligible as Spry (2001) states: "calls upon the body as a site of scholarly awareness and corporal literacy" (p. 727). In an article on field narratives, Laurent Demanze (2019) explains how footstepping and the immersed reenacting it entails engage "the body to determine the sensation concretely experienced by others. Such experimentation has a heuristic function, as in archaeology, where the reproduction of gestures does not merely consist of appropriating them but also of testing their validity" (p. 42).

Further in his article, Demanze addressed the historiographic practices of Philippe Artières, who deliberately blurs the boundaries between historical method, subjectivity, performance, and literary storytelling as exemplary of footstepping. To Philippe Artières, his great-uncle and Jesuit philosopher Paul Gény, was an unknown ancestor who only existed through familial archival material collected in a small plastic bag: letters, photographs, newspaper clippings of a traumatic event. In October 1925, Paul Gény was murdered in Rome by Bambino. For a year, Philippe Artières, then a resident at the Villa Medici, undertook historical research on his unknown ancestor. In an interview with Librairie Mollat, Paul Artières explained that his aim was to "write about this event, but to write it *in situ*" (Librairie Mollat, 2013). Therefore, the scholar did not hesitate to wear a cassock to reenact the murder of a Jesuit great-uncle as part of a well described performance (Artières, 2013a; Artières, 2013b). His historical investigation took shape as a situated embodied practice: the historian chose to walk the very streets of Rome where the murder had taken place, to embody the gestures, clothing, and trajectory of his unknown ancestor. He literally walked in the footsteps of Paul Gény—spatially, temporally, and affectively—crafting an inquiry rooted in the inhabited body, in the *soma*, rather than distanced analysis. The archival material—letters, photographs, clippings—served as a catalyst for this embodied epistemology, but the heart of the investigation lay in the corporeal proximity he sought with the past. Philippe Artières was inspired by the performances of Massimiliano Furlan, who reproduced, without a ball, Michel Platini's movements during the 1982 World Cup in the Parc des Princes stadium, Demanze (2019) elaborates that

> *this resembles something akin to "experimental archaeology" allowing one to experience for oneself what people of the past lived. Reproducing gestures, feeling the weight of a garment, reenacting what took place, this not only generates an excess of intelligibility by enabling one to feel what might have occurred but also establishes a reflexive protocol: in doing so, the historian highlights and explores the contacts, the intimacies, the intermittencies of identification between the historian and their subject (p. 43).*

I applied the same reflexive protocol of the footstepping enacted in the art project *Looking for my Japanese Family*, where footstepping did not aim at retrieving factual knowledge. Footstepping helped cultivate an embodied intimate understanding of what might have been lived and felt by another person. Through the act of walking, an evolving relationship emerged with my long-absent grandfather. His presence had remained far, but his traces started to resurface through gesture and landscape. The practice of footstepping became a tool of posthumous connection, a form of co-presence in which togetherness was made possible, not through simultaneity, but through shared experienced. With the walk, the figure of the absent grandfather began to take form, not through memory or archive, but by gaining a body through mine. His life in Japan gradually materialized through the photographs I captured, and his experiences became entangled with my own. I began to write not as a surrogate for his voice, but from his position, *in situ*, grounded in the place where he once stood.

And as I walked, I wondered:
Did my grandfather meet his Japanese lover near this bridge where koinobori, carp-shaped windsocks, fluttered in the breeze?
Did they dream of marrying in this fake wedding chapel?
Did they stroll together?
No record of a child.
Was he with her when she waited for him?
When he was back home in Belgium, to his family.
When his return became impossible.
Might haves.
Could haves.
Never been.

SILENCES REWRITTEN: NOVELISTIC FICTION AS A SHARED NARRATIVE SPACE

In the context of family memory and storytelling, fiction is not merely a creative representation of reality. Fictional narratives can become sites of epistemological inquiry, as well as of relational transformation and healing. In the art project *Looking for My Japanese Family* (2019) and in particular the prequel visual poem *I am a cloud* (Duro, 2014), in which I gave voice to the Japanese lover in the form of imagined postcards, certain figures gradually ceased to be approached as historical individuals. My grandfather, his Japanese lover, and their child began to emerge instead through what Laurent Demanze describes as *romanesque* or "novelistic" lives. As Laurent Demanze (2014) explains, this concept implies

> *to build one's existence in the manner of a novel's hero, master of his destiny and protagonist of multiple adventures, but it is also to identify the lived life by an excess of passions and events that are cruelly lacking in ordinary life (p. 9).*

In this sense, I regard *I am a cloud* to possess the characteristics of a novelistic fiction, insofar as it stages imagined lives and amplifies them beyond the mere recovery of historical facts. Shifting from the factual to the fictional does not negate reality; rather, it reconfigures it. It opens a heuristic space for alternative forms of narration, particularly those that cannot easily be expressed within the constraints of inherited family discourses. The visual poem *I am a cloud* (Duro, 2014), composed of fifteen fictional postcards, exemplifies this process. I chose postcards, which hold a longstanding significance in both familial narratives in general and in my own family in particular, as the narrative support for imagined messages the Japanese lover might have wished to send to my grandfather. These imaginary postcards functioned as sensitive and hermeneutic objects, not only as narrative devices, but as tangible supports for meaning-making. They mediated between creation and reception, transmission and interpretation. As shared surfaces, they offered a space where meaning remained unfixed, mobile, and co-constructed. By combining narrative and emotion, these cards allowed their viewers not only to see, but also to feel the traces of past events. They offered a form of knowledge where sensation and information intersect. Through these postcards, literally held in my hands and those of my family, my grandfather, his Japanese lover, and their child gradually transformed into the characters of a novel. Although they were real people, the moment I identified my grandfather and his Japanese family in the characters on the postcards, I made them fictional characters with whom my family and I could interact, in the sense that we could explore them in order to create an interpretive narrative about what they might have been like in reality. While discussing the real individuals who inspired these characters remained almost impossible, the imagined versions became a shared point of dialogue. Gradually, this fictional space allowed us to shift back our focus from the imagined characters to the real people behind them. It was precisely by passing through the detour of fiction that we could return to the real figures, no longer as silenced or inaccessible, but as individuals about whom a dialogue could now be sustained.

This perceptual shift, triggered by fiction, finds an echo with what Viktor Chklovski (2008) describes as *ostranenie*, defamiliarization: the literary technique of disrupting automatic perception to renew the experience of the familiar. Chklovski famously illustrates this with Tolstoy's narrative strategy of presenting familiar situations from the unexpected viewpoint of a horse, compelling the reader to perceive the ordinary as if encountering it for the first time. As Chomsky observed, such narrative displacement revives attention to the texture of lived reality, rendering the known strange enough to be seen anew. The familiar ceased to be a transparent surface, it withdrew from recognition and required a new mode of engagement. However, in *I am a cloud*, the movement does not only proceed from over-familiarity to estrangement, but also from opacity and silence to renewed intelligibility. It is not to see what was unseeable, but to speak about what was unspeakable. The novelistic fiction allows to get away from the facts only to circle back to them. It acted as an intermediary frame that rendered the real, once silenced or emotionally blocked, again perceptible and open to discourse. It enables a renewed access to reality, not by reinstating prior knowledge, but by transforming the emotional and perceptual terms of that access. In that sense, this novelistic fiction carries a heuristic transformative power: it acts as a tool to access sensitive knowledge, through emotion, storytelling, and perceptual displacement. In this way, it opened up a new space where the weight of silence and avoidance was lessened, and where more factual stories could begin to emerge. This narrative fiction did not simply produce an illusion; it made visible what could not be said otherwise. It destabilized what had been imposed as an unquestioned state of silence, and in doing so rendered the past momentarily graspable, not through facts, but through fiction. In that sense, *ostranenie* in my work is not a detour away from reality, but a way of approaching it sideways through a misalignment of the gaze that opens a space for reconfiguration and meaning.

The novelistic fictional postcards contributed to a relational form of well-being. It allows to re-inhabit family memory and family narratives differently, not by erasing its gaps or traumas, but by creating a space where its silence could be held, reimagined, and shared. Fiction, in this sense, became a form of narrative care: a way to soften the sharp edges of what had remained unspoken, and to transform the solitary weight of uncertainty into a shared possibility for sense-making through storytelling. The well-being it fostered was not abstract or purely psychological; it was somatically anchored. Holding the postcards, engaging with their textures and silences, activated a form of body-mind resonance where meaning could be felt as much as thought. But perhaps more importantly, these postcards were not only held, but they were also passed from hand to hand, from body to body, in a gesture of shared attention. This tactile circulation enacted a mode of exchange that exceeded verbal expression. It embodied memory in the gesture itself, anchoring remembrance and recognition in somatic relationality. Through such affective and material contact, family memory became not only speakable, but inhabited anew—relationally, corporeally, and sensitively.

Family secrets, whether the existence of a hidden child or the murder of a Jesuit ancestor, carry an inherent paradox: while they serve to protect certain individuals, they often do so at the cost of harming others, typically across generational lines (Tisseron, 2011). In such contexts, novelistic fiction holds a distinctive epistemological potential. Precisely because it suspends the imperative of factual verification, it creates a space where silence becomes narratable. Rather than revealing truth in a forensic sense, fiction reconfigures the conditions under which something *can* be said. It enables indirect, affectively attuned forms of access to the unspeakable. As such, its significance lies less in what it discloses than in how it modulates proximity, allowing what was emotionally or socially blocked to become once again perceptible and shareable. In this regard, novelistic fiction acts not as a substitute for truth but as a catalyst for reengagement within the living family memory.

Anne Muxel (2007) identifies three functions of living family memory, each intrinsically linked to a corresponding role of forgetting: transmission, reminiscence, and reflexivity. First, the function of transmission, oriented toward the past, is perhaps the most readily associated with family memory. It evokes the transfer of knowledge from elders to descendants, forming a shared repertoire of norms, rituals, and references. It is the memory that enables "the recognition of a generational inscription within the long temporal continuity of a family group's existence, as well as the desire to perpetuate a set of attributes specific to its identity" (Muxel, 2007, p. 14). Nevertheless, when overly rigid, this function risks depriving memory of its adaptive potential. To remain relevant across generations, memory requires a space for reinterpretation and appropriation. This flexibility can emerge through the complementary role of forgetting, which introduces the necessary blank space for renewal and transformation. Secondly, the function of reminiscence seeks to bridge or even dissolve temporal boundaries, reactivating past experiences and emotions within the present. By reconnecting with past feelings, reminiscence creates a continuity of lived experience. Where the individual finds its own truth, family memory is "a way for each individual to evaluate their life. It is, strictly speaking, the consciousness of a past" (Muxel, 2007, p. 200). Yet forgetting, in this context, plays a protective role: it preserves the autonomy of individuals by shielding them from the perpetual rumination of unresolved or traumatic memories. Footstepping is a good example of the reminiscent function of memory. It represents the attempt of future generations to reconstruct and embody their emotional connections to the past in the absence of direct memories. Lastly, the function of reflexivity instrumentalizes memory to interrogate and explain personal destinies. Memory here becomes a tool for self-understanding and narrative construction. Forgetting, however, acts as a safeguard, protecting certain aspects of the past through silence. Among the Manouches, for instance, the practice of forgetting is deliberately exacerbated: the dead are never spoken of, and their belongings are burned (Williams, 1993). This silence is framed as an ethical act, a way to preserve the dignity of the deceased by avoiding the risk of misrepresentation or falsehoods. Through these interrelated functions, Muxel highlights the dynamic interactions between memory and forgetting. She emphasizes that both are essential in shaping the ways families navigate their stories across generations. Fiction, I argue, can perform functions analogous to those of forgetting, particularly when silence does not emerge from the natural fading or evolution of healthy memories but is instead experienced as a source of pain or trauma. This is especially relevant when the space left by silence is not merely blank but becomes vacant or inaccessible, an absence marked by the weight of family secrets or the unresolved traces of traumatic events. Fiction can act as a tool to bridge this void by creating a narrative framework through which the unspoken may be approached, reimagined, and eventually reintegrated into the web of family memory. Oscillating between what was and what wants to emerge, family memory is, as Anne Muxel (2007) observes "a personal history and its reconstruction. There is some novel in it. A true fiction through which the individual, mobilizing their past, gives themselves meaning—more or less voluntarily" (p. 9).

MOVED BY RESISTANCES: THE AGENCIES OF COUNTERFACTUAL FICTION AND MEDIATION

I had titled my narrative I Am a Cloud.
And there we were, literally, floating on them.
It was romance.
It was dreamscape.
But, on an autumn day, my alarm clock rang reality.
In the office of a Kyoto company, the human resources manager left the office only to come back with a crestfallen expression on her face.
I headed back to the shared house I had rented for a month near the bamboo forest of Arashiyama, empty-handed.
On that day, I wrote on Instagram[9]:
"My grandfather worked here.
My mother works with their products.

I went inside and was told that if there is one place where they would have information about my grandfather it would be in their plant in Germany ...
My astrology might be right ...
Maybe now is not the moment to go east."
A few days later, an unexpected email arrived from the West: "Julie, you're on the wrong track. Let's meet." My family is a web of complicated threads. I had never met the younger daughter of my grandfather.
Yet.

This event was more than just a turning point in the story. It showed how fiction can play an active role in family inquiry and family memory. Unlike *I am a cloud*, which openly presented itself as fiction, this other narrative claimed to tell the truth. Yet it turned out to be counterfactual, a story based on mistaken information. Precisely because of this mistake, it disrupted inherited silences and opened the way to unexpected encounters. It was inaccurate, but it was inaccurate in the very attempt to tell the truth.It is important, when dealing with fiction, to distinguish between different forms of non-knowledge. Although in a very different context, I would like to transpose the ethical concept of *méconnaissance* conceptualized by Vladimir Jankélévitch (1963). The French philosopher explains how ignorance refers to a simple lack of information or instruction. Ignorance produces a straightforward *I don't know*. In contrast, *méconnaissance*, best translated as misrecognition, is not born from an absence of knowledge but from a distortion, a misuse, or a misinterpretation of knowledge already present. What is misrecognized is not unknown; it is known in a twisted or partial way, often without awareness of this deformation. Unlike a lie, which deliberately conceals or falsifies what is known, *méconnaissance* operates under the guise of sincerity. When I claimed, "My grandfather worked here", I was not lying. I was unknowingly expressing a form of *méconnaissance*: a false statement that I believed to be true. And yet, paradoxically, this misrecognition became the trigger for a deeper truth to emerge, precisely because it disrupted the fragile equilibrium of silence that surrounded the family story. It made it act. The "mis-" in misrecognition, acted as a somatic trigger, almost like knee reflexes, to restore cognition. From that moment, fiction was no longer just a way of telling stories; it also became a method of inquiry and a means of reshaping relationships. This counterfactual narrative, embedded within the larger framework described with the novelistic narrative, disrupted the family's equilibrium and catalyzed movement within it. It served as a bridge, reconnecting two previously estranged branches of the family: in an effort to restore the truth, new bonds were formed or rediscovered through this process.

For speech to break out of silence, two things were essential. First, there had to be a space where expression was possible, which the initial fiction, *I am a cloud* helped to open. Second, there needed to be an impulse, a spontaneous and almost visceral force, which came from the counterfactual story and the need to restore the truth. Together, these fictions not only invited dialogue but also reshaped the contours of family memory, enabling a reconfiguration of relationships and shared understanding.

Although I photographed extensively, I did not really capture the first meeting with my aunt.
Just a timid picture, from the car.
A bad one.
We can see the McDonald afar.
The car window, a screen with no added value.
The camera, a shield I refused.

Choosing not to photograph my aunt raises broader methodological and ontological questions about the decisive role of photography, both as an object and as an act. In this situation, refusing to take a picture during our first encounter, and keeping only an unsatisfactory one, becomes another kind of index. The untaken photograph, and the narrative I later made out of this failed "capture", neither proves nor tells anything about the encounter itself. However, it does tell other stories. It speaks of the precarity of the situation and of my unease, but more importantly, it reveals my will to resist photography as a straightforward record. A single well-composed image might even have told us less. As John Tagg reminds us "if the Photograph is unarguable, like the name, it nevertheless teaches us nothing" (Tagg, 2009, p. 230). Building on the evidential force of photography theorized by Roland Barthes (1980), Tagg argues that what is ontologically guaranteed by photography is only that "something has been." The photograph may impose a proximity to a past presence that has vanished but cannot be denied. What "was there" was there, yet everything else remains untold unless and until the image is inscribed within an apparatus of discourse.

One of the specificities of photography relies in the fact that while calling necessarily a direct connection, a presence to a past reality through indexicality, it also acts as a medium. It is not only a possible trace, but a way of mediating experience. Photography acts as mediation, it introduces a frame, a screen, a distance, an interpretive layer between subject and experience. In certain contexts, this mediated distance may be productive: it can enable reflection, open space for interpretation, or provide protection against emotional overwhelm. This protective function of mediation is particularly significant when we consider what Marianne Hirsch (2008) calls post-memory, the specific memory of the second generations of survivors (victims or perpetrators) of massive traumatic event, such as genocides. Post-memory describes the "structure of inter- and trans-generational transmission of traumatic knowledge and experience" (Hirsch, 2008, p. 106). It is the conflictual incorporated memory of those who cannot recall a traumatic event, because they are not the ones who actually lived it, but on to whom some of its consequences were transmitted, and mediated to the past "by imaginative investment, projection and creation" (Hirsch, 2008, p. 107). Due to the nature of those traumatic events, photographs

> *thus become screens—spaces of projection and approximation and of protection. Small, two-dimensional, delimited by their frames, photographs minimize the disaster they depict and screen their viewers from it. But in seeming to open a window to the past and materializing the viewer's relationship to it, they also give a glimpse of its enormity and its power (Hirsch, 2008, pp. 116–117).*

While Marianne Hirsch develops this argument in relation to the specific and incomparable context of Holocaust postmemory, I draw on her notion of photographs as "screens" in a more modest, analogical way. The emotional magnitude and historical stakes of the particular events and family conflicts discussed in this chapter are not of the same order as those associated with Holocaust postmemory. What I retain from her work is not the scale of trauma but the mechanisms she identifies, which I suggest can be extended, by analogy, to other postmemory situations. In the case of *I am a cloud*, photographic mediation opened a space for dialogue within the family about previously taboo events and family members. It showed how photographs can create a space in which to think, feel, and transmit what is otherwise unavailable or emotionally difficult to access. In this sense, mediation through fiction, photography, or other artistic representation[10] can function as a shield, a lens, and/or a bridge.

The mediations discussed above act as bridges: they connect, evoke, and transmit, but they also impose distance, which is the second reason why I chose not to "capture" my aunt's portrait on that day. The camera materializes this double movement, functioning both as a shield and a facilitator. To photograph demands more than the movement of the body; it requires the full engagement of one's physical presence in every capture. The eyes, of course, are involved, as are the hands and fingers operating the camera. But beyond these, the entire body participates, entering into a multisensory, embodied relationship with the surrounding environment. Photography is not just about seeing, it is about being in the environment, learning from it, and allowing oneself to be transformed by it. Yet this bodily immersion is interrupted by the act of capture itself. Photography and narration alike introduce a frame, a screen, a distance, an interpretive layer between subject and experience. In certain contexts, this mediation enables reflection, provides protection, or opens a space for deferred understanding. In others, however, it may obstruct the immediacy required for relational engagement. The gesture of photographing, like that of narrating, entails a structuring of the real that may preclude full presence. Choosing not to photograph can therefore be understood not as a gesture of withdrawal, but as one of situated engagement, an embodied engagement in the nexus of life itself. In this sense, the decision not to produce a clear, legible image of my aunt, and to leave only an oblique and unsatisfactory trace of that day, is the core aesthetic operation through which this difficult inheritance is mediated: the family wound is approached by inscribing a gap and a limit in the visual archive rather than by offering a full visual record. This dynamic reappears in other fields of inquiry, notably in ethnographic contexts, where presence precedes interpretation and where embodiment becomes the primary vector of access to meaning.

Jeanne Favret-Saada (1977) demonstrates this dilemma perfectly. While conducting research on witchcraft in the Bocage, she discovered that engagement was only possible if she participated not merely as an observer, but as an active participant. Before she herself was ensnared by witchcraft, it was impossible for her to fully engage in the investigation or to liberate the speech of her interlocutors. True engagement required being physically and existentially present, a holistic engagement of the body-mind. This is the precondition for knowledge production and implies two disjointed but interconnected temporalities. Presence in the moment and then, reflection and critical analysis. Clearly, one cannot take a photograph retrospectively, as it would be the case with storytelling. Therefore, it is the absence of image that speaks for itself. Photography, whether it is captured or viewed, has the peculiar property of, in the same gesture, immersing us in the present while simultaneously distancing us from the past.

FROM FAMILY MEMORY TO INDIVIDUAL TRAJECTORY: THE REFLEXIVE POWER OF FIGURATION

Was I going to uncover the truth about my grandfather's hidden Japanese son? That remained more than uncertain. But something more important happened in the process. I was no longer alone in my project, leaning under the heavy silences of family memory. I was supported by some, critiqued by others. Through the fictions I had constructed, the photographs I had taken, voices started to be heard. And the entire family became connected, speaking to one another about my grandfather, about all and everything else.

After meeting my aunt for the first time, my investigation shifted from Kyoto to Tokyo. It was there, she taught me, that my grandfather had actually worked. It was there I met his Japanese colleagues. I visited his workplace. Near Shinagawa Station, I visited the Prince Hotel where he used to stay. At this point, I was tracing his actual footsteps. The blossoming mountains of my imagination were far away. Under my feet, the asphalt of Roppongi. The doors of its numerous bars, jazz clubs, and hostesses' lounges were all closed to me, this time, limited by my gender and limited resources.

I struggled. How to withhold judgment? My European, feminist, and postcolonial perspective revealed tensions. Yet another rupture in the flow of my experiences.

As I was learning about my grandfather's lifestyle in Tokyo, I inherited a guilt that was not mine to bear, faults that I felt an implicit responsibility to address. For some family members, however, it was the other way around. Family memory is complex, and it is not solely mine to control or define. A hidden son was acceptable to me, perhaps because I infused the narrative with a sense of romanticism. Under the flashy neon lights, I was facing other issues.
My grandfather had never been heard thanking anyone with a simple arigato. I would learn Japanese. I would eat the entire fish starting from its head, practice tea ceremony, arrange flowers, learn the culture of the land that had accepted our walks. As an act of transgenerational reconciliation. As an effort to understand the legacy he had left behind. The legacy I had chosen to become the heir of.
My paths had switched. None of them brought me closer to discovering the whereabouts of my Japanese uncle. But as I walked, I started observing the thresholds of houses, allowing my imagination to roam freely. Again.

Figure 2. Looking for my Japanese Family

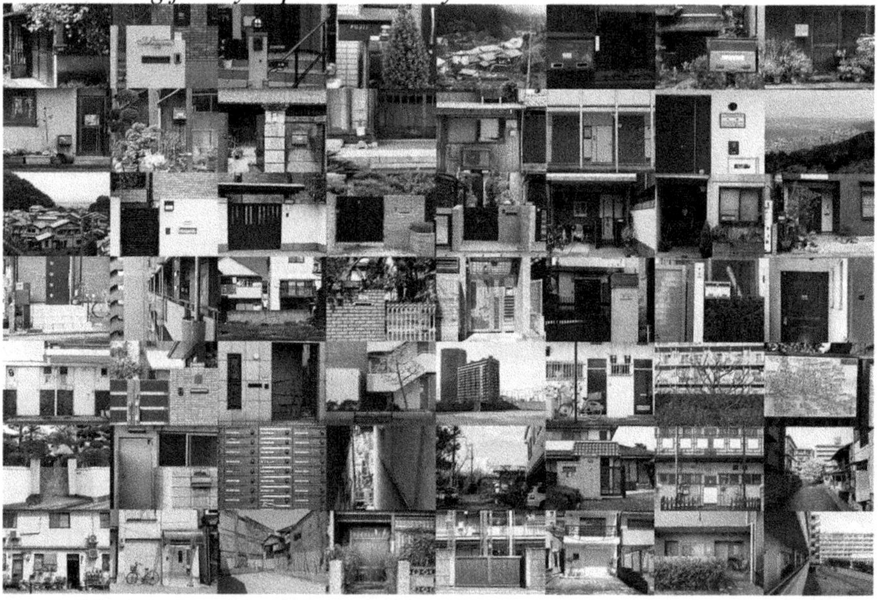

photograph by the author (Julie-Marie Duro, 2019)

Does my uncle live in a modest apartment like the one near the station? Or perhaps in a house like this one? What kind of life might he have had, had he lived here or there? Did he study at this school, then move on to this university? I was moved by the long absence of any tangible lead. With the help of statistics from public records, history books, testimonies, I had constructed an entire life for my uncle.

I had even given him a name.

Figure 3. Looking for my Japanese Family

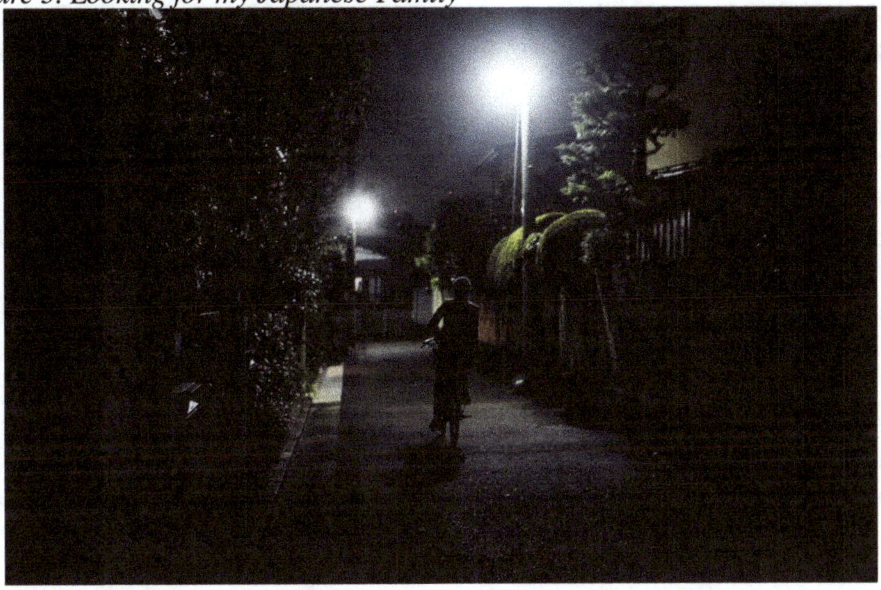

photograph by the author (Julie-Marie Duro, 2019)

And in that instant, another type of fiction emerged.

This third fictional narrative was neither novelistic nor counterfactual. It strayed too far from factual reality, presenting a deviation that was, in its own way, revealing of the situation. Although there was almost no available information about the main character in the story, this narrative cannot be considered a pure fantasy entirely disconnected from reality. This visual and textual fictional narrative is inscribed in the mode of what Dominique Viart calls *figuration*. Based on what could have existed, "what is globally true is so in a general way, without knowing whether, for such or such particular existence, events happened as we know they happened for most people" (Viart, 2009, p. 9). The sources used are no longer in the past, in the family memory and the stories of its direct recollections. The sources of the figuration narrative are drawn from books written by others, works of literature, sociology and similar works.

Gradually, the walk began to shift away from retracing footsteps and the urge to revive the past through an embodied attempt to feel what was once felt by another person. Instead, the act of walking became the requirement of the use of photography as a narrative medium. Each step is engaged with the present moment, engaged with the field and the quest. Step by step, image after image, I started distancing path from my uncle's life as I became the main character of the narrative I was writing.

Writing, photographing, walking, all of these narrative processes had become another embodied tool of knowledge. They narrated their own process through the meanderings and uncertainties of its creation.

The third narrative oscillates between figuration and what Laurent Demanze (2019) and Dominique Viart (2019) refer to as *littérature de terrain*, or field literature. Situated at the intersection of literature and the humanities, these narratives are "far from merely representing reality (…) [they] consider literature as a means to feel, study, and even experiment with reality" (Viart, 2019, p. 2). In field literature, the narrative that emerges is not only the outcome of the inquiry. It also narrates the reflexive process of both the search itself and of the transformation of the searcher. The embodied epistemological process was similar to the footstepping present in the novelistic narrative, but what was there to experience had shifted. This third narrative also fully embraced what Anne Muxel (2007) identifies as the reflexive function of family memory. No longer merely recounting or reconstructing the past but actively engaging with it as a tool for self-reflection and transformation, forging connections between memory, present actions, and the possibilities of what lies ahead. In the end, to work on family memory implies an act of separation where "memory contributes to the autonomy of the subject" (Muxel, 2007, p. 203).

CONCLUSION

Through these personal narratives, this chapter demonstrates the critical role of verbal and visual storytelling in shaping family memory and in fostering both individual and collective well-being. As I have shown in this chapter, the three narratives have different relationships to fact and fiction and therefore act in different ways on the family, on family memory, and on myself.

The first narrative, *I am a cloud*, gave a novelistic shape and a voice to a story that had fallen silent. By offering a coherent yet imagined version that others could read and respond to, *I am a cloud* made that family past accessible again. The use of fiction acted as a shield that protected what needed to remain unsaid while helping to reopen conversations about my grandfather's and the Japanese side of the family. Until then, the inquiry remained far removed from the facts. Once speaking became possible, however, it only needed a trigger to move away from novelistic narration and closer to what had actually happened. That trigger was the counterfactual story, the one that wrongly claimed my grandfather had worked in a factory where he never did. This second narrative unsettled the newly shared memory. It exposed gaps. It created discomfort. And precisely because it was "wrong", the story I wrote prompted my aunt to speak up and correct it. Her intervention opened the way for a more factual inquiry in an area where the lack of information had previously made this impossible. More importantly, it helped restore family relationships. To restore reality, we had to talk, and to be able to talk, we had to meet.

The third narrative is grounded in meeting my aunt and walking through the places where my grandfather actually lived. It confronts the gap between the life I had imagined for him and the life he actually led. The earlier stories had filled the blanks with conjecture. They produced a relatively smooth, even comforting version of his trajectory, largely disconnected from the facts. Listening to my aunt, seeing the places, and facing dates and documents forced that imagined life to crack. Family memory was reshaped once again when factual corrections partially gave way to embodied experience. As this narrative unfolded, it gradually moved beyond what could be factually known. It developed into an imagined life for my uncle, in what also may have been a way for me to cope with the failure of my inquiry. This is probably one of the reasons why this narrative had a particularly deep impact on me. It helped me locate myself within the fabric of family memory, understood not only as a past to be recovered but as a living web of ongoing relations. At the same time, it shifted my project. What had started as a biographical search focused on family members became an epistemological inquiry into what different materials and body-mind practices allow us to create knowledge. In this sense, the path it opened is both personal and epistemological. Ultimately, these narratives led to this chapter, which constitutes a fourth, reflexive narrative whose full effects remain to be explored.

Each narrative examined embodies a distinct meliorative potential. The novelistic narrative opened a space for dialogue, allowing previously silenced topics to resurface. The counterfactual narrative catalysed action and supported reconnections and revelations. The third one reshaped my personal trajectory, leading me to settle in Japan and to pursue embodied inquiry through doctoral research in arts and art science. For me, this journey has also been a healing process. It did not erase past wounds or contradictions, but it made them speakable and livable in new ways. By weaving walking, photographing, and writing into a sustained artistic practice, it allowed me to hold together grief, attachment, and curiosity, and to inhabit my family's history with less fragmentation and more continuity.

Taken together with this present reflection, these four narrative moments correspond to the theoretical, practical, and pragmatic dimensions of somaesthetic experience. They invite us to think of embodied forms of knowledge in which inquiry grows out of experience, affect, and situated practice rather than abstraction alone. As a partial, situated, embodied, and personal account, this inquiry helps restore a sense of holistic coherence by reconnecting the researcher with her own being as a whole person and by treating narrative not only as a mode of expression but as a way of knowing.

REFERENCES

Adams, T. E., Ellis, C., & Jones, S. H. (2015). *Autoethnography. Understanding qualitative research.* Oxford University Press.

Artières, P. (2013a). *Reconstitution, jeux d'histoire*. Manuella éditions.

Artières, P. (2013b). *Vie et Mort de Paul Gény*. Seuil.

Bahloul, J. (1992). *La maison de mémoire, ethnologie d'une demeure judéo-arabe en Algérie (1937-1961)*. Editions Métailié.

Barthes, R. (1980). *La Chambre claire: Note sur la photographie*. Gallimard.

Borgdorff, H. (2012). *The Conflict of the Faculties: Perspectives on Artistic Research and Academia*. Leiden University Press.

Chang, H. (2008). *Autoethnography as Method.* Routledge., DOI: 10.4324/9781315433370

Chklovski, V. (2008). *L'art comme procédé*. Editions Allia.

Demanze, L. (2014). *Les vies romanesques d'Emmanuel Carrère*. Roman 20-50, 57(1), 5–14. https://doi.org/DOI: 10.3917/r2050.057.0005

Demanze, L. (2019). *Expériences de terrain, terrain d'expérimentation*. Revue critique de fixxion française contemporaine, 18, Article 18. https://doi.org/DOI: 10.4000/fixxion.1513

Descartes, R. (1996). *Meditations on first philosophy: With selections from the objections and replies* (Cottingham, J., Ed. & Trans.). Cambridge University Press.

Despret, V. (2009). *Penser comme un rat*. Editions Quae.

Despret, V. (2015). *Au bonheur des morts. Récits de ceux qui restent*. La Découverte.

Despret, V. (2021). *Our Grateful Dead. Stories of Those Left Behind.* University of Minnesota Press.

Dewey, J. (1938). Logic: The theory of inquiry. In Boydston, J. A. (Ed.), *The later works of John Dewey, 1925–1953* (Vol. 12, pp. 1–528). Southern Illinois University Press.

Dewey, J. (1997). *How we think.* Dover publications.

Dewey, J. (2005). *Art as Experience*. Penguin.

Duke, M. P., Lazarus, A., & Fivush, R. (2008). Knowledge of family history as a clinically useful index of psychological well-being and prognosis: A brief report. *Psychotherapy (Chicago, Ill.)*, *45*(2), 268–272. DOI: 10.1037/0033-3204.45.2.268 PMID: 22122420

Duro, J.-M. (2014). *I am a cloud*. Self-published.

Duro, J.-M. (2019). *Looking for my Japanese Family*. Self-published.

Elias, A., & Brown, A. D. (2022). The role of intergenerational family stories in mental health and wellbeing. *Frontiers in Psychology*, *13*. Advance online publication. DOI: 10.3389/fpsyg.2022.927795 PMID: 36237680

Favret-Saada, J. (1977). *Les mots, la mort, les sorts*. Gallimard.

Fivush, R. (2008). Remembering and reminiscing: How individual lives are constructed in family narratives. *Memory Studies*, *1*(1), 49–58. DOI: 10.1177/1750698007083888

Frayling, C. 1993. Research in Art and Design. *Royal College of Art Research Papers* 1(1). https://researchonline.rca.ac.uk/id/eprint/384

Gariglio, L. (2024). On fieldwork in the hybrid field: A "methodological novel" on ethnography, photography, fiction, and creative writing. *Qualitative Research*, *24*(2), 444–456. DOI: 10.1177/14687941221149584

Gouirir, M. (1998). L'observatrice, indigène ou invitée? Enquêter dans un univers familier. *Genèses*, *32*(1), 110–126. DOI: 10.3406/genes.1998.1527

Haraway, D. (1988). Situated Knowledges: The Science Question in Feminism and the Privilege of Partial Perspective. *Feminist Studies*, *14*(3), 575–599. DOI: 10.2307/3178066

Harding, S. (1986). *The Science Question in Feminism*. Cornell University Press.

Harding, S. (1991). *Whose Science? Whose Knowledge? Thinking from Women's Lives*. Cornell University Press.

Harding, S. (2015). *Objectivity and Diversity. Another Logic of Scientific Research*. The University of Chicago Press.

Havelange, C. (2014). *Plaidoyer pour une recherche-compagne* [conference presentation]. 9e édition des Ateliers de la Recherche en Design (ARD), Liège, Belgium. https://hdl.handle.net/2268/175916

Havelange, C. (2018). *Gaspard – Une écriture ouvrière au XIXe siècle*. Les presses du réel.

Havelange, C. (2022). *La recherche-création: remarques rétrospectives sur le doctorat en art et sciences de l'art* [Conference presentation]. La recherche-création avec Yves Citton, Louvain-la-Neuve, Belgium. https://hdl.handle.net/2268/297848

Hirsch, M. (2008). The Generation of Postmemory. *Poetics Today*, *29*(1), 103–128. DOI: 10.1215/03335372-2007-019

Jankélévitch, V. (1963). La méconnaissance. *Revue de Metaphysique et de Morale*, *68*(4), 389–406. https://www.jstor.org/stable/40900772

Librairie mollat (Director). (2013, January 31). *Philippe Artières—Vie et mort de Paul Gény* [Video]. *YouTube*. https://www.youtube.com/watch?v=-cHibcs3lrY

Michell, H. (2015). *Bush Cree Storytelling Methodology: Northern Stories that Teach, Heal, and Transform*. In Education, 21(2), Article 2. https://doi.org/DOI: 10.37119/ojs2015.v21i2.213

Muxel, A. (2007). *Individu et mémoire familiale*. Hachette.

Orvell, M. (1992). Writing Posthistorically: Krazy Kat, Maus, and the Contemporary Fiction Cartoon. *American Literary History*, *4*(1), 110–128. https://www.jstor.org/stable/489940

Richardson, L. (2005). Writing: A Method of Inquiry. In E. A. St. Pierre (Ed.), *The Sage handbook of qualitative research, 3rd ed* (pp. 959–978). Sage Publications Ltd.

Rosenthal, R., Rosnow, R. L., & Alan, E. Kazdin. (2009). *Artifacts in Behavioral Research: Robert Rosenthal and Ralph L. Rosnow's Classic Books*. Oxford University Press. https://doi.org/DOI: 10.1093/acprof:oso/9780195385540.001.0001

Shusterman, R. (2008). *Body Consciousness. A philosophy of Mindfulness and somaesthetics*. Cambridge University Press.

Shusterman, R. (2012). *Thinking through the body. Essays in Somaeasthetics*. Cambridge University Press.

Spatz, B. (2017). Embodied research: A methodology. *Liminalities: A Journal of Performance Studies, 13*(2). http://liminalities.net/13-2/embodied.pdf

Spry, T. (2001). Performing Autoethnography: An Embodied Methodological Praxis. *Qualitative Inquiry*, *7*(6), 706–732. DOI: 10.1177/107780040100700605

Tagg, J. (2009). *The Disciplinary Frame: Photographic Truths and the Capture of Meaning*. Univ Of Minnesota Press.

Thiault, F. (2009). *Recherche indigène et familiarité avec l'objet de recherche.* Études de communication. langages, information, médiations, 32. https://doi.org/ DOI: 10.4000/edc.914

Tisseron, S. (2011). *Les secrets de famille.* Presses Universitaires de France.

Viart, D. (2009). Le silence des pères au principe du « récit de filiation ». *Etudes Francaises (Montreal, Quebec)*, *45*(3), 95–112. DOI: 10.7202/038860ar

Viart, D. (2019). *Les littératures de terrain.* Revue critique de fixxion française contemporaine, 18, Article 18. https://doi.org/DOI: 10.4000/fixxion.1275

Williams, P. (1993). *Nous, on n'en parle pas, les vivants et les morts chez les Manouches.* Editions de la Maison des sciences de l'homme.

ENDNOTES

1 "You always told me not to open /Pandora's box. /I, I'm the one filling it."

2 As human beings, all our experiences are embodied, since we cannot live without being our bodies. In this sense, speaking of "embodied experience" might appear pleonastic. And it is. Yet the term signals an important distinction: whereas ordinary experience may use the body without awareness, embodied experience (which Shusterman also calls somatic experience) brings into focus the body itself. It designates an experience in which the body is not only the medium through which things happen, but the object of conscious attention, reflection, and cultivation as a source of perception, action, knowledge and thought.

3 A fuller comparison between Dewey's conception of inquiry (Logic: The Theory of Inquiry, 1938) and his account of aesthetic experience (Art as Experience, 1934/2005) would certainly be valuable, since both share a similar structure of transformation from indeterminacy toward a unified whole. Such a discussion, however, exceeds the scope of this chapter.

4 Richard Shusterman does not just write about the body/soma. He is involved in different body-mind disciplines such as zen or yoga and is a certified Feldenkrais Method instructor. These practices are informing his writings as embodied philosophy.

5 Rosenthal, Rosnow, & Kazdin (2009) republish and comment on Rosenthal's earlier works from 1963 and 1966, including the classic rat experiments.

6 In this chapter, reflexive, sensitive and narrative sections are indicated in italics, while analytical sections are presented in regular font.

7 In the French original, Despret writes "ce qui nous touche nous requiert" (Despret, 2015, p. 98). The English translation renders this as "what touches needs us" (Despret, 2021, p. 56). However, the French *requiert* carries a stronger connotation than "need": it suggests a demand or requisition, a call to act, rather than a mere dependency.

8 For a more detailed treatment, see Havelange, C. (2018). *Gaspard – Une écriture ouvrière au XIXe siècle.* Les presses du réel.

9 See https://www.instagram.com/p/vZXiA_PX71/

10 Graphic memoirs such as Art Spiegelman's *Maus* (2003) have become paradigmatic for thinking about how visual and narrative mediation can both shield and expose second-generation subjects to inherited Holocaust trauma, while opening a space for dialogue between survivors and their children (Hirsch, 2008; Orvell, 1992).

Chapter 10
Silver Lining of Adversity:
Role of Gratitude

Poonam Khurana
http://orcid.org/0000-0001-5134-9147
Vivekananda Institute of Professional Studies-TC, India

Deepika Chhikara
http://orcid.org/0000-0003-3009-9999
Vivekananda Institute of Professional Studies-TC, India

Renuka Kapoor
http://orcid.org/0009-0006-8138-4625
Amity University, Noida, India

ABSTRACT

The expression "every cloud has a silver lining" focuses on identifying a positive aspect in a gloomy or negative situation. Traumatic events can have long-lasting and adverse impacts, but some individuals may experience growth. The personal growth aftermath of adverse or traumatic events is referred to as adversarial growth. While experiencing trauma, cultivating gratitude may help to foster a positive outlook. This research analysed the role of gratitude on adversarial growth following chronic illness in India. A survey method was employed to collect responses from individuals who have experienced chronic illness in the last year. An updated version of SLQ-38 and GQ-6 was employed to measure constructs. A total of 368 respondents filled out the survey, and PLS-SEM on SmartPLS was employed to analyse the data. The findings of the study established a positive and significant association between gratitude and adversarial growth. In conclusion, theoretical contributions, interventional implications and future directions were discussed.

DOI: 10.4018/979-8-3373-3521-6.ch010

INTRODUCTION

In life, we experience a wide range of emotions, events and circumstances that shape our life journey. These experiences can be positive, like joy, wins, love, learning, hope, and gratitude or negative, like hardships, loneliness, losses, and adversity. As human beings, we are naturally inclined to seek out more positive emotions and avoid negative ones. The term "finding silver lining" describes this psychological process of deriving positive meaning from negative circumstances (Barr et al., 2024). In the psychology domain, such outcomes reflect what is often referred to as adversarial or post-traumatic growth, the positive psychological shifts experienced due to engaging in highly challenging life events (Tedeschi et al., 2018). While often used synonymously, it is critical to distinguish between the various constructs of positive adaptation. *Adversarial growth* serves as an umbrella term encompassing the positive psychological changes due to any life struggle (Blackie et al., 2023; Bride et al., 2008). Adversarial growth occurs as a natural process, rather than as a result of intentional action or therapy. In contrast, *post-traumatic growth* specifically refers to a fundamental seismic shift in an individual's worldview following a trauma that challenges their core beliefs (Tedeschi & Calhoun, 1996, 2004).

Building on previous research, a primary contribution of this research is the conceptual shift from post-traumatic growth to adversarial growth in finding silver linings in the case of recent health issues (Bride et al., 2008; McBride et al., 2009). While the term post-traumatic often implies that the negative event has concluded, adversarial growth more accurately captures the positive psychological shifts that occur *during* ongoing stressors, such as illness (Bacon et al., 2023; Drewes et al., 2020). This study argues that in the context of persistent health challenges, growth is not a post-event outcome but a continuous process of adaptation and meaning-making (Bacon et al., 2023; Blackie et al., 2023). Hence, in the present context, researcher refer to finding a silver lining as adversarial growth, because the term post-traumatic suggests that the negative situation has ended.

One of such positive changes is also feeling more gratitude towards life. Gratitude is defined in the literature as "the appreciative functioning that involves appraisals of benefits and support" (Rusk et al., 2016). Through gratitude, individuals can process their experiences, find silver linings, and discover new strength and positive transformation in the aftermath of hardships. Various previous studies have reflected that gratitude can act as a catalyst for an individual's adversarial growth in different difficult life-threatening situations in life, like cancer (Parikh et al., 2015), natural disasters (Henson et al., 2021), and terrorist attacks (Fredrickson et al., 2003). Despite a sufficient body of data supporting the relationship between these two variables in a Western setting, less number of researches has been conducted in the Indian context. The Indian context offers a unique socio-cultural lens for studying these constructs, as traditional Indian values often emphasise collectivism and spiritual fatalism, which may influence how blessings (gratitude) and suffering (adversity) are perceived. Additionally, most of the previous empirical studies studied adversarial growth as a unidimensional concept. The present research examined adversarial growth as a five-factor dimensional concept of silver lining (Bride et al., 2008). By examining adversarial growth as a multidimensional construct within this population, this study addresses a significant geographical gap in positive psychology literature (Zhou & Wu, 2015).

Furthermore, this study adopts a novel methodological approach by utilizing the Silver Lining Questionnaire to resolve the conceptual ambiguity surrounding silver linings in psychological literature (Barr et al., 2024; Bride et al., 2008). By employing the SLQ-38, researchers transition from using silver linings as a vague metaphor to treating it as a measurable, multidimensional framework for adversarial growth (Barr et al., 2024; McBride et al., 2009). This scale allows for a rigorous evaluation of five distinct growth dimensions, including improved personal relationships and inner strength, directly linked to the experience of illness (Bride et al., 2008; McBride et al., 2008). By examining the relationship between gratitude and these specific facets of growth, this study provides a pioneering look at how an appreciative disposition enables individuals to identify silver linings and cultivate resilience while still navigating the complexities of an illness (Bacon et al., 2023).

The current study aims to examine the relationship between gratitude and finding silver linings as adversarial growth in people who have recently faced hardship, such as illness, in India.

LITERATURE REVIEW

Considering adversarial growth as a multidimensional phenomenon, this study operationalises the construct of "silver linings" to capture the diverse domains of positive psychological shifts occurring within the context of illness (Barr et al., 2024; Brewer et al., 2017; Drewes et al., 2020). Unlike singular or linear models of adaptation, the multidimensionality of silver linings, as measured through the SLQ-38, allows for a granular assessment of growth across distinct facets such as improved personal relationships, enhanced inner strength, and changes in life philosophy (Bacon et al., 2023; Barr et al., 2024; Bride et al., 2008). This multidimensional framework distinguishes silver linings from broader constructs like post-traumatic growth by emphasising the iterative, ongoing nature of finding benefits during persistent health-related stressors rather than after a resolved event (Barr et al., 2024; Şenol-Durak et al., 2023). This process is fundamentally driven by gratitude, which serves as the cognitive catalyst for meaning-making and cognitive reappraisal, enabling individuals to transcend the limitations of their illness and reconstruct a more resilient, multi-faceted worldview (Armenta et al., 2017; Blackie & McLean, 2021; Lin, 2022; Nie et al., 2024). Central to this transformation is the Broaden-and-Build theory, which posits that positive emotions like gratitude expand an individual's thought-action repertoire, thereby building the personal and social resources necessary for resilience (Fredrickson, 2004).

Adversarial Growth

Adversarial growth refers to positive changes that individuals experience after adversity in their identity, relationships, and world views during ongoing stressors (Blackie et al., 2023). Due to the persistent health challenges observed during illness, adversarial growth has been studied as a catalyst for finding silver linings by previous researchers. In the extant literature, a special focus is given to adversarial growth during illness lsuch as multiple sclerosis (MS), cancer, cardiac and renal diseases (Bride et al., 2008; McBride et al., 2009; Cormie et al., 2017), and more recently, COVID-19 (Bacon et al., 2023). A study found that HIV-positive patients experience adversarial growth, and this enhances their mental health, treatment adherence and reduces risk behaviour (Boals et al., 2019). According to a recent research on breast cancer patients (Parikh et al., 2015), adversarial growth develops after the diagnosis and course of treatment, while post-traumatic stress disorder is identified within the early stages. Thus, there is enough evidence to explore whether adversarial growth helps to overcome different illnesses positively through present research.

A meta-analysis (Wu et al., 2019) of 26 studies highlighted that 52.58% individuals reported adversarial growth after a traumatic event; hence, the prevalence of adversarial growth is not rare (Ning et al., 2023). Adversarial growth is an umbrella term (Bride et al., 2008) used in the literature to refer to stress-related growth (Park et al., 1996), positive consequences (Sodergren & Hyland, 2000), benefit-finding (Affleck & Tennen, 1996), finding meaning (Folkman, 1997), and positive changes (Collins et al., 1990). In research, adversarial growth has been explored for various difficult phases like car crashes (Nishi et al., 2010), grief (Taku et al., 2008), and physical abuse (Kleim & Ehlers, 2009). Adversarial growth is seen as a significant experience that impacts a person's entire life in multiple ways (Confino et al., 2023). Hence, adversarial growth should be considered as a multi-dimensional construct rather than unidimensional. Various factors, such as positive coping strategies, personality traits, sharing negative emotions, rumination, resilience, growth actions, and experiencing multiple sources of traumatic events, promote adversarial growth (Henson et al., 2021). The extant literature considered various factors for measuring adversarial growth like positive life changes after hardships include improved personal relationships, a change in life philosophy (McBride et al., 2009; Calhoun & Tedeschi,

1999), personal inner strength (Joseph & Linley, 2006), greater appreciation for life (Bellizzi & Blank, 2006) and spiritual development (Henson et al., 2021). To ensure measurability of this multi-dimensional constructs, researchers follow the previous research where SLQ-38 (Sodergren and Hyland, 2000) is considered to measure how finding silver linings ensures adversarial growth operationalised into the five-factors, which are 1) improved personal relationships, 2) greater appreciation for life, 3) positive influence on others, 4) personal inner strength and 5) changes in life philosophy (Barr et al., 2024; McBride et al., 2009, Bride et al., 2008).

Gratitude

Having gratitude is a morally good feeling that comes from being appreciative (Khoury-Malhame et al., 2023; McCullough et al., 2004). It enables a person to remember and concentrate on prior happy occasions and experiences (Watkins et al., 2003). It is a tendency to express appreciation for benefits and positive aspects of life (Fagley, 2012). It encompasses recognising and appreciating the worth of positive events, experiences, and actions along with fostering emotional bonds with them(Adler & Fagley, 2005). Gratitude enhances the enjoyment of ordinary everyday occurrences (McCullough et al., 2002) and has various positive effects on one's physical, mental, and emotional health (Jans-Beken & Wong, 2021). Grateful people generally experience higher life satisfaction and lower levels of anxiety and depression (Butler & Jaffe, 2021; Lambert et al., 2009). It also increases positive relations and motivates prosocial behaviour, social support and positive social relations (Ruini & Vescovelli, 2013; Wood et al., 2010). Both a trait and a state are reflected in gratitude (Strzeminski & Ferreira, 2020). Gratitude as a "state" is an affective-cognitive or attribution-dependent condition that is predicated on valuing favourable results and acknowledging their external source. "Trait" gratitude refers to a more expansive way of living that involves appreciating and observing the good things that happen in the world (Confino et al., 2023; Jans-Beken et al., 2020).

Adversarial Growth and Gratitude

The association between gratitude and adversarial growth has been a topic of interest in psychology research. The study (Confino et al., 2023) examined the role of gratitude in Israeli adults who experienced a recent (past year) traumatic event, and the results showed a positive association between gratitude and adversarial growth. Another study (Ruini & Vescovelli, 2013) observed the role of gratitude in breast cancer patients and its strong correlation with adversarial growth. Fredrickson et al. (2003) found that gratitude is positively associated with resilience and growth after a terrorist attack and is considered a positive emotion by traumatised people. Another study investigated the role of gratitude and resilience in adversarial growth following the campus shooting at Seattle Pacific University, USA, and the results suggested that both resilience and gratitude can act as protective mechanisms, with gratitude promoting growth after trauma (Vieselmeyer et al., 2017). El Khoury-Malhame et al., 2023 examined the variables linked to antagonistic development following the trauma experienced by 252 Lebanese individuals. The findings showed that enhanced gratitude was substantially linked to increased growth. When combined, these results imply that thankfulness may play a significant role in antagonistic development. As a result, the current study makes the following claim.

H1: Gratitude has a significant impact on adversarial growth.
H1a: Improved personal relationships have a significant impact on adversarial growth.
H1b: A greater appreciation for life has a significant impact on adversarial growth.
H1c: Changes in life philosophy have a significant impact on adversarial growth.
H1d: Positive influence on others has a significant impact on adversarial growth.
H1e: Personal inner strength has a significant impact on adversarial growth.

Figure 1. Proposed model

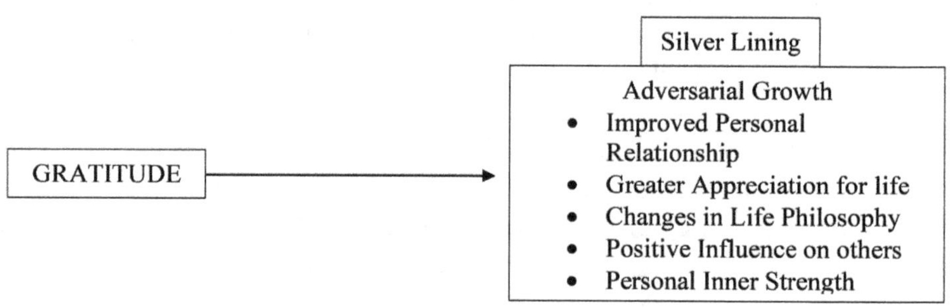

Research Methodology

Participants

The data is collected by administering a standardised questionnaire through an online survey. The positive sides of illness were asked in the questionnaire, and further, the impact of gratitude on their adversarial growth was asked. The survey was floated through WhatsApp and emails to ensure appropriate respondents filled the form. The sampling technique utilised for the study is a criterion for selecting individual that fulfilled the criterion of being ill in the last year **(Palinkas, et al. 2015)** through convenience sampling. Questionnaires were sent online to 450 respondents; however, 368 completed the form. Their demographic profile is given in Table 1.

Measures:

Gratitude Questionnaire: The gratitude questionnaire-6 (GQ-*6) by* McCullough et al., 2002 GQ-6 has six items to measure gratitude. The measure evaluates individual variations in the likelihood of feeling thankful in day-to-day experiences. Items 3 and 6 were reverse-coded among those. Gratitude is measured on a 7-point Likert scale in the GQ-6 (1 being strongly disagree and 7 being strongly agree). The scale calculates the degree of thankfulness, and a respondent's total score can vary from 6 to 42. The GQ-6 has been evaluated for construct validity, internal consistency, and reliability. It has strong psychometric qualities too.

Silver Lining Questionnaire: The silver lining questionnaire SLQ-38, developed by Sodergren and Hyland (2000), was later updated by Bride et al., 2008 into 24 items factored into a five-subscale: "improved personal relationships, greater appreciation for life, positive influence on others, personal inner strength and changes in life philosophy" measured the adversarial growth. The scale considered adversarial growth as a multi-dimensional construct. The scale was rated on a 7-point Likert scale (range from 1=strongly disagree to 7= strongly agree).

Demographics: The respondents were asked demographic questions like gender, age and education.

Data Collection

Data was collected by online survey methods. The questionnaire was sent to those who agreed to participate. Participants were initially asked to provide demographic details like gender, age and education and further asked to rate remaining measures assessing gratitude and adversarial growth. The questionnaire takes 15-20 minutes to respond to 35 questions. A total of 368 respondents completed the questionnaire. It fulfilled the minimum sample required for CFA as suggested by Hair et al. (2006), that is, to have at least ten times as many observations as there are variables to be analysed. The total number of items to measure all variables in this study are 30, and 10 times of 30 equals 350. Therefore, the present sample size of 368 is more than sufficient.

Data Analysis and Results

To ensure the findings are both rigorous and accessible for a book chapter, the data were analysed using Partial Least Squares Structural Equation Modelling. A systematic two-step approach was employed, first validating the measurement model to ensure the accuracy and reliability of the psychological scales, followed by the structural model to test the hypothesised relationships between the constructs. This sequence ensures that all interpretations are based on a stable and verified psychometric foundation.

The participant profile (N=368) consists primarily of educated emerging adults, with 81% of the sample under the age of 30 and 83% holding university-level degrees.

Table 1. Depicting the demographic profiles of the respondents

Items	*Categories*	*Frequency*
Age	15-25	245
	26-35	92
	36-45	9
	45 and above	22
Gender	Male	202
	Female	166
Highest level of Degree	12th passed	61
	Graduation	202
	Post-Graduation	88
	PhD	17

Source: Prepared by authors

The Measurement Model

The initial step involved refining the scales to ensure each item accurately reflected its intended psychological construct. Two items (GR3 and GR6) were excluded due to low factor loadings, a process that improves the content validity and precision of the overall assessment. Following this refinement, all scales demonstrated high internal consistency, with reliability coefficients well within the recommended range for psychological measurement. This indicates that the instruments provide a stable and reproducible assessment of the participants' psychological experiences.

To ensure the theoretical integrity of the model, researchers verified that the items for each scale correctly converged to represent a single psychological concept (convergent validity) while remaining distinct from other unrelated concepts (discriminant validity). The results confirmed that while gratitude, adversarial growth, and silver lining perceptions are statistically related, they are conceptually distinct psychological processes. This clear differentiation is essential for the interpretation of the results, as it allows researchers to pinpoint which specific dimensions of adversarial growth are most influenced by gratitude. By establishing this robust psychometric foundation, one can confidently interpret the underlying mechanisms that facilitate positive adaptation in the face of struggle.

The Structural Model

After validating the psychological assessment tools, the analysis transitioned to the structural model to examine the actual pathways between gratitude and adversarial growth. This stage ensures the findings are practically relevant by measuring the explanatory power (R^2) and predictive accuracy (Q^2) outside of the immediate sample of these relationships, confirming that gratitude is a reliable driver of positive psychological change (Chicco et al., 2021; Hair et al., 2021; Riou et al., 2015). Statistical validation indices, the variance inflation factor, which confirm that the data are free from statistical bias, can be accessed in the Appendix Section. Finally, the path coefficients serve as a practical guide for triage, identifying which specific actions, such as helping a patient find a silver lining, will yield the strongest results for promoting long-term resilience and well-being. This robust framework allows practitioners to trust that the observed links are not merely coincidental but represent a stable foundation for understanding how individuals adapt to significant life challenges.

Hypothesis Testing

To ensure the results were reliable and not due to chance, the model utilised a bootstrapping procedure with 5,000 resamples (Hair et al., 2018). This robust stress test confirmed that gratitude is a powerful driver of adversarial growth across all five dimensions measured. The table below summarises these results, showing how gratitude directly facilitates specific positive changes in patients. All the hypotheses are accepted; hence, gratitude has a significantly positive impact on adversarial growth.

Table 2. Summary of Growth Outcomes Driven by Gratitude

Hypothesis	Dimension of Silver Lining as Adversarial Growth	Impact Level	Result
H1a	Improved personal relationships have a significant impact on adversarial growth.	**High**	Accepted
H1b	A greater appreciation for life has a significant impact on adversarial growth.	**Moderate**	Accepted
H1c	Changes in life philosophy have a significant impact on adversarial growth.	**Moderate**	Accepted
H1d	Positive influence on others has a significant impact on adversarial growth.	**Moderate/Low**	Accepted
H1e	Personal inner strength has a significant impact on adversarial growth.	**High**	Accepted

Prioritise Relationship Building: The highest explanatory power (R^2) was found in improved personal relationships. This suggests that gratitude-based interventions are most effective at helping patients reconnect with their support systems, which is crucial in the Indian socio-cultural context where family involvement is high.

Building Inner Fortitude: Gratitude explained nearly 40% (R^2) of the change in a patient's personal inner strength. Gratitude journaling or reflection as a tool can help patients recognise their own resilience, transforming their self-perception.

Shifting Perspectives: With a moderate R^2 of 0.348 for changes in life philosophy, focusing on gratitude helps patients find a silver lining or a new sense of purpose despite their diagnosis. This confirms that gratitude isn't just a fleeting emotion; it creates a lasting shift in how a patient views their world.

Reliable Results: The Q^2 values (all greater than 0) reassure practitioners that these findings are not specific only to this study group. There is strong predictive relevance, meaning a clinician can expect similar growth when applying these gratitude strategies to their own diverse patient populations.

Robustness Check

To confirm the reliability of the findings, a robustness check was conducted using the Gaussian copula technique to test for endogeneity, a statistical bias that occurs when independent variables are unintentionally correlated with hidden errors in the model. The statistical analysis output can be referred to in the Annexure. By verifying that all Gaussian Copula values were non-significant ($p > 0.05$), the results were relevant in confirming that the study is free from such biases and establishing the model's overall robustness. This means the study does not suffer from endogeneity issues. This ensures that the observed positive relationship between gratitude and adversarial growth is a true, direct effect rather than a statistical fluke caused by unmeasured factors. This result reinforces the idea that finding a silver lining identified in the psychological shift towards gratitude leads to adversarial growth.

The corresponding statistical outputs can be accessed in the Annexure Section.

DISCUSSION AND CONCLUSION

Understanding the nexus between gratitude and adversarial growth is crucial, given the perspective that by incorporating gratitude into life, individuals can emerge from adversity with greater wisdom, strength, and personal growth. In order to investigate the connection between gratitude and adversarial growth in individuals who had encountered any kind of illness over the past year, the current study used PLS-SEM. The findings indicated that gratitude has a positive significant impact on adversarial growth, which is consistent with the results of Ruini & Vescovelli, 2013; Vieselmeyer et al., 2017; Zhou & Wu, 2015.

Here, gratitude positively impacts personal relationships, the reason for this could be that patients acknowledge the social support they received in their adverse situation which consequently strengthens their relationships. Gratitude also made people appreciate their life by making them more tolerant, less concerned about the approval of others, less concerned about failure due to illness, more at ease with others, and less judgmental of others. By incorporating gratitude, individuals experience change in their life philosophy as well. Their illness makes them think about their true purpose in life, and their religious and spiritual beliefs deepen. Personal inner strength is also experienced because of the feeling of gratitude. They feel that their illness permits them to do things for themselves, makes them a more determined person, helps them to find themselves, discover a talent they did not know they had, makes them more aware of their strength, makes them face up to problems of life, and teaches them how to stand up to illness. Gratitude also opens up an individual to have a greater appreciation of life. Their illness gave them a new start in life, which made them feel much better than they felt before the illness, made them live life to the fullest, made them happier people, and more confident. Additionally, people experience a positive influence on others after adverse situations like illness by incorporating gratitude. Other people appreciate them more due to the internal gratitude resource during illness, find inspiration in them, can be more open with them and change their perception for the better.

The results of the investigation confirm the strong relationship between gratitude and adversarial growth. Gratitude helps to increase positive affect, optimism, and physical functioning and lowers depression and anxiety (Wood et al., 2010). According to the study, thankfulness intervention can be created for adversarial growth through daily gratitude lists, behavioural expressions of gratitude, and thankful thinking (Ruini & Vescovelli, 2013).

Implications

The findings of the study must be interpreted within the unique socio-cultural framework of India. In collectivistic cultures, gratitude is often intertwined with social harmony and a sense of relational indebtedness, which differs from an individualistic culture on individual autonomy (Srirangarajan et al., 2020). The results show that gratitude strongly impacts *Improved Personal Relationships*, which suggests that in the Indian context, growth is deeply social. Indian patients may perceive support from family and community as a blessing, which facilitates growth by reinforcing the sense of belonging (Dixit & Sinha, 2024; Unanue et al., 2019). Additionally, the prevalent cultural value of spiritual fatalism may allow individuals to accept their illness as a predetermined path, while gratitude helps them find silver linings within that path (Okuzono et al., 2025).

Theoretical Implications

The findings of the study significantly advance the knowledge of how gratitude fosters adversarial development in the Indian context. The theoretical frameworks of positive psychology of finding silver linings are supported by the positive relationships found between gratitude and various dimensions of adversarial growth, including enhanced interpersonal relationships, a greater appreciation for life, modifications to one's philosophy of life, positive influence on others, and inner strength. These results are consistent with earlier studies showing that psychological well-being and resilience are enhanced by thankfulness (Emmons & McCullough, 2003). The study supports the idea that fostering gratitude can be an essential strategy for people overcoming adversity by showing that it has a significant impact on these aspects (Fredrickson, 2004). This theoretical development broadens the understanding of the mechanisms by which thankfulness contributes to personal development and provides directions for further investigation.

This research clarifies the theoretical consideration of silver linings within the broader field of positive psychology. By distinguishing silver linings from posttraumatic growth, researchers argue that growth in illness is not a post-event outcome but a continuous process of adaptation (Barr et al., 2024; Drewes et al., 2020) as adversarial growth. The study confirms that gratitude is a stable predictive factor for this ongoing growth, supporting models that position appreciative functioning as a precursor to successful cognitive accommodation after adversity (Blackie & McLean, 2021; Drewes et al., 2020).

Practitioner Implications

From a practitioner's standpoint, the results point to useful implications for businesses, especially in terms of staff development and well-being initiatives. Improved interpersonal interactions result from fostering thankfulness in the workplace, and this promotes a friendly and cooperative work environment. Employees who participate in workshops or programs centred on thankfulness report higher job satisfaction and retention rates as a result of their increased appreciation for life (Watkins et al., 2003). Furthermore, by encouraging a culture of thankfulness, companies can persuade staff members to embrace an optimistic outlook on life and inner fortitude, improving their capacity to handle obstacles at work. Gratitude practices can be incorporated by managers into team-building exercises, which may enhance productivity and organisational culture in general. These interventions support employee engagement and organisational goals of employee growth while also contributing to personal growth.

For healthcare practitioners, these findings suggest that implementing gratitude-based interventions can serve as a potent clinical tool for fostering adversarial growth among patients managing illness. Specifically, incorporating daily gratitude lists, where patients record positive daily occurrences, facilitates cognitive reappraisal by systematically shifting a patient's focus toward beneficial experiences (Diniz et al., 2023). This approach can be deepened through meaning-focused coping exercises, such as thankful thinking sessions during therapy, which help patients reframe their diagnosis from a narrative of loss into a new start or a unique opportunity for personal and spiritual development. Furthermore, by encouraging the explicit behavioural expression of gratitude toward caregivers and family members, practitioners can help patients strengthen the vital social bonds that act as a buffer against psychological distress, ultimately promoting a more sustainable and resilient model for mental health care (Bohlmeijer & Westerhof, 2021).

Limitations

The present study has several limitations that need to be noted. Firstly, constructs were measured using a self-reported scale that is limited to assessing conscious content and lacks temporal resolutions, which may not capture all aspects of an individual's mental state. Secondly, the sample size of the study is small due to the limited set of people who fulfilled the criteria, which could affect its generalisation to a large audience. Thirdly, the impact of demographics of the respondent, like age and gender, has not been examined. Fourthly, whereas a variety of factors may influence adversarial growth, only the effect of appreciation has been examined in this study. Future researchers can explore additional factors impacting adversarial growth. Factors that can moderate the relation can be explored. Adversarial growth after a specific illness can also be studied.

DECLARATIONS

Conflict of Interest: The authors have no conflicts of interest to report.

Ethical Approval: Not Applicable

Informed Consent: Not Applicable

Funding: The authors declare that no funds, grants, or other support were received during the preparation of this manuscript.

Data Availability Statement: The spreadsheet of the survey data that supports the findings of this study is available from the corresponding author upon request.

REFERENCES

Adler, M. G., & Fagley, N. S. (2005). Appreciation: Individual differences in finding value and meaning as a unique predictor of subjective well-being. *Journal of Personality, 73*(1). Advance online publication. DOI: 10.1111/j.1467-6494.2004.00305.x PMID: 15660674

Atkinson, , RFlint, , J. (2001). Accessing hidden and hard-to-reach populations: Snowball research strategies. *Social Research Update, 33*(1). Retrieved from http://sru.soc.surrey.ac.uk/SRU33.html

Affleck, G., & Tennen, H. (1996). Construing Benefits from Adversity: Adaptational Significance and Dispositional Underpinnings. *Journal of Personality, 64*(4). Advance online publication. DOI: 10.1111/j.1467-6494.1996.tb00948.x PMID: 8956517

Bacon, , A. MCharlesford, , JHyland, , MPuskas, , THughes, , P. (2025). Finding silver linings in the covid-19 pandemic: A 2-wave study in the UK. *Psychological Reports,* 128(6), 4120-4138.

Barr, , E. ARaybin, , J. LBennett, , C. RSmith, , M. C. (2024). Silver Linings: A principle-based concept analysis examining the emergence of positive changes that accompany adversity. *International Journal of Nursing Studies Advances*, 7, 100243.

Bellizzi, K. M., & Blank, T. O. (2006). Predicting posttraumatic growth in breast cancer survivors. *Health Psychology, 25*(1). Advance online publication. DOI: 10.1037/0278-6133.25.1.47 PMID: 16448297

Blackie, , L. E. RWeststrate, , N. MTurner, , KAdler, , J. MMcLean, , K. C. (2023). Broadening our understanding of adversarial growth: The contribution of narrative methods. *Journal of Research in Personality, 103*. Advance online publication. DOI: 10.1016/j.jrp.2023.104359

Boals, , ABedford, , L. ACallahan, , J. L. (2019). Perceptions of change after a trauma and perceived posttraumatic growth: A prospective examination. *Behavioral Sciences, 9*(1). https://doi.org/10.3390/bs9010010

Bohlmeijer, , EWesterhof, , G. (2021). The model for sustainable mental health: future directions for integrating positive psychology into mental health care. *Frontiers in psychology, 12*, 747999.

Bride, O. M., Dunwoody, L., Lowe-Strong, A., & Kennedy, S. M. (2008). Examining adversarial growth in illness: The factor structure of the silver lining questionnaire (SLQ-38). *Psychology & Health, 23*(6). Advance online publication. DOI: 10.1080/14768320701356540 PMID: 25160809

Butler, J., & Jaffe, S. (2021). Challenges and Gratitude: A diary study of software engineers working from home during Covid-19 Pandemic. *Proceedings - International Conference on Software Engineering*. DOI: 10.1109/ICSE-SEIP52600.2021.00047

Calhoun, L. G., & Tedeschi, R. G. (1999). Facilitating Posttraumatic Growth: A Clinician's Guide. In *Personality and Clinical Psychology Series*.

Collins, R. L., Taylor, S. E., & Skokan, L. A. (1990). A Better World or a Shattered Vision? Changes in Life Perspectives Following Victimization. *Social Cognition, 8*(3). Advance online publication. DOI: 10.1521/soco.1990.8.3.263

Confino, D., Einav, M., & Margalit, M. (2023). Post-traumatic growth: the roles of the sense of entitlement, gratitude and hope. *International Journal of Applied Positive Psychology, 8*(2). Advance online publication. DOI: 10.1007/s41042-023-00102-9 PMID: 37361623

Cormio, , CMuzzatti, , BRomito, , FMattioli, , VAnnunziata, , M. A. (2017). Posttraumatic growth and cancer: a study 5 years after treatment end. *Supportive Care in Cancer, 25*(4). https://doi.org/10.1007/s00520-016-3496-4

Diniz, , GKorkes, , LTristão, , L. SPelegrini, , RBellodi, , P. LBernardo, , W. M. (2023). The effects of gratitude interventions: a systematic review and meta-analysis. *Einstein (Sao Paulo), 21*.

Dixit, S. K., & Sinha, J. (n.d.) Efficacy of Gratitude Intervention in India: Distinctive Cross-Cultural Conceptions of Gratitude Matter. *Psychological Studies*.

Drewes, , JLanger, , P. CEbert, , JKleiber, , D., & Gusy, B. (2021). Associations between experienced and internalized HIV stigma, adversarial growth, and health outcomes in a nationwide sample of people aging with HIV in Germany. *AIDS and Behavior, 25*(4), 1037-1046.

El Khoury-Malhame, M., Sfeir, M., Hallit, S., & Sawma, T. (2023). Factors associated with posttraumatic growth: Gratitude, PTSD and distress; one year into the COVID-19 pandemic in Lebanon. *Current Psychology (New Brunswick, N.J.)*. Advance online publication. DOI: 10.1007/s12144-022-04159-8 PMID: 36684466

Emmons, R. A., & McCullough, M. E. (2003). Counting blessings versus burdens: An experimental investigation of gratitude and subjective well-being in daily life. *Journal of Personality and Social Psychology*, *84*(2), 377–389. PMID: 12585811

Fagley, N. S. (2012). Appreciation uniquely predicts life satisfaction above demographics, the Big 5 personality factors, and gratitude. *Personality and Individual Differences*, *53*(1). Advance online publication. DOI: 10.1016/j.paid.2012.02.019

Folkman, S. (1997). Positive psychological states and coping with severe stress. *Social Science & Medicine*, *45*(8). Advance online publication. DOI: 10.1016/S0277-9536(97)00040-3 PMID: 9381234

Fornell, C., & Larcker, D. F. (1981). Fornell, C. and Larcker, D.F. (1981), "Evaluating structural equation models with unobservable variables and.pdf. *JMR, Journal of Marketing Research*, *XVIII*(February).

Fredrickson, B. L. (2004). The broaden-and-build theory of positive emotions. *Philosophical Transactions of the Royal Society of London. Series B, Biological Sciences*, *359*(1449), 1367–1378. PMID: 15347528

Fredrickson, B. L., Tugade, M. M., Waugh, C. E., & Larkin, G. R. (2003). What Good Are Positive Emotions in Crises? A Prospective Study of Resilience and Emotions Following the Terrorist attacks on the United States on September 11th, 2001. *Journal of Personality and Social Psychology*, *84*(2). Advance online publication. DOI: 10.1037/0022-3514.84.2.365 PMID: 12585810

Hair, J. F.Jr, Hult, G. T. M., Ringle, C. M., & Sarstedt, M. (2021). A primer on partial least squares structural equations modeling (PLS-SEM). Sage Publications. *Journal of Tourism Research*, *6*(2).

Hair, J. F., Risher, J. J., Sarstedt, M., & Ringle, C. M. (2019). When to use and how to report the results of PLS-SEM. In *European Business Review* (Vol. 31, Issue 1). DOI: 10.1108/EBR-11-2018-0203

Henson, C., Truchot, D., & Canevello, A. (2021). What promotes post traumatic growth? A systematic review. In *European Journal of Trauma and Dissociation* (Vol. 5, Issue 4). DOI: 10.1016/j.ejtd.2020.100195

Information, M., & Chin, W. W. (2013). Commentary Issues and Opinion on Structural Equation Modeling. *Management Information Systems Quarterly*, *22*(1).

Jans-Beken, L., Jacobs, N., Janssens, M., Peeters, S., Reijnders, J., Lechner, L., & Lataster, J. (2020). Gratitude and health: An updated review. *The Journal of Positive Psychology, 15*(6). Advance online publication. DOI: 10.1080/17439760.2019.1651888

Jans-Beken, L., & Wong, P. T. P. (2021). Development and preliminary validation of the Existential Gratitude Scale (EGS). *Counselling Psychology Quarterly, 34*(1). Advance online publication. DOI: 10.1080/09515070.2019.1656054

Jöreskog, K. G. (1971). Simultaneous factor analysis in several populations. *Psychometrika, 36*(4). Advance online publication. DOI: 10.1007/BF02291366

Joseph, S., & Linley, P. A. (2006). Growth following adversity: Theoretical perspectives and implications for clinical practice. *Clinical Psychology Review, 26*(8). Advance online publication. DOI: 10.1016/j.cpr.2005.12.006 PMID: 16473442

Kim, E., & Bae, S. (2019). Gratitude Moderates the Mediating Effect of Deliberate Rumination on the Relationship Between Intrusive Rumination and Post-traumatic Growth. *Frontiers in Psychology, 10*. Advance online publication. DOI: 10.3389/fpsyg.2019.02665 PMID: 31849774

Kleim, B., & Ehlers, A. (2009). Evidence for a curvilinear relationship between posttraumatic growth and posttrauma depression and PTSD in assault survivors. *Journal of Traumatic Stress, 22*(1). Advance online publication. DOI: 10.1002/jts.20378 PMID: 19230007

Lambert, N. M., Graham, S. M., Fincham, F. D., & Stillman, T. F. (2009). A changed perspective: How gratitude can affect sense of coherence through positive reframing. *The Journal of Positive Psychology, 4*(6). Advance online publication. DOI: 10.1080/17439760903157182

Leguina, A. (2015). A primer on partial least squares structural equation modeling (PLS-SEM). *International Journal of Research & Method in Education, 38*(2). Advance online publication. DOI: 10.1080/1743727x.2015.1005806

Linley, P. A., & Joseph, S. (2004). Positive Change Following Trauma and Adversity: A Review. In *Journal of Traumatic Stress* (Vol. 17, Issue 1). DOI: 10.1023/B:JOTS.0000014671.27856.7e

McBride, O., Schroevers, M. J., & Ranchor, A. V. (2009). The structure of adversarial growth in a sample of cancer patients 8 years post-diagnosis: A revision of the SLQ-38. *Psychology & Health, 24*(10). Advance online publication. DOI: 10.1080/08870440802108900 PMID: 20204988

McCullough, M. E., Emmons, R. A., & Tsang, J. A. (2002). The grateful disposition: A conceptual and empirical topography. *Journal of Personality and Social Psychology*, *82*(1). Advance online publication. DOI: 10.1037/0022-3514.82.1.112 PMID: 11811629

McCullough, M. E., Tsang, J. A., & Emmons, R. A. (2004). Gratitude in Intermediate Affective Terrain: Links of Grateful Moods to Individual Differences and Daily Emotional Experience. *Journal of Personality and Social Psychology*, *86*(2). Advance online publication. DOI: 10.1037/0022-3514.86.2.295 PMID: 14769085

Ning, J., Tang, X., Shi, H., Yao, D., Zhao, Z., & Li, J. (2023). Social support and posttraumatic growth: A meta-analysis. In *Journal of Affective Disorders* (Vol. 320). DOI: 10.1016/j.jad.2022.09.114

Nishi, D., Matsuoka, Y., & Kim, Y. (2010). Posttraumatic growth, posttraumatic stress disorder and resilience of motor vehicle accident survivors. *BioPsychoSocial Medicine*, *4*. Advance online publication. DOI: 10.1186/1751-0759-4-7 PMID: 20573276

Okuzono, S. S., Cowden, R. G., Padgett, R. N., Yancey, G., Johnson, B. R., & VanderWeele, T. J. (n.d.) Sociodemographic Variation in Gratitude Using a Cross-National Analysis with 22 Countries. *International Journal of Applied Positive Psychology*, *10*, 60.

Parikh, D., De Ieso, P., Garvey, G., Thachil, T., Ramamoorthi, R., Penniment, M., & Jayaraj, R. (2015). Post-traumatic stress disorder and post-traumatic growth in breast cancer patients - A systematic review. *Asian Pacific Journal of Cancer Prevention : APJCP*, *16*(2). Advance online publication. DOI: 10.7314/APJCP.2015.16.2.641 PMID: 25684500

Park, C. L., Cohen, L. H., & Murch, R. L. (1996). Assessment and Prediction of Stress-Related Growth. *Journal of Personality*, *64*(1). Advance online publication. DOI: 10.1111/j.1467-6494.1996.tb00815.x PMID: 8656319

Park, S., & Gupta, S. (2012). Handling endogenous regressors by joint estimation using copulas. *Marketing Science*, *31*(4). Advance online publication. DOI: 10.1287/mksc.1120.0718

Ruini, C., & Vescovelli, F. (2013). The Role of Gratitude in Breast Cancer: Its Relationships with Post-traumatic Growth, Psychological Well-Being and Distress. *Journal of Happiness Studies*, *14*(1). Advance online publication. DOI: 10.1007/s10902-012-9330-x

Rusk, R. D., Vella-Brodrick, D. A., & Waters, L. (2016). Gratitude or Gratefulness? A Conceptual Review and Proposal of the System of Appreciative Functioning. In *Journal of Happiness Studies* (Vol. 17, Issue 5). DOI: 10.1007/s10902-015-9675-z

Srirangarajan, , TOshio, , AYamaguchi, , AAkutsu, , S. (2020). Cross-Cultural Nomological Network of Gratitude: Findings From Midlife in the United States and Japan. *Frontiers in Psychology, 11*, 571. https://doi.org/10.3389/fpsyg.2020.00571

Sodergren, S. C., & Hyland, M. E. (2000). What are the positive consequences of illness? *Psychology & Health, 15*(1). Advance online publication. DOI: 10.1080/08870440008400290

Taku, K., Calhoun, L. G., Cann, A., & Tedeschi, R. G. (2008). The role of rumination in the coexistence of distress and posttraumatic growth among bereaved Japanese university students. *Death Studies, 32*(5). Advance online publication. DOI: 10.1080/07481180801974745 PMID: 18767236

Tedeschi, R. G., & Calhoun, L. G. (1996). The posttraumatic growth inventory: Measuring the positive legacy of trauma. *Journal of Traumatic Stress, 9*(3). Advance online publication. DOI: 10.1002/jts.2490090305 PMID: 8827649

Tedeschi, R. G., & Calhoun, L. G. (2004). Posttraumatic Growth: Conceptual Foundations and Empirical Evidence. In *Psychological Inquiry* (Vol. 15, Issue 1). DOI: 10.1207/s15327965pli1501_01

Tedeschi, R. G., Shakespeare-Finch, J., Taku, K., Calhoun, L. G. (2018). *Posttraumatic growth: Theory, research, and applications*. Routledge.

Unanue, , WGomez Mella, , M. ECortez, , D. ABravo, , DAraya-Véliz, , CUnanue, , JVan Den Broeck, , A. (2019). The Reciprocal Relationship Between Gratitude and Life Satisfaction: Evidence From Two Longitudinal Field Studies. *Frontiers in Psychology, 10*, 2480. https://doi.org/10.3389/fpsyg.2019.02480

Vernon, L. L., Dillon, J. M., & Steiner, A. R. W. (2009). Proactive coping, gratitude, and posttraumatic stress disorder in college women. *Anxiety, Stress, and Coping, 22*(1). Advance online publication. DOI: 10.1080/10615800802203751 PMID: 18791902

Vieselmeyer, J., Holguin, J., & Mezulis, A. (2017). The role of resilience and gratitude in posttraumatic stress and growth following a campus shooting. *Psychological Trauma: Theory, Research, Practice, and Policy, 9*(1). Advance online publication. DOI: 10.1037/tra0000149 PMID: 27548470

Watkins, P. C., Woodward, K., Stone, T., & Kolts, R. L. (2003). Gratitude and happiness: Development of a measure of gratitude, and relationships with subjective well-being. *Social Behavior and Personality, 31*(5). Advance online publication. DOI: 10.2224/sbp.2003.31.5.431

Wood, A. M., Froh, J. J., & Geraghty, A. W. A. (2010). Gratitude and well-being: A review and theoretical integration. In *Clinical Psychology Review* (Vol. 30, Issue 7). DOI: 10.1016/j.cpr.2010.03.005

Wu, X., Kaminga, A. C., Dai, W., Deng, J., Wang, Z., Pan, X., & Liu, A. (2019). The prevalence of moderate-to-high posttraumatic growth: A systematic review and meta-analysis. In *Journal of Affective Disorders* (Vol. 243). DOI: 10.1016/j.jad.2018.09.023

Zhou, X., & Wu, X. (2015). Longitudinal relationships between gratitude, deliberate rumination, and posttraumatic growth in adolescents following the Wenchuan earthquake in China. *Scandinavian Journal of Psychology, 56*(5). Advance online publication. DOI: 10.1111/sjop.12237 PMID: 26122407

APPENDIX

Scale for Gratitude

1. I have so much in life to be thankful for.
2. If I had to list everything that I felt grateful for, it would be a very long list.
3. When I look at the world, I don't see much to be grateful for.*
4. I am grateful to a wide variety of people.
5. As I get older I find myself more able to appreciate the people, events, and situations that have been part of my life history.
6. Long amounts of time can go by before I feel grateful to something or someone.*

* Items 3 and 6 are reverse-scored.

Updated Scale for Silver Lining (Adversarial Growth) -24 SLQ 382

1. My illness gave me a new start in life
2. My life is much better now than it was before my illness
3. My illness has made me live life to its fullest
4. My illness made me think about the true purpose of life
5. My religious/spiritual beliefs deepened because of my illness
6. I became a happier person because of my illness
7. My illness made me a more tolerant person
8. My illness gave me more confidence
9. I am less concerned about failure because of my illness
10. My illness gave me permission to do things for myself
11. My illness made me a more determined person
12. My illness helped me find myself
13. My illness made me more aware of my strengths
14. My illness made me face up to problem areas of my life
15. My illness strengthened my relationships with others
16. My illness made me less concerned with the approval of others
17. My illness made me more at ease with others
18. My illness taught me how to stand up for myself
19. My illness made me less judgemental of others
20. I have been an inspiration to others
21. People can be more open with me since my illness
22. My illness changed other people for the better

23. My illness changed other people's perception of me for the better
24. Other people appreciate me more because of my illness

The Measurement Model

Table 3. Measurement model result

Latent Variables	*Factors*	*Loadings*	*CA*	*CR*	*AVE*
Change in Life Philosophy	CLP1	0.911	0.641	0.843	0.730
	CLP2	0.794			
Greater Appreciation of life	GAL1	0.832	0.906	0.930	0.726
	GAL2	0.862			
	GAL3	0.888			
	GAL4	0.882			
	GAL5	0.792			
Gratitude	GT1	0.905	0.930	0.950	0.827
	GT2	0.929			
	GT4	0.897			
	GT5	0.907			
Improved Personal relationship	IPR1	0.765	0.802	0.858	0.504
	IPR2	0.641			
	IPR3	0.824			
	IPR4	0.735			
	IPR5	0.697			
	IPR6	0.570			
Personal Inner Strength	PIS1	0.818	0.936	0.949	0.757
	PIS2	0.889			
	PIS3	0.871			
	PIS4	0.906			
	PIS5	0.878			
	PIS6	0.856			
Positive Influence on Others	PIO1	0.767	0.860	0.897	0.637
	PIO2	0.708			
	PIO3	0.832			
	PIO4	0.799			

continued on following page

Table 3. Continued

Latent Variables	*Factors*	*Loadings*	*CA*	*CR*	*AVE*
	PIO5	0.875			

Source: *Smart PLS Output*

Table 4. Depicting the Discriminant Validity (Fornell- Lacker)

Constructs	*CLP*	*GAL*	*GT*	*IPR*	*PIS*	*PIO*
CLP	0.854					
GAL	0.740	0.852				
GT	0.590	0.541	0.909			
IPR	0.697	0.754	0.665	0.850		
PIS	0.720	0.672	0.631	0.823	0.870	
PIO	0.537	0.591	0.389	0.564	0.606	0.798

Source: Smart PLS Output

The Structural Model

Table 5. Variance Inflation Factor (VIF)

Constructs	**CLP**	**GAL**	**IPR**	**PIS**	**PIO**
Gratitude	1.000	1.000	1.000	1.000	1.000

Source: Smart PLS Output

Hypothesis Testing

Table 6. Hypotheses testing

hypothesis	Relationship	Sample mean	Standard deviation	T statistics	P values	Decision
H1a	**GT ⇒ IPR**	0.676	0.071	9.303	0.000	Accepted
H1b	**GT ⇒ GAL**	0.550	0.077	7.067	0.000	Accepted
H1c	**GT ⇒ CLP**	0.591	0.079	7.458	0.000	Accepted
H1d	**GT ⇒ PIO**	0.412	0.083	4.685	0.000	Accepted
H1e	**GT ⇒ PIS**	0.634	0.081	7.764	0.000	Accepted

Source: Smart PLS Output

Table 7. Explanatory and Predictive Power

Construct	R^2	Q^2
CLP	0.348	0.326
GAL	0.293	0.274
IPR	0.442	0.414
PIS	0.398	0.374
PIO	0.151	0.111

Source: Smart PLS Output

Figure 2. Model

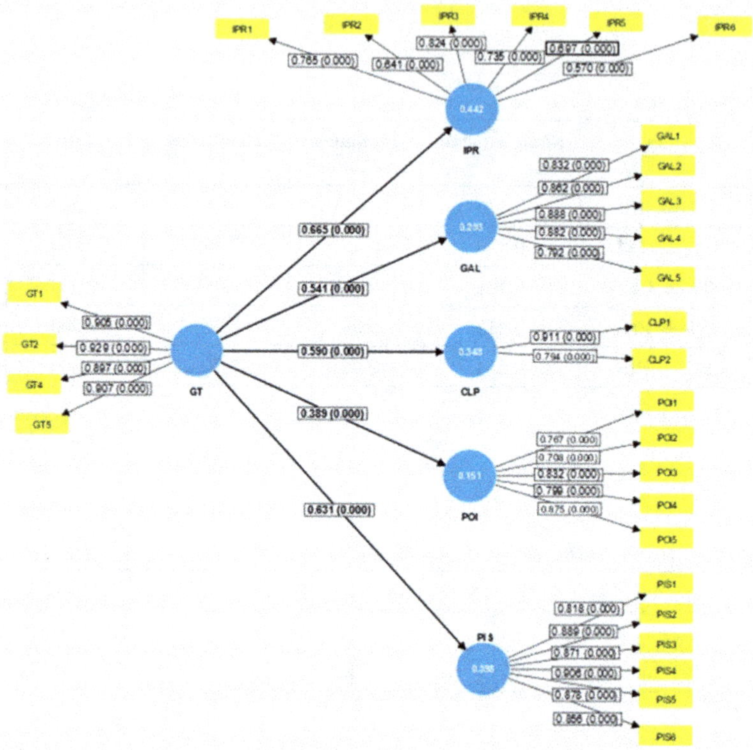

Source: Smart PLS output

Robustness Check

Table 8. Depicting Endogeneity Test (Gaussian copula(GC) approach)

Tests	Constructs	Coefficient	P values
GC of IPR	GT -> CLP	0.593	0
	GT -> GAL	0.549	0
	GT -> IPR	0.722	0.003
	GT -> PIS	0.636	0
	GT -> PIO	0.413	0
	GC (GT) -> IPR	**-0.047**	**0.913**
GC of GAL	GT -> CLP	0.593	0
	GT -> GAL	0.428	0.068
	GT -> IPR	0.676	0
	GT -> PIS	0.636	0
	GT -> PIO	0.413	0
	GC (GT) -> GAL	**0.115**	**0.37**
GC of CLP	GT -> CLP	0.672	0.002
	GT -> GAL	0.549	0
	GT -> IPR	0.676	0
	GT -> PIS	0.636	0
	GT -> PIO	0.413	0
	GC (GT) -> CLP	**-0.078**	**0.777**
GC of PIO	GT -> CLP	0.593	0
	GT -> GAL	0.549	0
	GT -> IPR	0.676	0
	GT -> PIS	0.636	0
	GT -> PIO	0.698	0.007
	GC (GT) -> PIO	**-0.278**	**0.224**
GC of PIS	GT -> CLP	0.593	0
	GT -> GAL	0.549	0
	GT -> IPR	0.676	0
	GT -> PIS	0.896	0
	GT -> PIO	0.413	0
	GC (GT) -> PIS	**-0.253**	**0.237**

Source: Smart PLS Output

Chapter 11
Ritual Recitation as a Mind-Body Practice for Trauma Recovery:
Exploring the Healing Power of Mantras

Aira Dutta
http://orcid.org/0009-0005-7171-9359
O.P. Jindal Global University, India

Kirti Tyagi
http://orcid.org/0000-0001-8454-335X
O.P. Jindal Global University, India

ABSTRACT

Ritual recitation, central to many religious traditions, is increasingly recognized as a promising mind-body intervention for trauma recovery. Trauma often disrupts the nervous system, leaving survivors in cycles of emotional dysregulation, hyperarousal, and loss of meaning. While conventional trauma therapies offer significant support, they may not fully address all the dimensions of trauma recovery. In this context, mantra-based meditation (MBM) emerges as a culturally grounded, low-cost practice that supports healing across physiological, cognitive, emotional, and spiritual dimensions. This chapter employs a theoretical approach and synthesizes existing research and conceptualizes the role of ritual recitation in trauma recovery. It further explores the neural mechanisms underlying mantra recitation and understands the integration of recitation-based interventions into trauma therapy. By bridging psychological, spiritual, cultural, and religious perspectives, this chapter positions ritual recitation as a holistic tool for fostering mental well-being in trauma survivors.

DOI: 10.4018/979-8-3373-3521-6.ch011

INTRODUCTION

Mind-body interventions emphasize the dynamic interaction between the brain and body, aiming to enhance overall well-being by improving mood, supporting physiological functioning, addressing sleep disturbances, and fostering relaxation. Such practices include biofeedback, spiritual practices, visual imagery, and expressive therapies through art, dance, and music (Lee & Moore, 2017). Spiritual practices are increasingly gaining attention in contemporary research due to their multifaceted benefits and widespread applicability. Many of these interventions are well embedded within religious and traditional practices that have long served society. They serve as a means of connecting with the divine, building community, and transforming interpersonal relationships.

Ritual recitation, particularly the chanting of mantras, is one such practice emerging as a powerful mind-body intervention for trauma recovery. Mantra chanting invites focused attention, rhythmic breath, and vocal resonance. Together, these elements foster emotional regulation and a felt sense of safety. Indulgence in religious practices encourages one to seek the sacred during times of stress, thereby further alleviating negative thoughts, emotions, and anxiety (Harper & Pargament, 2015).

This chapter employs an exploratory, narrative review approach. It synthesizes conceptual and empirical literature across multiple disciplines to explore the potential of mantra-based meditation for trauma healing. The goal is not to offer definitive conclusions but to identify emerging patterns, conceptual linkages, and promising avenues for future research. Given the heterogeneity of available studies and the limited number of randomized trials, this review positions MBM as an emerging integrative approach that requires future empirical validation. The chapter primarily focuses on the theoretical mechanisms through which Mantra-Based Meditation (MBM) may alleviate trauma-related symptoms, and does not aim to evaluate its empirical efficacy. It also proposes exploring mantra recitation not only as a religious or cultural tradition but also as a therapeutic modality with profound implications for healing trauma. This chapter uses the terms “ritual recitation” and “mantra-based meditation” interchangeably.

Methods and Scope

This chapter is a narrative, theory-integrating review of mantra-based meditation (MBM) in trauma contexts. Literature was identified through searches of MEDLINE/PubMed, PsycINFO, Embase, Cochrane Library, and Google Scholar (January 2000-December 2025), using keywords such as mantra, mantram repetition, chanting, Transcendental Meditation, PTSD, trauma, autonomic, vagal, heart rate variability, and default mode network.

Inclusion Criteria

Peer-reviewed empirical or review articles involving adults, focusing on trauma symptoms or mechanisms relevant to trauma (autonomic regulation, attentional/rumination processes, spiritual/existential dimensions).

Exclusion Criteria

Commentaries, opinion pieces, case reports without standardized measures, and meditation interventions not centered on linguistic repetition (e.g., breath-only practices, open-monitoring mindfulness).

Evidence is weighted according to study design (meta-analyses and randomized controlled trials > observational studies > qualitative studies), sample size, and relevance to trauma populations. Findings from small pilot studies (e.g., neuroimaging, HRV) are treated as preliminary and hypothesis-generating, not definitive.

This chapter, therefore, provides a conceptual synthesis, integrating empirical evidence while explicitly acknowledging limitations, heterogeneity, and the preliminary nature of many studies.

Ritual Recitation/Mantra-Based Meditation (MBM): A Contemplative Healing Tool

Mantra-Based Meditation (MBM) refers to practices in which a specific sound, word, or phrase is repeated silently or aloud as the primary attentional anchor. This includes standardized programs (e.g., Transcendental Meditation, Mantram Repetition Program) and culturally rooted chanting or prayer repetition. The term 'mantra' originates from Sanskrit, meaning "instrument of thought" or "sacred text" (Burke et al., 2017; Barnes, 2018; Orme-Johnson et al., 2024). MBM is distinct from mindfulness-based programs (e.g., MBSR, MBCT), which emphasize open monitoring or non-judgmental awareness without a fixed linguistic anchor. MBM is therefore categorized as a focused-attention family centered on linguistic repetition (Álvarez-Pérez et al., 2022). In studies where interventions combine multiple elements or where categories are blurred, these ambiguities are noted, and no MBM-specific effects are inferred.

Other forms of MBM include programs such as Benson's Relaxation Response and standardized mantra techniques. In contrast, practices such as breath-focused, body-scan, or loving-kindness (metta) meditation do not use mantra repetition as their core method. They are thus explicitly excluded from the MBM category (Álvarez-Pérez et al., 2022). MBM falls under Automatic Self-Transcending. In contrast, mindfulness practices are classified as Focused Attention (FA), which essentially means sustaining attention on a chosen object, or Open Monitoring (OM), which involves non-judgmental awareness of moment-to-moment experience (Orme-Johnson et al., 2024).

Mantra chanting as a practice is relatively easy to engage in. However, its complex interplay of breath, sound, rhythm, and focused attention guides one towards spiritual transformation and psychological and physical healing. Chanting the sound 'AUM' generates vibrations and sound frequencies that produce physical sensations directly affecting our whole body. The process stimulates the entire vocal and resonance system as 'A' resonates the stomach and chest, U' resonates the throat and chest, and finally 'M' stimulates the brain, nasal cavity, and skull, involving some body parts and organs (Acosta, 2020).

Reciting a mantra extends beyond fostering a state of rest; it also cultivates skills such as shifting and sustaining attention. As the human mind tends to wander, the possibility of the mind being devoid of any idea/ thought is nearly impossible. Through continuous repetition, chanting trains the practitioner to engage in focused attention and sustain it for an extended period. This routine restoration of attention, the moment it wavers, trains the mind to maintain focus and helps the individual develop the ability to shift it deliberately, reinforcing mental discipline and attentional control (Perry et al., 2022).

Understanding Trauma: Core Disruptions

Trauma has enduring effects on the nervous system, often leaving survivors caught in cycles of emotional dysregulation, hyperarousal, and a diminished sense of meaning (Center for Substance Abuse Treatment, 2014b). Trauma-related disturbance can be understood across three interacting domains:

Autonomic Dysregulation

Trauma frequently results in a chronic loss of homeostasis balance, leaving the individual caught between states of hyperarousal and hypoarousal. Additionally, the disruption of vagal balance impairs the body's natural capacity for physiological settling. This lack of autonomic flexibility is clinically evidenced by reduced Heart Rate Variability (HRV), a key metric indicating a diminished ability to regulate emotional and physical stress.

Cognitive-Emotional Dysregulation

The psychological and neurocognitive fragmentation is marked by persistent intrusions of memories and rumination, which prevent the individual from maintaining a stable orientation to the present. It is often manifested as attentional narrowing, survival-based 'tunnel vision' that prioritizes threat detection over broader environmental engagement. In addition, there is the experience of profound numbing as a protective defense against overwhelming distress. These symptoms are often compounded by negative self-appraisals and distorted beliefs about safety and self-worth, which further entrench the traumatic experience within the individual's mental architecture.

Existential, Spiritual, and Cultural Disruption

An individual's life meaning and social connectivity are often seen as significant markers of the trauma dysregulation framework, which is manifested in the form of rupture in identity, creating a disconnect between one's past and present selves. This disruption can manifest as moral injury, violating one's core ethical or spiritual values. Furthermore, trauma frequently serves ties to cultural or communal belonging, leaving the individual isolated from the social support systems and rituals that traditionally provide a sense of security. This existential displacement represents a collapse of the individual's worldview, necessitating a reconstruction of meaning that goes beyond simple symptom reduction.

This tripartite framework demonstrates that trauma is an integrated crisis of the body, mind, and spirit. By understanding these interacting domains, the application of Mind-Body Medicine becomes a targeted process of reintegration (Center for Substance Abuse Treatment, 2014b).

Why Mantra-Meditation for Trauma Recovery?

Mind-body interventions such as yoga, meditation, relaxation, and breathwork have demonstrated significant benefits for stress reduction, emotional balance, and activation of the parasympathetic nervous system. Amongst the most notable outcomes for these interventions is the reduction in severity of PTSD symptoms (Kim et al., 2013). These practices are supported by scientific evidence, indicating that alterations in physiological processes and activation of specific brain regions contribute to relaxation, mental clarity, grounding, and restorative states.

Trauma is not confined to the mind; it is also embodied within the body. Fear, anxiety, shame, and guilt often manifest as chronic physical tension, which results in being 'always on the edge', sleep difficulties, and difficulty concentrating (Lebow, 2023). Trauma may further be presented through a range of symptoms like muscle tension, panic attacks characterized by shortness of breath, chest tightness, and hyperventilation, digestive issues like stomach pain, fluctuations in appetite, cardiovascular difficulties like risk for high blood pressure, and heart diseases

(Center for Substance Abuse Treatment, 2014b). Such somatic issues may persist if not appropriately addressed. However, trauma has conventionally been addressed through cognitive and talk-based approaches like cognitive behavioral therapy (CBT), rational emotive behavior therapy (REBT), Beck's cognitive therapy, and narrative exposure therapy, which primarily target maladaptive cognitions and often overlook somatic dimensions, which thus remain unresolved (Lebow, 2023).

This fundamental limitation underscores the need for integrative approaches addressing psychological and physiological aspects. Empirical research reveals the effectiveness of non-clinical, less intrusive, and low-cost approaches like mantra chanting or similar traditional practices in reducing trauma-related symptoms. In contrast, psychotherapies like CBT and others often require clients to cognitively engage with the memories and aspects of the event, which leads to reliving them, thus resulting in significant distress. MBM allows one to enter the divine realm and experience relaxation as well as establish a sacred connection with a divine power or oneself, further facilitating a state of transcendence (Beshai et al., 2024)

Mantras have a religious connotation or sacred meaning, which makes mantra chanting both a spiritual and religious practice. Research indicates that such interventions reduce the intensity of trauma symptoms effectively. It has been brought to light that positive religious interventions, which essentially represent a strong spiritual connection, effectively contribute to post-traumatic recovery as well as growth. Results include finding hope and purpose, greater appreciation for life, and personal development. A body of research highlighted how repetition of mantras based on religious traditions over a period of 10 weeks was found to notably reduce intrusive thoughts, anger, symptoms of stress, and depression, which are common in PTSD, and improve overall perceived quality of life (Harper & Pargament, 2015; Larsen et al., 2025). This indicates that mantra recitation as a positive religious practice contributes to the reduction of post-traumatic symptoms. Based on the findings, it can be established that mantra recitation has therapeutic potential. Accordingly, this chapter explores how mantra-based meditation (MBM), a culturally grounded and accessible practice, addresses trauma healing at physiological, cognitive, emotional, and spiritual levels.

Three Pathways Model

The chapter is organized thematically to examine the trauma-healing process through mantra recitation. The first pathway investigates how MBM facilitates bodily regulation by engaging breath, rhythm, and sound. It highlights how these elements activate the parasympathetic nervous system and support emotional grounding, which is especially valuable for trauma survivors experiencing chronic hyperarousal and physiological dysregulation.

The second pathway explores the cognitive functions, emphasizing their role as cognitive anchors and creating pathways for emotional resilience and meaning-making in the wake of trauma. This section draws upon positive coping theory to illustrate how repetitive sacred sounds can help restructure traumatic experiences through patterns and cultivate inner stability.

The third pathway discusses existential and communal dimensions of healing. It addresses how mantra-based practices enable spiritual reconnection and reinforce cultural belonging, especially in non-Western and faith-oriented contexts.

Embodied Regulation Pathway

Traumatic events are highly stressful experiences that can disrupt the body's typical functioning. One of the most pronounced differences in functioning, post-trauma, is the dysregulated fight-or-flight response. Individuals often remain hypervigilant, indicating that their fight-or-flight response, a survival mechanism, is rarely deactivated after exposure. Hyperarousal impairs an individual's ability to respond appropriately to stimuli, often triggering exaggerated reactions to non-threatening events (Center for Substance Abuse Treatment, 2014b). For instance, an unexpected loud noise, such as a dog barking, may provoke a disproportionate fear response, such as an urge to hide. This indicates how their body is always prepared to fight or flee when it experiences a 'threatening' stimulus; it is the body's way of preparing for the future (Center for Substance Abuse Treatment, 2014b; Sherin & Nemeroff, 2011).

Mind-body practices such as chanting or mantra recitation are recommended to regain arousal, reduce stress to an optimal level, and activate the parasympathetic nervous system. Early research found that Transcendental Meditation elicits a "restfully alert" hypometabolic state, essentially the opposite of the sympathetic "fight or flight" response. A meta-analysis of 32 studies found that respiratory rate, skin conductance, and blood lactate decreased significantly during Transcendental Meditation practice compared with eyes-closed rest (Orme-Johnson et al., 2024). Additionally, Functional neuroimaging research suggests that mantra repetition exerts widespread inhibitory effects on cortical activity, particularly within the default mode network (DMN). A seminal fMRI study demonstrates that covert repetitive speech (an analog of silent mantra practice) resulted in a broad, unidirectional reduction in blood-oxygen-level-dependent (BOLD) signal, most prominently in the medial prefrontal, posterior cingulate, and precuneus regions. These areas are strongly implicated in self-referential cognition and autobiographical memory processes that are often hyperactive in trauma (Whitfield-Gabrieli & Ford, 2012).

Chanting, studied for its potential as a regulator of various bodily states, is woven into spiritual frameworks. Its impact has been found mainly on the autonomic nervous system, specifically the parasympathetic branch, as reflected by reductions in heart rate, respiratory rate, and blood pressure, and an increase in galvanic skin resistance (GSR) indicating subdued sympathetic tone (Telles et al., 1995).

A recent study demonstrated that mantra meditation can decrease HRV indices, indicating elevated stress. The study included subjects participating in an eight-week intervention, with pre- and post-intervention assessments using EEG and heart rate variability (HRV), enabling simultaneous evaluation of cortical oscillations and autonomic regulation. Following the intervention, participants demonstrated a significant increase in HRV indices. The metrics involved in this, namely the root mean square of successive differences (RMSSD) and the standard deviation of normal-to-normal intervals (SDNN), are gold-standard measures of parasympathetic activity. A reduction in resting heart rate and stress index was also observed, indicating a shift towards vagal dominance and improved autonomic regulation. The study also reports an increase in the correlation between EEG metrics and HRV after the intervention, indicating neural-cardiac synchrony, synchronization of brain oscillations, and autonomic function. These findings support the claim that MBM can mitigate sympathetic overactivation, a hallmark of PTSD and chronic hyperarousal (Singh et al., 2025).

Chanting is multifaceted, encompassing vibratory sensation, respiratory frequency, and rhythmic entertainment. Repeating sounds or specific phrases during chanting has been linked with reduced heart rate and breathing (Singhdeo, 2023), thereby activating the parasympathetic system. Vocalizing is associated with focused attention on the sound and the vibration, coupled with the physiological changes, leads to feelings of calmness and relaxation. Repetition helps ground one in the present moment, anchors attention, and creates a sense of peace (Perry et al., 2022).

Chanting supports the alignment of breathing and heart rate in a way distinct from everyday respiration. In daily speech or movement, exhalations tend to be brief. In contrast, chanting involves prolonged exhalations, further stimulating the parasympathetic system, optimizing physiological processes, and enhancing emotional resilience and mental clarity (Barbaresi et al., 2025). Its restorative nature makes it particularly valuable within the trauma recovery framework.

Synonymously used with it is another practice, mantra recitation. Mantra-based meditation (MBM) or mantra recitation has demonstrated rehabilitative effects, such as reducing stress, anxiety levels, and post-traumatic symptoms (Álvarez-Pérez et al., 2022). Practitioners may report experiences described as spiritual or transcendent.

While MBM is effective in isolation, integrating it into a collaborative therapeutic approach alongside complementary practices such as Trauma Sensitive Yoga (TSY) and breath-based techniques may amplify its effects. TSY generally includes low-impact forms guided by gentle directions coupled with trauma-informed language, helping trauma survivors cope with dissociation and intrusive symptoms by anchoring their attention to the somatic sensations, thus allowing them to remain grounded and aware (Oosterbroek & Dirk, 2021). Coupling these movements and forms with the chanting of mantras or humming 'OM' will likely synchronize bodily processes with their vibrations, allowing the individual to experience internal safety and the reconnection of mind and body. Using mantra chanting with breath-based therapies enhances its capacity to regulate hyperarousal and an activated parasympathetic nervous system (Malesu, 2025). These practices support the reestablishment of interoception, often altered due to trauma, propelling therapists to offer recovery frameworks that are holistic, spiritual, and sensitive, with minimal engagement with traumatic aspects. These findings are preliminary, small-sample, and not specific to the trauma population.

Cognitive-Emotional Reframing Pathway

Following trauma, individuals begin to view the world as unfair and dangerous, leading to helplessness and hopelessness. This disrupted belief system makes it difficult for them to trust others, impair the ability to build and maintain relationships, adjust to changes, lower self-esteem and self-confidence, and further create fragments within their identity, for instance, difficulty distinguishing between their past and present selves (Cruz et al., 2022). It underscores the importance of trauma interventions that aim to not only rebuild one's core beliefs and assumptions but also help them engage in adaptive coping strategies and piece back the puzzles of their identity.

Trauma symptoms reflect more than surface-level distress or mere consequences; they indicate a maladaptive utilization of cognitive resources, disrupting cognitive functions. Effective intervention, therefore, must address underlying difficulties, allowing the brain to regulate and obtain cognitive stability. The repetitive nature of mantra chanting aligns with this idea as it helps focus the mind in one direction and reduces the 'wandering' characterized by a constant stream of thoughts. The tunnel averts the mind from potentially discomforting thoughts and emotions, guiding it towards a state of harmony and a more desirable space (Bormann, 2010).

One widely used method to promote this growth is through positive affirmations. Inculcating them in daily life reinforces emotional healing (Finley et al., 2018). This has been a crucial part of trauma healing because it includes the development of neural pathways. The brain's neuroplasticity allows these positive pathways to strengthen over time, with repeated use, and eventually the negative circuits will wither as the positive ones take over. Additionally, activation of the prefrontal cortex, a brain region responsible for emotional regulation, cognitive control, and stress reduction, supports the formation of positive thought patterns and emotional resilience (Falk et al., 2015).

Trauma's impact on core beliefs and assumptions extends beyond personal identity, including spiritual frameworks and religious worldviews. In this light, coping through religious and spiritual means becomes central. Many individuals tend to have a constructive relationship with their spiritual and religious practices, which they use to navigate distress. This is known as positive religious coping, an adaptive strategy that involves faith and religious practices and may include feeling closer to the divine, experiencing a renewed sense of purpose, and fostering unity with a higher power (Larsen et al., 2025). Practices such as praying have been found to be effective for emotional regulation and healing.

Moreover, MBM or mantra chanting is preferable because conventional trauma therapy emphasizes narration to achieve cognitive integration and reprocessing, which can be intrusive and emotionally taxing for the client, especially during early recovery stages. The most significant part of narration is meaning-making. Repeatedly narrating traumatic events in detail can trigger the individual and overwhelm them in the process, resulting in potential re-traumatization. It is often accompanied by cognitive overload, which can lead to distress. Additionally, constant focus on storytelling can prevent the client from being grounded in the present and keep them stuck in the past (Center for Substance Abuse Treatment, 2014a).

Furthermore, mantra recitation has the potential to become a widely used self-regulation strategy to foster a sense of safety and reduce cognitive load. Familiarity is often comforting because it offers a respite from the unpredictability and the distress that comes with it. If one continues to practice chanting or MBM, the soothing familiarity of this practice may offer the required predictability and comfort. This is better explained by the 'mere exposure effect', which suggests that we like things we are more exposed to (Ungvarsky, 2024). It might also be why people rewatch the same shows and movies over and over again. It brings them comfort, familiarity, and predictability. Similarly, returning to a practiced mantra can serve as a cognitive anchor in distress, offering an immediate, accessible sense of safety and stability and further acting as a reliable emotional refuge.

Spiritual and Cultural Restoration Pathway

From the discussions in the previous sections, it is evident that trauma can inflict profound wounds, making it difficult for individuals to find their purpose in life, question their place in society, and experience an overarching sense of loss. For survivors of traumatic events that involve a brush with death, mortality becomes salient, often triggering existential reflection, leading them to engage in existential quests. It may include emphasizing and prioritizing small things that seem more important, like family, friends, and daily indulgences over material pursuits or long working hours. Such existential clarity results in more concrete and meaningful ways of living (Tedeschi et al., 2014).

Since trauma leads to fragmentation of different fabrics of an individual's life, feelings of hopelessness, worthlessness, and an overall sense of disconnection with one's own body are some commonly observed outcomes. These are particularly pronounced in the case of developmental trauma, which can include dysfunctional attachments, abuse or violence at a young age, bullying, chronic sibling discord, etc. Since early childhood is a formative period during which one is developing one's identity, beliefs, and assumptions, a discourse in that process is bound to cause significant damage to overall development, a dysfunctional view of oneself and others, and feelings of shame and guilt (Treisman, 2017).

Parallelly, communal experiences of trauma like oppression, discrimination, systemic violence, wars, pandemic, etc., can result in a diminished sense of belonging and a loss of shared values. These traumas remain within the collective memory of the survivors, which can persist for a long time, leading to transmission across generations (Heart, 2003). It causes significant damage to the group's identity and erodes their sense of belonging, leading to the loss of crucial associations with the community. This contributes to existential wounds, alienation from society, and dislocation.

Trauma, rooted in racism, colonialism, homophobia, and other systemic oppressions, is not just collective but also historical and enduring, resulting in shaping their perception of the world, fundamentally altering core beliefs and assumptions. This notion is also referred to as insidious trauma (Menhinick & Sanders, 2023). Grief arising from cultural trauma is not just a sum of individual traumas; it collectively impacts the entire fabric of culture for those individuals. The hopeful prospect in collective trauma is that they are not alone and can work together to reconstruct their identity, engage in collective meaning-making, and try to convert their loss experience into a renewed sense of purpose and shared identity. This allows them to believe they are not alone and can work as a group to reconstruct their identity, engage in collective meaning, and try to convert their experience into a renewed sense of purpose and belonging. Modalities drawn from traditional and spiritual concepts may offer relatively greater effectiveness for those who have endured cultural trauma.

Studies from psychology and neuroscience have recognized ritualistic practices like chanting and recitation as 'holistic health interventions' due to their efficacy and ability to establish connections and restore stability. These practices are particularly impactful in regulating the 'Default Mode Network (DMN)'- a network of brain regions facilitating mind-wandering and ruminations.

Somatic symptoms of trauma can also be addressed by engaging in breathwork and ritual practices, as they require utilizing energy, aiding in eliminating trauma stored within the body. Physiological and spiritual benefits come hand in hand with mantra recitation and similar practices. Rhythmic, loud, and communal chanting of mantras, often called 'divine utterance,' may induce a state of transcendence, provide mental clarity, heal the body and soul, and foster positivity (Perry et al., 2022).

. Group chanting is a powerful example of how individuals with similar experiences can come together to process their difficulties while simultaneously receiving and providing empathy and solace. It generates 'collective spiritual energy' and a sense of togetherness, enhancing unity. Chanting is relatively more effective when done within a group setting. It is highly relevant in the context of cultural trauma because chants, including traditional or religious content, connect practitioners to their heritage, honoring their ancestors and paying homage to their traditions (Saxena, 2023). These group-oriented practices create collective catharsis, transforming suffering into renewed strength and growth.

Furthermore, engaging in traditional and ancestral practices and ceremonies to heal collective trauma can be one of the best ways of healing (Angeli-Gordon, 2025). Amongst the most impactful of these traditions is storytelling, which engages people, helps them learn about their history, ancestry, and lineage, and brings cohesion within the group. It is a powerful tool for transmitting memory collectively and integrating narratives that oppressive perpetrators have buried. Sharing and listening to narratives about the culture and individual experiences of trauma, healing, and resilience allow communities to engage in group healing within their cultural context. Furthermore, sharing knowledge about one's culture helps retain it. It makes others aware of the ancestral way of life, which they can incorporate into their contemporary way of life (Ghanem, 2024).

These kinds of positive changes, such as reconciliation, reconstruction, and the integration of a lost culture, are drawn from the concept of Post Traumatic Growth, which refers to a level of recovery from a traumatic event, a significant crisis, or a highly stressful situation that may occur in its aftermath which are usually transformative (Tedeschi et al., 2014). Ceremonies and practices, on the other hand, have a similar yet dynamic impact on stimulating growth. They promote continuity and sustain practices, thus honoring their forefathers. Importantly, it is an effective method for healing cultural wounds, including through collective dialogue, memory, and the reintegration of suppressed traditions. An integral part of bringing back traditional practices is that they can be modified to meet contemporary needs while preserving their original essence and carrying on the legacy. This idea goes beyond retaining culture and involves healing, reconstructing, adapting, and paving the path towards a reclaimed future (Ghanem, 2024). The fact that communities can establish shared values, purpose, narratives, and make meaning of their experiences is PTG, characterized by increased strength and resilience and healed cultural wounds.

Evidence Snapshot - MBM for Trauma Meta-analyses:

- Mantra-based meditation shows small to moderate reductions in anxiety, depression, stress, and post-traumatic stress symptoms (e.g., $g \approx -0.59$), but evidence is limited by risk of bias and few long-term PTSD trials.
- Yoga-related meta-analyses show improvements in self-reported PTSD symptoms but not in clinician-rated outcomes; effects vary widely by modality and study quality.
- Transcendental Meditation trials show promising effects in some analyses, but require independent replication and direct comparisons with first-line PTSD treatments

Guidelines:

- The 2023 VA/DoD PTSD Clinical Practice Guideline rates trauma-focused psychotherapies (e.g., EMDR, CPT, PE) as first-line.
- Mindfulness-based stress reduction receives a "weak for" suggestion; mantram repetition currently has insufficient evidence as primary PTSD treatment.

Mechanisms:

- fMRI studies of mantra/repetitive speech indicate DMN deactivation, but samples are small and non-clinical.
- HRV studies of OM chanting suggest parasympathetic increases, but evidence is preliminary and not trauma-specific.

Safety:

- Across meditation research, 8–37% of participants report unpleasant or adverse effects; trauma history increases risk.
- Dissociation, panic spikes, and intrusive memories may occur; screening and monitoring are recommended.

Overall:

- MBM appears promising as a complementary, present-centered practice supporting stabilization and regulation. Current evidence does not justify its use as a standalone treatment for PTSD.

Integrative Model: Mantra Meditations as a Multilevel Intervention

Mantra recitation and Mantra-Based Meditation offer a comprehensive and holistic strategy for trauma recovery by simultaneously indulging cognitive, physical, spiritual, and emotional domains. In ritual ceremonies and practices, mantras are not merely sounds but highly meaningful expressions of sacred content, often representing devotion, loyalty, and a sense of connection with the Divine. This spiritual aspect enhances their healing potential.

Psychological, neurobiological, and scientific studies have shown that chanting or mantra repetition can reduce stress, modify mood, promote mental clarity, and bring the mind to rest. MBM has been shown to be beneficial for individuals and groups experiencing various forms of trauma, offering potential applicability across diverse populations. A review synthesizes 61 eligible longitudinal studies, including randomized controlled trials, controlled trials, and case series spanning January 1970 to June 2024. All studies involved participants diagnosed with PTSD from a variety of settings, such as veterans, refugees, survivors of violence, and medical clinics. The meta-analysis highlights how one type of MBM, that is, Transcendental Meditation, yielded significant improvements in PTSD symptoms. Treatment adherence amongst the population was 85% at the start of the course and 81% at completion. Higher adherence rate in this case suggests that meditation therapies are feasible across diverse trauma-affected groups (Orme-Johnson et al., 2024).

At a physiological level, mantras combined with synchronized breathing activate the parasympathetic nervous system, reducing cortisol levels, increasing prefrontal cortex activity, and reducing amygdala activity. These neurobiological changes support the regulation of hyperarousal symptoms, facilitating a stable platform for recovery (Boyd et al., 2017). Overall, it counteracts the body's stress response, which gets dysregulated post-trauma.

MBM also serves as a potential tool to manage difficult emotions and alter affective states by cultivating 'present-moment awareness', and reducing emotional exhaustion (Lynch et al., 2018). Intrusive symptoms such as negative thought patterns and ruminations, which are the hallmarks of trauma, are also addressed through this meditative practice. Employing focused attention on the sound helps decrease 'mind-wandering', which is often linked to depression and anxiety, as it causes ruminative narratives. Hence, decreasing mind-wandering ensures overall well-being (Perry et al., 2022).

For many, trauma can cause existential wounds that can be healed through meditation and chanting as practitioners develop a sense of hope, meaning, and purpose (Álvarez-Pérez et al., 2022; Harper & Pargament, 2015). Even without a religious connotation, this practice may induce one into a state of transcendence, the deepest meditative state with the highest level of calmness, further mediating mental endurance. Mantra-based meditation has been able to bridge the mind-body divide, which traditional trauma therapies lack due to their emphasis on cognitive dimensions, making it a practical and integrative mind-body intervention. In addition to that, psychotherapies for trauma have seen significant drop-out rates and relatively lower adherence to treatment, as many clients find it uncomfortable and are reluctant to go through exposure or cognitive therapies (Kaplan et al., 2024). Therefore, for those who do not wish to process trauma directly, Mind-Body Interventions like MBM can act as an entry-level treatment or even primary treatment strategy due to its 'present-centered' element, making it more efficacious and reducing drop-out rates (Boyd et al., 2017).

While these findings highlight promising therapeutic possibilities, it is essential to recognize that much of the current evidence remains preliminary and heterogeneous. Studies vary widely in methodology, population, and outcome measures, making it difficult to draw definitive causal inferences. Therefore, the following discussion should be considered conceptually exploratory, synthesizing existing trends rather than establishing clinical efficacy.

Comparison With Established PTSD Treatments

MBM and Other Mind-Body Practices. To fully grasp the unique therapeutic potential of MBM, it is critical to distinguish it from other mind-body practices commonly used in therapeutic contexts. The fundamental difference lies in its primary mechanism: focused attention meditation, whereas practices like Mindfulness-Based Stress Reduction are classified as open monitoring (Boyd et al., 2017). While mindfulness meditation cultivates a non-reactive awareness of the present moment by observing thoughts, feelings, and sensations without attachment, MBM directs the mind to a single, repetitive object of focus. This distinction is particularly relevant for trauma survivors; the structure and predictability of a focused attention practice can be more accessible and less overwhelming than the non-directive, open-ended nature of mindfulness, which may inadvertently lead to distressing thoughts or body sensations (Lynch et al., 2018).

Position Within the PTSD Treatment Landscape. The strongest evidence for treating PTSD comes from trauma-focused psychotherapies such as Prolonged Exposure (PE), Cognitive Processing Therapy (CPT), and EMDR. These remain first-line treatments according to major guidelines. MBM, when used, should be considered a complementary or adjunctive practice for regulation, stabilization, and meaning-making, especially for individuals who decline trauma-focused interventions. Moreover, evidence for MBM as a *primary* PTSD treatment remains insufficient.

Individual Differences and Moderators

Response to MBM may vary by trauma type (developmental vs. single-event), cultural background, religious identity, prior meditation experience, dissociation levels, and personal preference. These factors should guide mantra selection, session pacing, and whether MBM is introduced early (stabilization) or later (integration)

Cultural and Ethical Applications

Chanting is often perceived through a religious lens, obstructing its global acceptance as a therapeutic intervention. Despite this, it is a cross-cultural practice deeply rooted in many traditions worldwide. Although languages and interpretations may vary, every culture's fundamental objective remains unchanged. Be it vocalization or silent chanting, its core principle of stress reduction, cognitive resilience, and overall regulation is pervasive. For individuals deeply connected to their cultures and traditions, Mantra-Based Meditation (MBM) serves as a practice that caters to their individual needs, strengthens their cultural identity, and provides emotional comfort, contributing to positive health outcomes. Given the importance of cultural relevance, MBM should not be viewed solely as a therapeutic intervention devoid of its corresponding spiritual and religious significance (Kadri, 2024; Rao, 2024).

Mantra Meditation originates in non-Western spiritual traditions, such as Hinduism, and carries cultural meaning. In Western therapeutic settings, there is a risk of cultural appropriation if these practices are stripped of context or taught without respect (Surmitis et al., 2018). Counselors are urged to adopt a culturally responsible approach to meditation, which means recognizing the practice's heritage and guiding clients in an informed, ethical manner (Surmitis et al., 2018). For example, interventions should respect any religious or philosophical significance clients attach to a mantra and avoid portraying meditation as a decontextualized 'quick fix'. Some of the best practices include being aware of "spiritual bypass", meaning using meditation to avoid healing frameworks that include psychological work and strive to honor the practice's original purpose. Lack of spiritual bypass can lead to discrepancies in clinical application of such methods, where either clients do not experience the psychological effects of the practices or unconsciously suppress their emotional turmoil while asserting themselves as 'spiritual' (Surmitis et al., 2018).

Trauma Response and Trauma Care

Trauma response and meaning making are shaped by multiple variables such as developmental factors, cultural meaning, type of trauma exposure, reactions of others, available resources, support systems, and many more. They determine how one perceives their trauma and reacts to it. Culture, in particular, plays a vital role in shaping how trauma is processed and expressed, which many therapeutic approaches end up disregarding. For some, their traumatic experience may be deeply intertwined with cultural practices, and the loss involved could hold significant cultural meaning. In addition, cultural norms influence how distress is communicated, what is considered an 'acceptable' trauma response, who one turns to for support, and what constitutes healing (Center for Substance Abuse Treatment, 2014a). This points towards the need for trauma-informed care and trauma therapies to inculcate culturally responsive practices or strategies. It also increases the success rate and makes it more effective.

Culturally Responsible Use of Mantra-Based Practices

A culturally sensitive lens is specifically essential when dealing with historical trauma, collective trauma, or intergenerational transmission of trauma. Its implementation includes acknowledgement of the diverse historical and cultural origins of contemplative practices, particularly regarding the use of mantras. Practioners must recognize that such techniques are deeply rooted in specific religious lineages, including Hindu, Buddhist, Sikh, Christian and Islamic traditions. To avoid the pitfalls of cultural appropriation clinicians should offer interventions that are culturally congruent to the client. This might include Dhikr in Islamic contexts, the Jesus Prayer within Christian traditions or entirely secular phrases for those without a religious affiliation (Ohio Department of Job and Family Services, Office of Families and Children, 2024).

Furthermore, a culturally responsible framework must address the psychological phenomenon of spiritual bypassing wherein spiritual practices are inadvertently used to avoid addressing necessary emotional processing or unresolved trauma. Clinicians must ensure these tools do not act as replacements. Additionally, when utilizing culturally specific mantras or techniques it is essential for one to provide respectful contextualization that avoids decontextualization or commercialization. This allows for an inclusive therapeutic environment that honors the intersection of spirituality, identity and clinical efficacy.

Safety, Contraindications, and Monitoring

Meditation practices, including mantra-based practices, can cause unpleasant or adverse effects in a significant minority of practitioners (reported to range from 8% to 37% across studies). Trauma survivors show heightened vulnerability to dissociation, emotional flooding, panic, and intrusive memories during contemplative practices. To monitor for safety, it is important to carry out a screening procedure where one is assessed for dissociation, psychosis spectrum conditions, active suicidality, severe emotional instability, recent trauma exposure, and substance intoxication. This must be followed by informed consent, which involves explicitly discussing potential temporary unpleasant sensations (e.g., resurfacing memories, anxiety spikes) and the plan for managing them. Furthermore, monitoring can be done by providing "escape valves," such as eyes-open practice, grounding, switching to external focus, and stopping practice immediately in case of destabilization. For a professional to avoid contraindications, one must avoid intensive, unguided, or silent retreats for individuals with complex trauma. It is advisable to begin with brief, titrated sessions of 5–10 minutes. Finally, in case of any doubt, stabilization-oriented approaches may be prioritized, such as movement, grounding, and controlled breathing, before introducing linguistic repetition.

Practitioner Training Requirement

Effective delivery of MBM requires specialized practitioner training to ensure clinical safety and efficacy. The Mantram Repetition Program (MRP) uses a manual approach, structured into eight weekly sessions, to be delivered by either trained clinicians or supervised paraprofessionals. More specialized techniques, such as Transcendental Meditation (TM), require formal certification from accredited instructors to maintain the practice's integrity.

Beyond specific modalities, practitioners must pursue comprehensive trauma-informed meditation training. This emphasizes critical clinical competencies, including administering pre-intervention screenings, obtaining informed consent, and monitoring patients for signs of dissociation or adverse emotional reactions. Finally, practitioners must have consistent access to professional supervision when integrating MBM into trauma recovery or general clinical care. This oversight provides a necessary layer of ethical accountability and support, ensuring that the intervention remains responsive to the complex needs of the trauma survivor.

Implementation Guidelines

Illustrative MBM Implementation Protocol (Adjunctive Use)

Clinical implementation of MBM for trauma recovery follows a structured 6–8-week curriculum, with sessions lasting 60-90 minutes. The protocol begins with psychoeducation and informed consent, followed by the collaborative selection of a safe, culturally congruent mantra. Practice should be increased gradually, starting with 5–10-minute intervals and progressing to 15-20 minutes as the client's self-regulatory capacity stabilizes. To facilitate integration sessions, include grounding and orienting techniques, optional meaning-making through journaling, and 5-10 minutes of daily home practice.

Safety can be maintained through the establishment of 'stop' protocols that allow clients to shift to an external focus when internal sensations become overwhelming. Due to the high risk of dissociation and traumatization in early recovery, intensive silent retreats are generally contraindicated. This structure ensures that the intervention remains within the client's window of tolerance, systematically rebuilding autonomic and emotional stability.

Limitations of MBM as an Intervention

Although a significant body of research provides insights into the usefulness and effectiveness of mantra chanting, like any other practice, this also has certain limitations and challenges. Many studies on practices like meditation, mantra chanting, and mindfulness have been conducted on small samples, making it challenging to map the large-scale influence of MBM.

Effective implementation of MBM requires specialized education and rigorous commitment to professional standards (Champagne-Langabeer et al., 2025). Inappropriate or uninformed teaching may be counterproductive, undermining its benefits. Consequently, formal and professional training is a prerequisite for safe therapeutic application. Special modalities, such as transcendental meditation, require instruction from certified teachers who complete accredited, extensive programs. More broadly, therapists integrating MBM should seek formal training in both meditation instruction and trauma-informed care. This interdisciplinary approach ensures that the spiritual and physiological components of MBM are delivered within a robust ethical and clinical framework (Surmitis et al., 2018).

This chapter primarily centers on the theoretical underpinnings of how Mantra-Based Meditation (MBM) may contribute to the alleviation of trauma-related symptoms, rather than assessing its empirical effectiveness. Therefore, certain methodological and evaluative aspects remain beyond the scope of this discussion. Future research can clearly distinguish between well-established findings and preliminary research, incorporating effect sizes and confidence intervals when reporting outcomes, and include both positive and null findings to strengthen the evidence base. Additionally, greater attention is needed to identify for whom and under what conditions MBM is most appropriate, as effectiveness may vary according to trauma type, cultural background, and individual readiness. These dimensions represent important directions for future investigation rather than limitations of the present theoretical exploration.

Future Directions

Future research should include pre-registered randomized controlled trials comparing MBM with first-line PTSD treatments, using clinician-rated outcomes, larger samples, and long-term follow-ups. Additionally, mechanistic studies should examine autonomic and neural markers in trauma populations specifically. Moderators (trauma type, dissociation, spirituality, cultural background) should be explicitly tested. Finally, safety monitoring should be standardized in all contemplative studies.

Despite encouraging early evidence, the current research based on MBM and trauma remains methodologically limited. Most studies rely on small, non-representative samples and short–term outcomes. While much of the existing research on trauma and mind-body practices has focused on veterans, further studies should broaden their scope and explore different types of traumas, like childhood trauma, trauma from dysfunctional attachments, medical trauma, etc., across varying age groups. Longitudinal studies examining the influence of MBM and mind-body practices on survivors of these types of traumas will provide insight into whether these practices offer sustained healing over time or primarily yield short-term benefits. It should be systematically implemented to determine the clinical utility of mantra recitation, and its outcomes should be rigorously assessed.

Further, its effectiveness could be explored in combination with established trauma recovery modalities such as Narrative Exposure Therapy (NET), Internal Family System (IFS), Somatic Experiencing (SE), Cognitive Behavioral Therapy (CBT), Rational Emotive Behavioral Therapy (REBT), and Beck's Cognitive Therapy. Within the cultural context, researchers could also investigate whether the type of mantra aligned with an individual's cultural background versus those from other traditions affects therapeutic outcomes. Lastly, comparing the impact of mantra chanting in group versus individual settings can reveal significant differences in outcomes, providing further direction for clinical application.

CONCLUSION

This chapter offers an exploratory framework for understanding Mantra-Based Meditation as a multidimensional healing practice. Rather than presenting MBM as a definitive therapeutic intervention, it highlights emerging evidence, conceptual linkages, and culturally grounded pathways that warrant further empirical validation and ethical integration into trauma-informed care.

REFERENCES

Acosta, A. (2020, June 3). *The science and philosophy of OM.* Iyengar Yoga London. https://iyengaryogalondon.co.uk/the-science-and-philosophy-of-om-aum/

Álvarez-Pérez, Y., Rivero-Santana, A., Perestelo-Pérez, L., Duarte-Díaz, A., Ramos-García, V., Toledo-Chávarri, A., Torres-Castaño, A., León-Salas, B., Infante-Ventura, D., González-Hernández, N., Rodríguez-Rodríguez, L., & Serrano-Aguilar, P. (2022). Effectiveness of mantra-based meditation on mental health: A systematic review and meta-analysis. *International Journal of Environmental Research and Public Health, 19*(6), 3380. DOI: 10.3390/ijerph19063380 PMID: 35329068

Angeli-Gordon, J. M. (2025). Ancestral parenting: Reclaiming Māori child-rearing practices in the wake of colonial disruption. *Genealogy, 9*(2), 36. DOI: 10.3390/genealogy9020036

Barbaresi, M., Nardo, D., & Fagioli, S. (2025). Physiological entrainment: A key mind–body mechanism for cognitive, motor and affective functioning, and well-being. *Brain Sciences, 15*(1), 3. DOI: 10.3390/brainsci15010003 PMID: 39851371

Barnes, V. A. (2018). Transcendental Meditation and treatment for post-traumatic stress disorder. *The Lancet. Psychiatry, 5*(12), 946–947. DOI: 10.1016/S2215-0366(18)30423-1 PMID: 30449710

Beshai, S., Tesar, E., & Brown, L. (2024). Mindfulness and CBT: A conceptual integration bridging clinical science and contemplative meditation. *Frontiers in Psychology, 15*, 1489798. DOI: 10.3389/fpsyg.2024.1489798 PMID: 39723397

Bormann, J. E. (2010). Mantram repetition: A "portable contemplative practice" for modern times. In Plante, T. G. (Ed.), *Contemplative practices in action: Spirituality, meditation, and health* (pp. 78–99). ABC-CLIO.

Boyd, J. E., Lanius, R. A., & McKinnon, M. C. (2017). Mindfulness-based treatments for post-traumatic stress disorder: A review of the treatment literature and neurobiological evidence. *Journal of Psychiatry & Neuroscience : JPN, 43*(1), 7–25. DOI: 10.1503/jpn.170021 PMID: 29252162

Burke, A., Lam, C. N., Stussman, B., & Yang, H. (2017). Prevalence and patterns of use of mantra, mindfulness and spiritual meditation among adults in the United States. *BMC Complementary and Alternative Medicine, 17*(1), 316. DOI: 10.1186/s12906-017-1827-8 PMID: 28619092

Center for Substance Abuse Treatment. (2014a). *Trauma-informed care: A sociocultural perspective (Chapter 1).* In *TIP 57: Trauma-informed care in behavioral health services* (Treatment Improvement Protocol [TIP] Series, No. 57). Substance Abuse and Mental Health Services Administration. https://www.ncbi.nlm.nih.gov/books/NBK207195/

Center for Substance Abuse Treatment. (2014b). *Understanding the impact of trauma (Chapter 3).* In *TIP 57: Trauma-informed care in behavioral health services* (Treatment Improvement Protocol [TIP] Series, No. 57). Substance Abuse and Mental Health Services Administration. https://www.ncbi.nlm.nih.gov/books/NBK207191/

Champagne-Langabeer, T., Ratcliff, C. G., Bakos-Block, C., Vega, F., Cardenas-Turanzas, M., Malik, A., & Korupolu, R. (2025). Evaluating the meditation practices and barriers to adopting mindful medicine among physicians. *American Journal of Lifestyle Medicine*. Advance online publication. DOI: 10.1177/15598276251323850 PMID: 40092531

Cruz, D., Lichten, M., Berg, K., & George, P. (2022). Developmental trauma: Conceptual framework, associated risks and comorbidities, and evaluation and treatment. *Frontiers in Psychiatry*, *13*, 800687. DOI: 10.3389/fpsyt.2022.800687 PMID: 35935425

Falk, E. B., O'Donnell, M. B., Cascio, C. N., Tinney, F., Kang, Y., Lieberman, M. D., Taylor, S. E., An, L., Resnicow, K., & Strecher, V. J. (2015). Self-affirmation alters the brain's response to health messages and subsequent behavior change. *Proceedings of the National Academy of Sciences of the United States of America*, *112*(7), 1977–1982. DOI: 10.1073/pnas.1500247112 PMID: 25646442

Finley, A. J., & Crowell, A. L. (2018). Self-affirmation enhances processing of negative stimuli among threat-prone individuals. *Social Cognitive and Affective Neuroscience*, *13*(6), 569–580. DOI: 10.1093/scan/nsy045 PMID: 29873770

Ghanem, Z. Y. (2024). The process of healing individual and communal traumatic experiences through natural and cultural reconnection in Silko's *Ceremony. International Journal of Undergraduate Research and Creative Activities*, *16*(1), 6. DOI: 10.61809/2168-0620.1339

Harper, A. R., & Pargament, K. I. (2015). Trauma, religion, and spirituality: Pathways to healing. In Pargament, K. I. (Ed.), Vol. 2, pp. 349–367). APA handbook of psychology, religion, and spirituality. Springer., DOI: 10.1007/978-3-319-18866-9_19

Heart, M. Y. H. B. (2003). The historical trauma response among natives and its relationship with substance abuse: A Lakota illustration. *Journal of Psychoactive Drugs*, *35*(1), 7–13. DOI: 10.1080/02791072.2003.10399988 PMID: 12733753

Kadri, R. (2024, June 30). Repetition of spiritual mantra meditation: A review. *Jurnal Kajian Islam dan Turath Antara, 1*(1), Article 5204. https://doi.org/DOI: 10.51200/kitab.v1i1.5204

Kaplan, J., Somohano, V. C., Zaccari, B., & O'Neil, M. E. (2024). Randomized controlled trials of mind–body interventions for post-traumatic stress disorder: A systematic review. *Frontiers in Psychology, 14*, 1219296. DOI: 10.3389/fpsyg.2023.1219296 PMID: 38327501

Kim, S. H., Schneider, S. M., Kravitz, L., Mermier, C., & Burge, M. R. (2013). Mind-body practices for post-traumatic stress disorder. *Journal of Investigative Medicine, 61*(5), 827–834. DOI: 10.2310/JIM.0b013e3182906862 PMID: 23609463

Larsen, S. E., Hopkins, S., & Harris, I. (2025). Addressing religious or spiritual dimensions of trauma and PTSD. *U.S. Department of Veterans Affairs*. https://www.ptsd.va.gov/professional/treat/txessentials/spirituality_trauma.asp

Lebow, H. I. (2023, January 21). How your body remembers trauma. *Psych Central*. https://psychcentral.com/health/how-your-body-remembers-trauma

Lee, R. T., & Moore, J. A. (2017). Integrative oncology and ethics. In *Integrative oncology* (pp. 101–119). Elsevier., DOI: 10.1016/B978-0-12-803831-4.00006-3

Lynch, J., Prihodova, L., Dunne, P. J., Carroll, Á., Walsh, C., McMahon, G., & White, B. (2018). Mantra meditation for mental health in the general population: A systematic review. *European Journal of Integrative Medicine, 23*, 44–49. DOI: 10.1016/j.eujim.2018.09.010

Malesu, V. K. (2025). The science behind breathwork and stress reduction. *News Medical Life Sciences*. https://www.news-medical.net/health/The-Science-Behind-Breathwork-and-Stress-Reduction.aspx

Menhinick, K. A., & Sanders, C. J. (2023). LGBTQ+ Stress, Trauma, Time, and Care. *Pastoral Psychology, 72*(3), 367–384. DOI: 10.1007/s11089-023-01073-z PMID: 37313005

Ohio Department of Job and Family Services, Office of Families and Children. (2024). *QRTP infosheet issue four: Culturally responsive trauma-informed approach* [PDF]. https://dam.assets.ohio.gov/image/upload/jfs.ohio.gov/ofam/QRTP-InfosheetIssueFour-CulturallyResponsiveTrauma-InformedApproachFinal.pdf

Oosterbroek, T., & Dirk, B. (2021). The experience of Trauma Center–Trauma Sensitive Yoga training on professional practice of mental health professionals and yoga instructors. *Complementary Therapies in Clinical Practice, 43*, 101365. DOI: 10.1016/j.ctcp.2021.101365 PMID: 33819832

Orme-Johnson, D. W., Barnes, V. A., Rees, B., Tobin, J., & Walton, K. G. (2024). Effectiveness of meditation techniques in treating post-traumatic stress disorder: A systematic review and meta-analysis. *Medicina, 60*(12), 2050. DOI: 10.3390/medicina60122050 PMID: 39768929

Perry, G., Polito, V., Sankaran, N., & Thompson, W. F. (2022). How chanting relates to cognitive function, altered states, and quality of life. *Brain Sciences, 12*(11), 1456. DOI: 10.3390/brainsci12111456 PMID: 36358382

Rao, P. D. (2024). Mantra-based cognitive resilience: Evaluating the viability of ancient sound practices as a culturally embedded mental health intervention. *Frontiers in Health Informatics, 13*(7), 805–823.

Rastogi, R., Rao, P. D., & Mehta, S. (2020). Mantra-based cognitive resilience: Evaluating the viability of ancient sound practices as culturally embedded mental health intervention. *Health Informatics Journal, 26*(4), 2792–2804. DOI: 10.1177/1460458220948748 PMID: 32691659

Saxena, R. (2023). Significance of religious chanting in various religions. *International Journal of Creative Research and Thoughts, 11*(12). https://ijcrt.org/papers/IJCRT2312100.pdf

Sherin, J. E., & Nemeroff, C. B. (2011). Post-traumatic stress disorder: The neurobiological impact of psychological trauma. *Dialogues in Clinical Neuroscience, 13*(3), 263–278. DOI: 10.31887/dcns.2011.13.2.jsherin PMID: 22034143

Singh, S., Gupta, K. V., Behera, L., & Bhushan, B. (2025). Elevated correlations in cardiac–neural dynamics: An impact of mantra meditation on stress alleviation. *Biomedical Signal Processing and Control, 99*, 106813. DOI: 10.1016/j.bspc.2024.106813

Singhdeo, A. (2023, August 28). *What are the benefits of mantra chanting?* Shvasa Yoga Blog. https://www.shvasa.com/yoga-blog/what-are-the-benefits-of-mantra-chanting

Surmitis, K. A., Fox, J., & Gutierrez, D. (2018). Meditation and appropriation: Best practices for counselors who utilize meditation. *Counseling and Values, 63*(1), 4–16. DOI: 10.1002/cvj.12069

Tedeschi, R. G., Calhoun, L. G., & Groleau, J. M. (2014). Clinical applications of post-traumatic growth. In Calhoun, L. G., & Tedeschi, R. G. (Eds.), *Handbook of post-traumatic growth* (pp. 291–310). Routledge., DOI: 10.4324/9781315805597

Telles, S., Nagarathna, R., & Nagendra, H. R. (1995). Autonomic changes during "OM" meditation. *Indian Journal of Physiology and Pharmacology*, *39*(4), 418–420. PMID: 8582759

Treisman, K. (2017). *Working with relational and developmental trauma in children and adolescents: The impact of complex trauma on children's sense of selves, relationships and development*. Routledge.

Ungvarsky, J. (2024). *Mere-exposure effect*. EBSCOhost. https://www.ebsco.com/research-starters/psychology/mere-exposure-effect

Whitfield-Gabrieli, S., & Ford, J. M. (2012). Default mode network activity and connectivity in psychopathology. *Annual Review of Clinical Psychology*, *8*, 49–76. DOI: 10.1146/annurev-clinpsy-032511-143049 PMID: 22224834

Chapter 12
The Effectiveness of Art Therapy in Addressing Social Anxiety in Contemporary Japan:
Two Case Studies

Sofia Rossatelli
http://orcid.org/0000-0002-6924-7998
University of Milan, Italy

ABSTRACT

This study investigates art therapy as a culturally embedded, non-pharmacological approach to mental well-being in contemporary Japan. It examines how visual and plastic art practices function within therapeutic contexts, contributing to identity formation, emotional expression, and social inclusion. Emphasising the embodied and relational dimensions of art therapy, the research highlights its potential to foster psychophysical transformation through sensory, symbolic, and intersubjective experiences. Adopting an interdisciplinary approach, it explores how local traditions, institutional structures, and socio-cultural values shape access to art-therapeutic practices – particularly concerning social anxiety disorder, one of Japan's most prevalent and socially debated mental health conditions. Fieldwork was conducted at two art therapy ateliers selected for their engagement with this issue. The methodology combines socio-cultural analysis with qualitative tools, including on-site visits, semi-structured interviews, and a visual research component featuring therapeutic artworks.

DOI: 10.4018/979-8-3373-3521-6.ch012

INTRODUCTION

Recent studies have documented a marked increase in common mental disorders in Japan—particularly depression, anxiety, and eating disorders—alongside a growing implementation of mental health services from the early 2000s through the 2010s (Nishi et al., 2019). Despite rising demand for psychological support, stigma surrounding mental distress remains pervasive, and care is still largely pharmacological (Kasahara-Kiritani et al., 2018).

This paper investigates the intersection of mental health and holistic therapeutic practices, with particular attention to the ways in which body-mind interactions contribute to subjective well-being. The latter is conceptualised not merely as the absence of psychopathology, but as a dynamic process in which emotional, somatic, and expressive dimensions are integrally interrelated. Within this framework, the integration of corporeal and mental experience denotes the bidirectional influence between psychological states and bodily experience, especially as manifested through creative and expressive activity.

Anxiety disorders, and notably Social Anxiety Disorder (SAD), exemplify the significance of such interactions. Although frequently comorbid with other conditions, anxiety exerts a pervasive influence on individuals' physical perception, emotional regulation, and social functioning, thereby shaping both everyday experience and engagement in therapeutic processes (Kutty, 2022).

This study adopts a qualitative approach, privileging semi-structured interviews and the analysis of creative works to elucidate the nuanced dynamics of body-mind processes, rather than emphasising quantitative clinical outcomes.

The first part of the paper considers social anxiety in contemporary Japanese society, highlighting socio-cultural influences such as *tatemae/honne* (public versus private self), the culturally embedded orientation of *amae*—reflecting dependence and interpersonal expectations—and the implicit categorisation of individuals as *kachigumi* or *makegumi* (winners and losers), all of which can contribute to social withdrawal (Hofmann et al., 2010; Nippoda, 2012).

The second part explores the potential of art therapy, particularly visual and plastic arts, to alleviate social anxiety and reduce internalised stigma (Koike et al., 2017; Kanesaki et al., 2023). To investigate this potential, two art therapy ateliers—one in Tokyo and one in Kyoto—were selected. Two users from each centre participated in semi-structured interviews, and three artworks per person were analysed qualitatively. This triangulated approach integrates user testimonies, visual analysis, and contextual data, offering a nuanced understanding of how creative practice can facilitate psychological relief, self-expression, and identity reconfiguration within the Japanese socio-cultural framework.[1]

SOCIAL ANXIETY IN JAPAN

Among the most prevalent forms of mental distress in Japan, recently exacerbated by the COVID-19 pandemic, are anxiety disorders, adjustment disorders, and depression, which, while distinct diagnostic entities, may present overlapping or sequential symptoms (Casey & Bailey, 2011; Cuijpers et al., 2014). Although anxiety can contribute to suicide risk (Tanji et al., 2018), its primary impact in Japan is often expressed through social withdrawal, absenteeism from school or work, and, in severe cases, *hikikomori* (Koyama et al., 2010; Teo & Gaw, 2010).

The DSM-5-TR (Diagnostic and Statistical Manual of Mental Disorders, Fifth Edition, Text Revision) defines anxiety disorders as conditions characterised by excessive fear, anxiety, avoidance, and hypervigilance. In contrast to short-term stress reactions, these symptoms typically persist for six months or longer and are frequently accompanied by physiological manifestations such as muscle tension and autonomic hyperarousal. Anxiety disorders often co-occur with other anxiety conditions (frequently involving panic attacks), as well as with depressive, neurodevelopmental, and substance use disorders (American Psychiatric Association, 2022).

Social Anxiety Disorder (SAD), or social phobia, is characterised by persistent fear or anxiety in social situations in which an individual may be exposed to scrutiny by others. Core features include fear of negative evaluation, embarrassment, humiliation, or rejection, leading to avoidance behaviours and functional impairment in social, academic, or occupational domains. SAD often begins in childhood or adolescence and follows a chronic course if untreated (American Psychiatric Association, 2022). Cultural factors can shape symptom expression and prevalence of SAD, and in some cases may give rise to culture-bound syndromes. In Japan, this is exemplified by *taijin kyōfushō* (TKS), a condition marked by the fear of offending or embarrassing others.[2]

A 2016 study, which refers to a World Mental Health Japan Survey conducted between 2002 and 2006, indicates that the incidence of social anxiety was 8.1% of a total estimate of 20.3% for all common mental disorders present in Japan at that time (Ishikawa et al., 2016), and the situation got worse during the Covid-19 pandemic (Kutty, 2022). Furthermore, some research findings suggest that the cultural climate and societal understanding of mental illness play a significant role in perpetuating disorders like SAD (Pescosolido et al., 2008; Kanesaki et al., 2023).

Within the sociocultural framework of Japan, a multitude of psychosocial tendencies are in evidence, and these coexist alongside clearly delineated hierarchies. The *tatemae* (external behaviour)-*honne* (inner feelings) distinction has been shown to influence social interactions and self-presentation, thereby creating implicit pressure to separate public and private selves (Kitayama, 2004). This dynamic may potentially exacerbate stress and contribute to anxiety-related symptoms. Another pervasive feature is the categorisation of individuals into *kachigumi* (winners) and *makegumi* (losers) across education, sports, and workplace settings. This has been shown to reinforce social evaluation anxieties (Ando et al., 2013; Hao et al., 2025) and generate emotional tensions that may hinder care delivery (Nippoda, 2012).

In contemporary Japan, the concept of the public and collective self appears to hold sway (Hofstede, 2001; Sugimoto, 2020), a view that is also supported by the definition of the "interdependent self" proposed by scholars Markus and Kitayama (1991). Their investigations have defined the "interdependent self" as a typical phenomenon in many cultures in East Asia (including those of China and Japan) and Latin America (e.g., El Salvador, Brazil, Chile and Argentina). This concept is characterised by individual human identities that exist only as the result of social relations and connections with the community to which they belong. The concept of the "interdependent self" is antithetical to the notion of the "independent self", which is prevalent in European (e.g., Italian, Spanish, Finnish, and German) and North American societies. The latter is characterised by a strong emphasis on individuality and analytical thinking (Markus & Kitayama, 1991).

Furthermore, introduced by Doi (1973) and discussed in subsequent studies (de Almeida & Nakao, 2021; Miike, 2003), *amae* refers to an orientation towards indulgence and acceptance that shapes the Japanese interdependent self, influencing relational security, communication, and social behaviour. The model under discussion involves two complementary functions: message-expanding, which relies on indirectness and interlocutor sensitivity, and message-accepting, which allows openness within trusted relationships. While promoting restraint in some interactions, *amae* also supports trust and assertiveness. Maladaptive forms, such as unmet expectations of acceptance, have been demonstrated to result in social withdrawal and heightened sensitivity to social evaluation (Behrens, 2004).

Considering the socio-cultural elements previously outlined, the Japanese mental healthcare system has historically sought to address anxiety-related (and depressive) symptoms through a range of conventional treatments. However, these approaches have not yielded optimal outcomes, as it will be discussed below in detail.

CONVENTIONAL AND NON-CONVENTIONAL TREATMENTS

In Japan, mental healthcare is predominantly hospital- and clinic-based (*seishinka shinryōsho*), yet persistent concerns remain regarding its effectiveness and responsiveness to patients' needs. Physical restraint continues to be a common practice in Japanese psychiatric hospitals, with substantially higher rates than those observed in other developed countries, including the United States, Australia, and New Zealand (Misawa, 2020; Azuma, 2020; Kawai et al., 2023; Savage et al., 2024). Involuntary admissions, often initiated by relatives, usually restrict patients' ability to discharge themselves. At the same time, the clinics, staffed by medical specialists, frequently operate under funding limitations and structural financial pressures, which restrict the quality and duration of care, reinforcing a predominantly pharmacological model focused on symptom management and work exemption (Nippoda, 2012). Together, these factors underscore the ongoing reliance on coercive, medically driven, and at times economically motivated approaches within Japan's psychiatric care system.

Despite an increase in awareness, the implementation of professional mental health services remains limited, with care often sought only in severe cases (Klein, 2024). As Nishi et al. (2019) and Kanesaki et al. (2023) have demonstrated, structural barriers, including cost and access issues within both public and private systems, are compounded by cultural reluctance to engage in psychotherapy. The notion of discussing personal difficulties with an unknown individual is incongruent with prevailing social norms that prioritise discretion and collective harmony. In addition, cultural constructs such as *gaman*, which values endurance, in conjunction with nationalist rhetoric following the 2011 Fukushima disaster, have fostered a form of stoic resilience termed "ganbarism" (Gebhardt & Masami, 2014).

The treatment of social anxiety is comparable to that of general anxiety, encompassing the administration of drugs such as anxiolytics, antidepressants, and beta-blockers. However, it should be noted that responses to treatment can vary, and the potential for dependency persists (Fritscher, 2023). Indigenous methods, including the Morita therapy, are still widely practiced, prioritising acceptance through a series of structured regimens which include talk therapy in later stages. Other modalities, such as cognitive behavioural therapy (CBT) and self-help strategies, have also gained traction. However, these interventions may not completely address the underlying systemic shortcomings.

Consequently, national efforts have been directed towards deinstitutionalisation and service decentralisation, as evidenced by the Ministry of Health's 2010 public education initiative.[3] This development can be traced back to the 2003 report On Social and Health Care in Mental Health, which made the case for a shift from institutional psychiatric care towards community-based models and the empowerment of patients (Ministry of Health, Labour and Welfare of Japan, 2003). Subsequent developments include the implementation of the Community-Based Integrated Care System (CICSM) and the enactment of the 2024 Act on Mental Health and Welfare for Persons with Mental Disorders or Disabilities (Ministry of Health, Labour and Welfare of Japan, 2024b). The objectives of these two legislative acts are to consolidate community support networks and to improve service quality. These reforms are consistent with Japan's overarching commitment to global health objectives, including Universal Health Coverage (UHC), as set out in the 2024 Japanese Report on Global Health Vision (Ministry of Health, Labour and Welfare of Japan, 2024a).

Recent years have also seen a diversification of psychotherapeutic practices, including the rise of narrative therapy, which has been found to be particularly effective with children, through culturally resonant mediums such as comics (Scarlet, 2017; Ono, 2024). Similarly, the efficacy of art therapy (visual and plastic arts) has been demonstrated for individuals with impaired verbal communication. Art therapy provides a non-verbal medium for alleviating socially induced distress, which may be exacerbated by sociocultural pressures (Nippoda, 2012). The government has demonstrated support for non-traditional interventions, including life skills coaching and community-based outreach initiatives, for conditions such as *hikikomori* (Yoshida & Ito, 2012).

Multifunctional centres located outside clinical settings have emerged as inclusive spaces for creative expression, particularly benefiting those with psychiatric or cognitive impairments. These centres facilitate exploration of artistic practices by individuals of diverse ages and identities, unencumbered by hierarchical constraints. They provide therapeutic alternatives rooted in embodied, symbolic interaction (Case, Dalley & Reddick, 1992/2022). The efficacy of art therapy is not solely attributed to its creative component, but also encompasses periods of therapeutic pause, which bears similarity to silence in verbal therapy.[4]

The domain of art therapy can be suitable for a wide range of conditions, including motor and cognitive impairments, as well as social withdrawal. This practice is employed across a variety of clinical, educational, and community settings. The present study is rooted in the theoretical framework of embodied cognition, which posits the externalisation of internal states and the facilitation of psychophysical integration (McNiff, 2004; Malchiodi, 2020). The process facilitates (abreactive) catharsis through the symbolic elaboration of repressed emotions, thereby aligning with Freud's theories of psychic conflict resolution (Freud, 1924).

Taking a holistic approach, this research considers art therapy as an integrative practice that engages with the physical, emotional, cognitive and existential aspects of a person. Here, well-being is conceptualised as a dynamic balance and meaningful expression, which is consistent with humanistic and integrative health frameworks (Rogers, 1961; WHO, 2001). Rather than adding further to the review of conventional and non-conventional approaches, the study now turns to an in-depth examination of two contemporary Japanese art therapy centres, located in Tokyo and Kyoto respectively.

ART THERAPY: TWO CENTRES AS CASE STUDIES

Participants displayed diverse clinical profiles, encompassing anxiety disorders as well as cognitive and social difficulties. This section emphasises therapeutic processes and the role of art as a medium for body-mind regulation, rather than focusing strictly on clinical diagnoses. Two independent ateliers in Japan, serving individuals with physical, cognitive, or psychological disabilities, were selected for in-depth investigation. Selection criteria included operational longevity (at least five years), accessibility and willingness of coordinators to participate, geolocation (urban periphery), and the predominant type of disability among users. Tokyo Soteria foregrounds artistic and aesthetic expression, while Kokoro-karada-art emphasises therapeutic and rehabilitative practices, reflecting their distinct missions. Ethical approval for the study was obtained in accordance with standard guidelines for research involving human participants.

A qualitative approach was adopted, combining dialogic exchanges with coordinators, semi-structured interviews with coordinators and selected users, and analysis of user-produced artefacts. Initial contact was conducted remotely, followed by two on-site visits per atelier: one outside operational hours and one during active sessions. To ensure user privacy and uphold the integrity of creative processes, extended interviews were mediated by coordinators, with informed consent allowing participants to respond freely and at their own pace. Coordinators selected two users per atelier whose experiences exemplified the atelier's activities, ensuring diversity in trajectories and outcomes. Analysis aligned with each atelier's mission: Kokoro-karada-art emphasised therapeutic pathways, whereas Tokyo Soteria highlighted users' artistic identities without prioritising a pathological framework. Accordingly, anonymity was not applied to Soteria participants, who have achieved international recognition as outsider artists.[5]

Both centres admit new users on the basis of recommendations from hospitals, medical practitioners, and local social services. Participants may engage in activities regardless of the severity of their original conditions, and sessions can be tailored or reduced when necessary. No evidence was found that any user was explicitly excluded, although access in some cases may not have been directly suggested by referring sources.

Following the selection of the two centres, the semi-structured written interview was conducted. This choice, noted on multiple qualitative social research (Corrao, 2005), is mainly motivated by the intention to avoid other time-consuming methods in the acquisition of the necessary information, given the delicate nature of the interlocutors. The interview was divided into two sections. The first aimed to collect general information on the centre, including details of its history, the staff employed, the users and the therapeutic approach. The second section aimed to collect information on the therapeutic path of two users selected as representatives.[6] Furthermore, in addition to the interview, at least three artworks produced by each of the selected users were studied to gain a deeper understanding of the therapeutic process. While the subject is undoubtedly intriguing, this study does not focus on the classification of drawings and their associated interpretations. For instance, it does not address whether abstract illustrations are more prevalent at specific levels of social anxiety symptoms. Instead, it presents a unique combination of verbal and artefactual testimonies, which collectively offer a comprehensive insight into the investigation.

In addition to the intrinsic value of such elements within a study contemplating the discipline of art therapy, there has recently been a growing generalised interest in similar qualitative approaches integrated with visual or graphic sources (Sandelowski, 2004). As Kearney and Hyle (2004) assumed, the act of drawing appears to facilitate the internalisation of feelings and associated emotions, thereby making these elements more accessible for expression. Similarly, Guillemin (2004) stated that: "The utilisation of an integrated methodology, encompassing both visual and verbal research techniques, provides the means of investigating the multifaceted and intricate aspects that underpin a considerable proportion of social research pertaining to human experience" (p. 273). Long employed by psychologists to assess cognitive development (Jolly, 2010), drawings are also utilised as a projective technique (with adults and children) to investigate conscious and unconscious issues and experiences. They serve to make visible aspects of the self and/or levels of development.

The two ateliers under examination are the NPO Tokyo Soteria Art Circle and Kokoro-karada-art, situated in Tokyo and Kyoto respectively. The following section presents a summary of the qualitative study conducted in each of the ateliers,[7] by means of the interpretative categories of the disciplines of art therapy (psychodynamics), psychological sciences and neuroscience.

It is important to underline that the act of creating artworks in these ateliers cannot be reduced to a purely cognitive or symbolic activity. Rather, it is a process in which gesture, movement, and sensory engagement play a central role. The tactile encounter with paper, the kinaesthetic rhythm of brushstrokes, or the haptic resistance of materials such as ink or collage fragments exemplifies how the body emerges as both the site and the medium of expression. This dimension highlights that the therapeutic impact of art is enacted not only through mental reflection but also through somatic interaction with materials, making visible the inseparability of body and mind in processes of healing and self-reconfiguration (Regev & Cohen-Yatziv, 2018).[8]

The non-governmental organisation Tokyo Soteria was established in 2009 in Edogawa by Noguchi Hirofumi, who, upon learning of the Soteria method[9] in Switzerland a few years earlier, resolved to introduce it to Japan. Among the various territorial services, the one offered by the NPO Tokyo Soteria Art Circle, an atelier that aims to recognise the talent of outsider artists in users suffering from psychiatric pathologies through art collective sessions, thus providing them with the necessary recognition and eliminating the social stigma that afflicts them, is particularly noteworthy. A significant proportion of the workforce at the centre comprises professionals from a range of disciplines, including psychology and social work. The atelier is led by an artist who has undergone training and who has a background in philosophy. The range of materials available to users is extensive, encompassing a diverse array of options such as acrylics, pastels, markers, Japanese paper, and canvases. Over time, a significant number of users have developed a particular expertise in a specific artistic technique, acquiring their own materials to use during sessions at the centre. The following section presents illustrative case studies of user experiences that were subjected to investigation.

Sasaki K., a non-binary individual between thirty and forty years of age, regularly visits the studio. Sasaki consistently experienced significant social pressure and an overwhelming stigma surrounding gender identity. As an individual challenging conventional norms in the Japanese society, Sasaki was categorised as a *makegumi* (loser) due to gender nonconformity. This position was associated with persistent anxiety, heightened self-consciousness, and periods of emotional dysregulation, reflecting the psychological impact of chronic social marginalisation.

Sasaki typically engages in a period of contemplation and reflection on the subject and technique before embarking on the creation of a work. The creative process evokes ambivalent sentiments in Sasaki, manifesting as a dichotomy of intense joy and profound frustration. However, the artist declares to experience a profound sense of fulfilment upon the completion of a work, stating: "The process of creation is, at times, painful, and sometimes fun. (However), upon completion of the work, a sense of elation mixed with fatigue is often experienced".[10] Moreover, Sasaki articulates the communicative capacity of artistic creativity as the singular medium through which one can express one's *honne* (true feelings): "(It is only through artistic means that) I want to express the feminine feelings hidden inside my heart due to fear of the judgement of others." The artist employs a series of elegant strokes, imbued with a discernible sensitivity, to represent female figures (Figures 1 and 2) and cats (Figure 3). These are rendered with the use of a ballpoint pen or Indian ink, encompassing shades of black, red, and green. It is noteworthy that Indian ink is seldom employed in art therapy studios, where not all participants possess a confident approach towards this medium. Indeed, the ink can readily result in unintended and irreversible stains, both on the paper and on the artist's hands.[11] On occasion, however, given the use of a nib that is easily gripped and direct on surfaces, it can be selected by users as a means of approaching painting (Albertini, 2012). Over time, engagement in the atelier, a safe and nonjudgmental space, appears to have enabled Sasaki to express previously constrained emotions, gradually reinforcing a sense of agency and contributing to the alleviation of anxiety linked to social stigma.

Sato M., a woman in her sixties, also visits the studio on a weekly basis. Sato attempts to adhere to the peculiar aesthetic standards of Japanese society, which engenders a state of chronic emotional distress and severe social anxiety. Sato employs pastels and watercolours to depict natural elements (Figures 4 and 5) or animals (Figure 6) in bright colours, especially red. She asserts a profound affinity with nature, particularly flowers, which has been formally validated by a license obtained at an *ikebana* school. Sato finds that sketching provides a means of relaxation prior to the creation of her works. The pressure to conform to societal aesthetic norms appears to generate persistent emotional strain and heightened vigilance toward social judgement. Immersing herself in preparatory sketching and the creation of vibrant compositions seems to offer Sato a way to channel and modulate these tensions, providing a structured yet flexible space for emotional exploration. Furthermore, she engages in the process of confrontation with others, which may entail the seeking of advice. Sato states: "At the outset of my art-therapeutic path, my goal was simply to become proficient in painting, but after two years of attending the atelier, my doctor told me, 'You can continue attending the atelier until you're about 90 years old', which has motivated me to continue creating while enjoying it." In the interview, M. stated: "I conceptualise and execute my designs my own way." In some of Sato's works, subjects and styles of renowned artists such as Marc Chagall (1887–1985) are discernible. In most cases, audiovisual materials and books serve as supplementary sources, facilitating users' acquisition of knowledge about art and inspiration. The image created embodies thoughts and emotions that are externally expressed in an unspoken way, which is only made explicit graphically. Each work circumscribes a space that is related to the outside and to other forms, between fractures and continuities (Albertini, 2012). Regular engagement in artistic creation appears to have helped Sato regulate emotions and alleviate social anxiety symptoms, suggesting that sustained participation in the atelier may contribute to mitigating chronic psychological distress.

Both users achieved recognition as outsider artists, exhibited their work at national and international levels, and occasionally sold their creations. Within the domain of creative therapy ateliers, it is not unusual to encounter artworks bearing the artist's signature, even though authorship is often underestimated or overlooked in therapeutic contexts. In the cases examined, authorship was established not only by the works' technical and thematic uniqueness but also through the conscious and voluntary act of signing one's name. This ostensibly modest gesture carries considerable therapeutic significance: the act of affixing a signature can be interpreted as a symbolic reclaiming of identity, a public assertion of authorship and personal agency. Such affirmation is particularly meaningful in social contexts where individuals with psychological vulnerabilities are frequently marginalised or rendered invisible. As Malchiodi (2020) highlights, the conscious authorship of creative output within therapeutic settings plays a crucial role in reinforcing self-worth, supporting emotional processing, and fostering pathways towards social reintegration.

The creative activity carried out at the NPO Tokyo Soteria Art Circle atelier suggests that it may provide participants with valuable opportunities for free individual identity expression beyond social pressure, while also potentially alleviating severe social anxiety symptoms and facilitating processes of social reintegration. Comparable tendencies have been noted in the case of the Kyoto centre, although the aims pursued and the characteristics of its users differ substantially. While Tokyo Soteria Art Circle primarily addresses users with psychiatric disorders within a collective framework, Kokoro-karada-art offers a more intimate, individually tailored therapeutic environment for users with cognitive impairments or emotional distress. Kokoro-karada-art, a project of the NPO Link Link Kyoto, is an art-therapeutic atelier established in 2009. Its staff consists solely of the atelier conductor, who is a clinical psychologist affiliated with Utano Hospital in Kyoto, and also an artist who channelled her passion into obtaining a nationally recognised qualification in art therapy. As it is detached from any purely clinical or hospital context, users are required to pay a fee for its services, art therapy and artistic rehabilitation.[12] From the perspective of the therapeutic approach, a significant focus is placed on the value of creative expression, encouraging participants, both in individual and collective (two to eight people) sessions, to explore their emotions in a free and uninhibited way. In terms of materials, the centre offers a comprehensive range of artistic tools, including pastels, watercolours, coloured chalks, clay, pens, pencils, white and coloured sheets of different size (including canvas and Japanese paper), as well as paper crafts.

The first Kokoro-karada-art user selected as case study, designated as A., is a male in his thirties. Given his psychophysical conditions, he typically participates in individual sessions for a limited time. A., who had previously suffered from alcohol addiction and a high level of social anxiety, exhibited significant cognitive impairment, including memory loss and a reduction in motor skills.[13] Consequently, he underwent extensive periods of rehabilitation in medical facilities. Upon his return to the community, he commenced an art therapy programme. A. was unable to speak and thus experienced significant difficulty in expressing himself. At the outset of his participation in art therapy sessions, his communication was largely limited to indicating assent or dissent in response to closed questions. In this phase, A. devoted himself almost exclusively to collage (Figures 7 and 8), a technique known to be highly effective for those who are reluctant to express themselves orally (Albertini, 2012). After approximately six months, A. began to interact more with the instructor, to the extent that he was able to formulate complete sentences, such as: "This is too difficult for me." The gradual emergence of speech and expression reflected an increase in self-efficacy and a growing capacity to reconcile *honne* and *tatemae*. In view of the observed improvement in A.'s communication and interrelation skills from session to session, the instructor also proposed some laboratory sessions in pairs with B., the second case study selected. The process was lengthy but yielded highly favourable outcomes. However, beginning with a purely artistic comparison, a sharing of ideas and comments on the works created during the sessions, the exchanges between the two intensified to the point of developing a solid friendship. In this phase, A. engaged in a more spontaneous and independent graphic artistic creation, utilising pastels to represent subjects of his own choosing, predominantly geometric shapes or abstract figures, on A4 sheets of paper (Figures 8 and 9). The man began to engage in jocular discourse, even addressing topics other than those pertaining to art. In the presence of the instructor, the dialogue was minimal, characterised by shyness and infrequency. Conversely, A. exhibited a gradual softening in the presence of others. He was even able to acknowledge and explicitly express his own difficulties, a notable change in his communicative behaviour, as evidenced by the following expressions: "I don't understand", and "Can you help me?". Upon completion of the art therapy programme, A. reported an enhanced awareness of his potential capabilities. His newly acquired self-confidence enabled him to resume his career, even though in an environment that was specifically designed for individuals with disabilities. At the time of the interview, A. holds positions of responsibility and is recognised and remunerated. As evidenced by both the descriptions of his works and A.'s own reflections on his experience with art therapy, this practice provided a channel of expression that had previously been almost inaccessible to him—obstructed for years by his pathological condition—and contributed to a noticeable reduction in anxiety-related symptoms. Moreover, art therapy also facilitated A.'s process of identity rebirth, which began to be acknowledged both in interpersonal and professional contexts. As his engagement deepened, the reconciliation fostered confidence, alleviated socially induced distress, and enabled fuller social and professional participation.

The second selected user, B., is a woman of a similar age to the first case. Upon arrival at the atelier, she was exhibiting symptoms of depression and severe panic attacks, symptomatologic traits of social anxiety, which had resulted in her inability to work. Due to the failure of pharmacological therapies and traditional psychotherapy to provide relief, B. was spending her daily life in bed. At this particularly critical juncture, she approached the world of art therapy. B. had even experienced a complete loss of appetite and stated: "Regardless of the food I consume, I feel like chewing sand." B. started the sessions with a certain degree of curiosity and a certain level of distrust. The initial artistic output produced by B. in the atelier was, indeed, collage work (Figure 10). B. then indicated a desire to engage in creative activities over an extended period.

During the initial phase, B. was compelled to forgo several appointments due to discomfort experienced during the hour-long train journey from her house to the atelier. This discomfort was likely attributable to the idea that the art therapy sessions would provide her the opportunity to fully express her inner self, thereby also releasing long-repressed emotional distress. B. stated: "While drawing pictures of those sensations, I danced, cried, laughed, and learned how to change my mindset." The flow of B.'s emotions often translated into an unstoppable creative impulse that produced works such as those in figure 11, extremely dynamic abstract drawings, made with chalks or watercolours in bright colours. The continuous choices made in the creation of the works have gradually led B. to the acquisition of confidence and independence. B. herself described her art therapy process as follows, divided into three distinct phases: before, during and after the sessions.

Before: It's painful, and I feel like I'm being dragged into an antlion pit. No matter how hard I struggle, I feel like I'm getting buried deeper and deeper in the sand. Is there any way to escape this situation?

During: I think art therapy suits me. Art therapy speaks for what's inside my heart.

After: I feel refreshed. It's fun. I want to continue art therapy. I'm glad I discovered art therapy.

Taken together, these phases suggest a cautious progression in which B. initially exhibited tendencies indicative of maladaptive *amae*, such as heightened dependency, fear of social evaluation and social withdrawal. Over time, the supportive environment of the atelier appears to have enabled a more regulated and constructive experience of *amae*, allowing safe expression of emotions, gradual negotiation between private feelings and social façade, and modest increases in agency, confidence, and social engagement.

In addition to the individual appointments, after a few months, B. also began to participate in group art therapy (of two or three people), with enthusiasm. This was perceived as a small step towards re-entering society. During this period, B. attempted to learn the fundamentals of drawing, with a particular focus on floral motifs, using coloured pastels. She prioritised natural elements as her preferred subject and proceeded to define her own distinctive representational style, characterised by the dynamic lines that had first emerged in her art therapy work (Figure 12). Subsequently, B. resumed professional activity, progressively decreasing the frequency of her art therapy sessions while maintaining a partial involvement in the practice.

The two Kokoro-karada-art users analysed showed that art therapy provided a means of self-expression, helping to mitigate their symptoms and reduce the burden of social stigma they experienced. A. enhanced verbal expression, social engagement, artistic autonomy, and fine motor skills through art therapy, fostering self-confidence, reducing anxiety, and supporting his reintegration into professional and interpersonal contexts. B. was able to resolve many of her internal conflicts, which were encouraged by her engagement with art, allowing her to resume an active role within society.

All of these case studies show that artistic production goes beyond cognitive or symbolic activity, unfolding as a deeply sensorimotor practice. Gestures such as sketching, painting, or collaging engage sensory, affective, and motor processes, connecting participants both to the materiality of their work and to their own corporeal presence. Therapeutic effects thus emerge not only from reflection but through active physical involvement and interaction with artistic media. In the art-therapeutic setting, this becomes especially evident. In Soteria, Sasaki's sustained use of ink, whose unpredictable flow marks both paper and the artist themselves, illustrates the risks and irreversibility of expressive mark-making. Sato's drawings reveal rhythmic gestures that regulate affect and induce relaxation. In Kokoro-karada-art, A.'s collages show how manipulating fragments enables communication when verbal language is limited, while B.'s vigorous chalks drawings channel emotional turbulence through kinaesthetic intensity.

Research highlights that embodiment is central to meaning-making and selfhood, with the lived body functioning as both a site of vulnerability and a resource for resilience and transformation (Koch & Fuchs, 2011). Viewed in this light, art-making exemplifies how corporeal presence shapes and grounds personal meaning. These cases underscore how art therapy operates at the intersection of body and mind, allowing participants to reclaim agency, negotiate trauma, and reconfigure identity. Ultimately, the body acts as an active agent in the therapeutic process, mediating psychological insight, resilience, and healing, and the integrated engagement of body and mind may also help attenuate symptoms of anxiety.

FINAL REMARKS

The case studies presented in this research, which focus on both the ateliers and their users, demonstrate the diverse outcomes of creative practices embedded within holistic therapeutic frameworks. These activities are not merely artistic exercises but structured processes that promote healing and foster the development of identity through embodied self-expression. Within the atelier setting, well-being is cultivated as a dynamic and integrative state that emerges through the interrelation of emotional and physical dimensions.

The analysis of the four users' testimonies reveals that each atelier operates as a secure and supportive environment where empathy and communication can flourish—often through non-verbal modalities that engage both cognitive and somatic processes. As already shown by Braun and Clarke (2006), the results of this study similarly reveal recurring themes, including personal transformation, the rediscovery of aesthetic value, and the articulation of previously unexpressed emotions. The findings underscore the pivotal role of creative processes in re-establishing a sense of coherence between psychological and physical experience. The ateliers under scrutiny can be conceptualised as "holding environments" in the Winnicottian sense (1971): nurturing and transitional spaces where individuals feel sufficiently safe to explore, reconnect, and reintegrate aspects of their identity that may have become fragmented or dissociated.

Within this paradigm, creative activity functions as a holistic practice wherein the interplay between body and mind becomes a wellspring of resilience, reparation, and agency. One participant, for instance, reported feeling accepted in the atelier—a sentiment that stood in stark contrast to the judgement previously encountered in other contexts. Another described how artistic practice enabled forms of self-expression beyond the limits of verbal language. Most of the users explored the aesthetic potential of discarded materials, transforming them into artworks and thus generating new perspectives on value, transformation, and meaning. Others discovered the expressive capacity of colour in conveying affective states that had previously remained difficult to be accessed.

These experiences underscore the atelier's distinctive impact as a catalyst for both individual well-being and embodied self-exploration. Despite the structural and cultural constraints that continue to limit the development of art therapy in contemporary Japan, these practices appear particularly effective in the co-treatment of anxiety-related disorders, especially social anxiety. The atelier, as a non-judgemental space, encourages participants to express themselves freely, thus fostering empathic understanding and collective meaning-making. This relational dimension supports broader processes of social reintegration, as demonstrated by the users of Kokoro-karada-art who returned to professional roles, and by former Soteria users who have since gained international recognition as artists.

While some participants begin the therapeutic process already aware of the roots of their psychophysical condition, others acquire increasing insight into the body-mind dynamics underpinning their symptoms over time. This progression yields two significant outcomes: enhanced internal clarity and greater external visibility of the therapeutic process and its effects.

For individuals whose social withdrawal was precipitated by anxiety and psychosomatic distress, the atelier provides a structured yet adaptable path towards re-engagement—with the self, with others, and with the wider social world. The restoration of psychophysical equilibrium attained through artistic creation frequently empowers participants to re-enter the workforce, often resuming the very professional roles they had once abandoned.

The therapeutic outcomes highlighted in these case studies may contribute to the destigmatisation not only of mental illness, but also of holistic and non-pharmacological forms of care. The growing visibility and legitimacy of art-based interventions are further bolstered by the ongoing efforts of the ateliers themselves to promote broader cultural acceptance. In this sense, creative therapeutic practices are shown to constitute viable pathways to well-being within the Japanese context.

REFERENCES

Albertini, C. (2012). *Arteterapia nel trattamento delle psiconevrosi. Fobie e situazioni traumatiche trattate in un contesto arteterapeutico e psicoterapeutico* [Art therapy in the treatment of psychoneurosis. Phobias and traumatic situations treated in an art-therapeutic and psychotherapeutic context]. Cleup.

American Psychiatric Association. (2022). *Diagnostic and statistical manual of mental disorders, text revision DSM-5-TR. English edition.* American Psychiatric Association Publishing.

Ando, S., Yamaguchi, S., Aoki, Y., & Thornicroft, G. (2013). Review of mental-health-related stigma in Japan. *Psychiatry and Clinical Neurosciences, 67*(6), 471–482. DOI: 10.1111/pcn.12086 PMID: 24118217

Azuma, N. (2020). Seishinka ni okeru shintai kousoku: jinken no shiten kara (Physical restraint in psychiatry: human rights considerations). *Seishin Shinkeigaku Zasshi. Psychiatria et Neurologia Japonica, 122*(12), 946–954.

Behrens, K. Y. (2004). A multifaceted view of the concept of *amae*: Reconsidering the indigenous Japanese concept of relatedness. *Human Development, 47*(1), 1–27. DOI: 10.1159/000075366

Braun, V., & Clarke, V. (2006). Using thematic analysis in psychology. *Qualitative Research in Psychology, 3*(2), 77–101. DOI: 10.1191/1478088706qp063oa

Campbell, J. (1993). *Creative art in groupwork.* Speechmark Publishing.

Case, C., Dalley, T., & Reddick, D. (2022). *The handbook of art therapy.* Routledge. (Original work published 1992)

Casey, P., & Bailey, S. (2011). Adjustment disorders: The state of the art. *World Psychiatry; Official Journal of the World Psychiatric Association (WPA), 10*(1), 11–18. DOI: 10.1002/j.2051-5545.2011.tb00003.x PMID: 21379346

Ciompi, L., & Hoffmann, H. (2004). Soteria Berne: An innovative milieu therapeutic approach to acute schizophrenia based on the concept of affect-logic. *World Psychiatry; Official Journal of the World Psychiatric Association (WPA), 3*(3), 140–146. PMID: 16633478

Corrao, S. (2005). L'intervista nella ricerca sociale [The interview in social research]. *Quaderni di Sociologia, 38*, 147–171.

Cuijpers, P., Karyotaki, E., Weitz, E., Andersson, G., Hollon, S. D., & van Straten, A. (2014). The effects of psychotherapies for major depression in adults on remission, recovery and improvement: A meta-analysis. *Journal of Affective Disorders, 159,* 118–126. DOI: 10.1016/j.jad.2014.02.026 PMID: 24679399

de Almeida, I., & Nakao, G. (2021). Amae, an emotion to understand the Japanese psyche. [Otemon Gakuin University Business Society.]. *Otemon Business Management Review*, *27*(1), 145–154.

Doi, T. (1973). *The Anatomy of dependence.* Kodansha International.

Freud, S. (1924). *Further recommendations in the technique of psycho-analysis: recollection, repetition, and working-through. Collected papers: clinical papers, papers on technique* (Riviere, J., Trans.). Hogarth Press.

Fritscher, L. (2023, November 9). Taijin kyofusho, a culture-bound social phobia. This form of anxiety is mostly found in Japan. *Verywellmind.* https://www.verywellmind .com/taijin-kyofusho-2671839

Gebhardt, L., & Masami, Y. (2014). *Literature and art after Fukushima. four approaches.* EBVerlag.

Guillemin, M. (2004). Understanding illness: Using drawings as a research method. *Qualitative Health Research, 15*(2), 272–289. DOI: 10.1177/1049732303260445 PMID: 14768462

Haibloom, S. (2012). *Taijin kyofusho: what clinicians need to know* [Doctoral dissertation, Alliant International University–Los Angeles]. DOI: 10.13140/2.1.4420.2249

Hao, Y., Zhao, H., Bai, R., Xu, Z., Feng, Y., & Gu, H. (2025). Thirty–year trends in anxiety disorders incidence across China, Japan, and Republic of Korea: An age–period–cohort analysis based on GBD 2021. *Health Care, 13*(12), 1376. DOI: 10.3390/healthcare13121376 PMID: 40565403

Heeren, , AMcNally, , R. J. (2016). An integrative network approach to social anxiety disorder: the complex dynamic interplay among attentional bias for threat, attentional control, and symptoms. *Journal of Anxiety Disorders, 42*, 95–104. https://doi.org/10.1016/j.janxdis.2016.06.009

Hofmann, S. G., Asnaani, A., & Hinton, D. E. (2010). Cultural aspects in social anxiety and social anxiety disorder. *Depression and Anxiety*, *27*(12), 1117–1127. DOI: 10.1002/da.20759 PMID: 21132847

Hofstede, G. (2001). *Culture's consequences: comparing values, behaviors, institutions, and organizations across nations.* SAGE Publications.

Ishikawa, H., Kawakami, N., & Kessler, R. C. (2016). Lifetime and 12-month prevalence, severity and unmet need for treatment of common mental disorders in Japan: Results from the final dataset of world mental health Japan survey. *Epidemiology and Psychiatric Sciences*, *25*(3), 217–229. DOI: 10.1017/S2045796015000566 PMID: 26148821

Iwata, Y., Suzuki, K., Takei, N., Toulopoulou, T., Tsuchiya, K. J., Matsumoto, K., Takagai, S., Oshiro, M., Nakamura, K., & Mori, N. (2011). Jiko-shisen-kyofu (Fear of One's Own Glance), but not taijin-kyofusho (Fear of Interpersonal Relations), is an east Asian culture-related specific syndrome. *The Australian and New Zealand Journal of Psychiatry*, *45*(2), 148–152. DOI: 10.3109/00048674.2010.534068 PMID: 21091156

Jolly, J. (2010). Florence L. Goodenough: Portrait of a psychologist. *Roeper Review*, *32*, 98–105. DOI: 10.1080/02783191003587884

Kanesaki, H., Watanabe, K., Osugi, K., Ohara, H., Takada, K., & Kinoshita, M. (2023). Utility of scratch art therapy in adult epilepsy patients with difficulties in social adaptation. *Epileptic Disorders: International Epilepsy Journal with Videotape*, *25*(5), 702–711. DOI: 10.1002/epd2.20127 PMID: 37518932

Kasahara-Kiritani, M., Matoba, T., Kikuzawa, S., Sakano, J., Sugiyama, K., Yamaki, C., Mochizuki, M., & Yamazaki, Y. (2018). Public perceptions toward mental illness in Japan. *Asian Journal of Psychiatry*, *35*, 55–60. DOI: 10.1016/j.ajp.2018.05.021 PMID: 29787953

Kawai, K., Yamada, H., Tomioka, H., Iwanami, A., & Inamoto, A. (2023). Factors associated with physical restraints in a psychiatric unit in Japan: A retrospective study. *East Asian Archives of Psychiatry: Official Journal of the Hong Kong College of Psychiatrists*, *33*(4), 120–125. DOI: 10.12809/eaap2334 PMID: 38955784

Kearney, K., & Hyle, A. E. (2004). Drawing out emotions in organizations: The use of participant-produced drawings in qualitative inquiry. *Qualitative Research*, *43*, 361–383. DOI: 10.1177/1468794104047234

Kitayama, O. (2004). Cross-Cultural Varieties in Experiencing Affect. In Akhtar, S., & Blum, H. (Eds.), *The language of emotions: development, psychopathology, and technique* (pp. 155–174). Jason Aronson.

Klein, C. (2024, January). *Mental health in Japan - statistics and facts*. Statista Japan Research Department. https://www.statista.com/topics/8609/mental-health-in-japan/#topicOverview

Koch, S. C., & Fuchs, T. (2011). Embodied arts therapies. *The Arts in Psychotherapy, 38*(4), 276–280. DOI: 10.1016/j.aip.2011.08.007

Koike, S., Yamaguchi, S., Ohta, K., Ojio, Y., Watanabe, K., & Ando, S. (2017). Mental-health-related stigma among Japanese children and their parents and impact of renaming of schizophrenia. *Psychiatry and Clinical Neurosciences, 71*, 170–179. DOI: 10.1111/pcn.12423 PMID: 27470981

Koyama, A., Miyake, Y., Kawakami, N., Tsuchiya, M., Tachimori, H., & Takeshima, T.World Mental Health Japan Survey Group, 2002-2006. (2010). Lifetime prevalence, psychiatric comorbidity and demographic correlates of "hikikomori" in a community population in Japan. *Psychiatry Research, 176*(1), 69–74. DOI: 10.1016/j.psychres.2008.10.019 PMID: 20074814

Kramer, E. (1971). *Art as therapy with children.* Schocken Books.

Kutty, N. (2022, October 17). Why making mental health care more accessible is particularly challenging in Japan. *World Economic Forum.* https://www.weforum.org/agenda/2022/10/japans-challenges-in-making-mental-health-more-accessible/

Malchiodi, C. A. (2020). *Trauma and expressive arts therapy: brain, body, and imagination in the healing process.* The Guilford Press.

Markus, H. R., & Kitayama, S. (1991). Culture and the self: Implications for cognition, emotion, and motivation. *Psychological Review, 98*(2), 224–253. DOI: 10.1037/0033-295X.98.2.224

Martins, L. A., Schiavo, A., Paz, L. V., Xavier, L. L., & Mestriner, R. G. (2024). Neural underpinnings of fine motor skills under stress and anxiety: A review. *Physiology & Behavior, 282*, 114593. DOI: 10.1016/j.physbeh.2024.114593 PMID: 38782244

McNiff, S. (2004). *Art heals: how creativity cures the soul.* Shambhala Publications.

Miike, Y. (2003). Japanese enryo-sasshi communication and the psychology of amae: Reconsideration and reconceptualization. *Keio Communication Review, 25*, 93–115.

Ministry of Health, Labour and Welfare of Japan. (2003). *Seishin hoken ni okeru shakaiteki iryō-teki kea ni kansuru hōkokusho* [Report on social and health care in mental health]. https://www.mhlw.go.jp/topics/2003/bukyoku/syougai/dl/j4a.pdf

Ministry of Health, Labour and Welfare of Japan. (2010). *Minna no mentaru herusu: Seishin shōgai, sābisu, seisaku ni kansuru sōgō saito* [Minna no mental health: comprehensive website on mental illness, services, and policies]. https://www.mhlw.go.jp/kokoro/

Ministry of Health, Labour and Welfare of Japan. (2024a, August 26). *Global health vision of the Ministry of Health, Labour and Welfare of Japan*. https://www.mhlw.go.jp/content/10501000/001295190.pdf

Ministry of Health, Labour and Welfare of Japan. (2024b). *Seishin shōgaisha no hoken fukushi ni kansuru hōritsu* [Act on mental health and welfare for persons with mental disorders or disabilities]. https://www.mhlw.go.jp/english/wp/wp-hw3/dl/Part02-06.pdf

Misawa, F. (2020). Yamanashi Kenritsu Kita Byoin ni okeru shintai kousoku (Physical restraint in Yamanashi Prefectural Kita Hospital). *Seishin Shinkeigaku Zasshi. Psychiatria et Neurologia Japonica, 122*(12), 955–961.

Mosher, L. R., & Hendrix, V. (2004). *Soteria. Through madness to deliverance*. Xlibris.

Nippoda, Y. (2012). Japanese culture and therapeutic relationship. *Online Readings in Psychology and Culture, 10*(3). DOI: 10.9707/2307-0919.1094

Nishi, D., Ishikawa, H., & Kawakami, N. (2019). Prevalence of mental disorders and mental health service use in Japan. *Psychiatry and Clinical Neurosciences, 73*(8), 458–465. DOI: 10.1111/pcn.12894 PMID: 31141260

Ono, K. (2024). *Genba de katsuyō suru hyōgen ātoserapi no jissai* [Expressive art therapy in the field]. Seishin Shobo.

Pescosolido, B. A., Martin, J. K., Lang, A., & Olafsdottir, S. (2008). Rethinking theoretical approaches to stigma: A framework integrating normative influences on stigma (FINIS). *Social Science & Medicine, 67*, 431–440. DOI: 10.1016/j.socscimed.2008.03.018 PMID: 18436358

Potash, J. S. (2020). We the art therapists: Democracy through creative action. *Art Therapy: Journal of the American Art Therapy Association, 37*(1), 3–5. DOI: 10.1080/07421656.2020.1724592

Regev, D., & Cohen-Yatziv, L. (2018). Effectiveness of art therapy with adult clients in 2018 – What progress has been made? *Frontiers in Psychology, 9*, 1531. DOI: 10.3389/fpsyg.2018.01531 PMID: 30210388

Rogers, C. R. (1961). *On becoming a person: a therapist's view of psychotherapy*. Houghton Mifflin.

Sandelowski, M. (2004). Using qualitative research. *Qualitative Health Research, 14*(10), 1366–1386. DOI: 10.1177/1049732304269672 PMID: 15538005

Savage, M. K., Lepping, P., Newton-Howes, G., Arnold, R., Staggs, V. S., Kisely, S., Hasegawa, T., Reid, K. S., & Noorthoorn, E. O. (2024). Comparison of coercive practices in worldwide mental healthcare: Overcoming difficulties resulting from variations in monitoring strategies. *British Journal of Psychiatry Open*, *10*(1), e26. DOI: 10.1192/bjo.2023.613 PMID: 38205597

Scarlet, J. (2017). *Superhero therapy: mindfulness skills to help teens and young adults deal with anxiety, depression, and trauma*. New Harbinger Publications.

Sugimoto, Y. (2020). *An introduction to Japanese society*. Cambridge University Press.

Tanji, F., Tomata, Y., Zhang, S., Otsuka, T., & Tsuji, I. (2018). Psychological distress and completed suicide in Japan: A comparison of the impact of moderate and severe psychological distress. *Preventive Medicine*, *116*, 99–103. DOI: 10.1016/j.ypmed.2018.09.007 PMID: 30219687

Teo, A. R., & Gaw, A. C. (2010). Hikikomori, a Japanese culture-bound syndrome of social withdrawal? *The Journal of Nervous and Mental Disease*, *198*(6), 444–449. DOI: 10.1097/NMD.0b013e3181e086b1 PMID: 20531124

Winnicott, D. W. (1971). *Playing and reality*. Routledge.

Yoshida, K., & Ito, J. (2012). Recovery-oriented community-based mental health service in Japan: The development of outreach services. *International Journal of Mental Health*, *41*(2), 29–37. DOI: 10.2753/IMH0020-7411410203

ENDNOTES

1 The therapeutic impact of art in these ateliers emerges not only through cognitive or symbolic processes but also via embodied engagement with materials, gestures, and movement, reflecting the inseparability of body and mind in creative practice (Regev & Cohen-Yatziv, 2018).

2 TKS is characterised by apprehension about causing discomfort to others rather than oneself and it is further classified into four subtypes: *sekimen kyōfu* (fear of blushing), *shūbō kyōfu* (fear of bodily deformity), *jiko shisen kyōfu* (fear of one's gaze), and *jiko shū kyōfu* (fear of body odour) (Hofmann et al., 2010; Iwata et al., 2011). Japanese psychiatric literature additionally distinguishes four forms of TKS based on severity and chronicity (Haibloom, 2012).

3 On 10 September 2010, the Japanese Ministry of Health, Labour and Welfare launched a portal titled "Minna no Mental Health" (Mental health for all) within its official website (Ministry of Health, Labour and Welfare of Japan, 2010). The website was established with the stated objective of providing a comprehensive range of information on mental health, including explanations of psychiatric disorders, guidance on available support services, and references to nationwide policies and guarantees.

4 The following sources are recommended for further reading on this subject: Campbell, J. (1993). *Creative art in groupwork*. Speechmark Publishing; Case, C., Dalley, T., & Reddick, D. (1992/2022). *The handbook of art therapy*. Routledge; Kearney, K., & Hyle, A. E. (2004). Drawing out emotions in organizations: the use of participant-produced drawings in qualitative inquiry. *Qualitative Research*, *43*, 361–383; Potash, J. S. (2020). We the art therapists: democracy through creative action. *Art Therapy*, *37*(1), 3–5.

5 The term "Outsider Art", as introduced by the critic Roger Cardinal, is rooted in the concept of "Art Brut" as pioneered by Jean Dubuffet. This term denotes artistic expression distinguished by its raw, uninhibited nature, often emerging from inner turmoil. Such works frequently embody intense psychological states, unconventional thought processes, or surreal visions, and are typically produced by individuals largely detached from mainstream art institutions.

6 The participants were selected based on their engagement in therapeutic and artistic pursuits, albeit through a variety of methods and with divergent outcomes, which serve to exemplify the vision and mission of the specific atelier. Furthermore, all individuals exhibited a strong willingness to participate in this research project.

7 It should be noted that this survey forms part of a wider research project of a qualitative and comparative nature, which encompasses both Italy and Japan.

8 While diagnostic information was provided by the centres, the present analysis emphasises the qualitative aspects of creative practice—such as self-expression, identity exploration, and emotional engagement—rather than numerical or clinical outcomes.

9 Soteria is a method initially conceived in the Seventies by American psychiatrist Loren Mosher (1933–2004) in San José, California. His objective was to demonstrate the possibility of treating psychosis, generally caused by anxiety or depression, even in acute phases, without resorting to restraint, while upholding the basic needs and existential dignity of psychiatric patients (Mosher & Hendrix, 2004; Ciompi & Hoffmann, 2004).

10 All direct quotes from ateliers' users are collected and translated from Japanese into English by the author.

11 In the domain of art therapy, Indian ink is esteemed for its bold, permanent lines and intense black tone, while *sumi* ink is held in high regard for its subtle tonal variations and the meditative process involved in its production, which allows for more expressive and nuanced creative exploration (Kramer, 1971).

12 The distinction between the terms "art therapy" and "artistic rehabilitation" is a defining characteristic of Kokoro-karada-art. The first comprises unstructured creative activity, with the constant presence of the atelier leader, for users who have psychological difficulties, generally social anxiety, or motor disabilities, including those caused by degenerative diseases such as Parkinson's. The objective is to either ameliorate or, in the most favourable cases, to resolve the pathological condition of the users. The second comprises an artistic trajectory designed to enhance memory, attention, concentration, planning, motivation, and the lack of realism observed in users, which are often the result of cognitive deterioration caused by diseases, particularly dementia (arguably one of the most prevalent pathological conditions currently in Japan). To ascertain the most appropriate course of action for users who have opted for artistic rehabilitation, a neuropsychological assessment is conducted to determine the extent of cognitive impairment and its progression.

13 Research suggests that social anxiety is associated with difficulties in memory and attention, and under heightened stress, may also affect fine motor skills. Individuals with elevated social anxiety tend to recall positive social events less accurately and demonstrate reduced attentional control (Heeren & McNally, 2018). Anxiety has also been shown to impair motor performance by disrupting the underlying neurobiological mechanisms (Martins et al., 2024).

APPENDIX I

This appendix presents a selection of artworks, mainly paintings, created by the user-artists of the two Japanese ateliers examined in this study. Images 1 to 6 showcase pieces produced at Soteria, while images 7 to 12 feature works from Kokoro-karada-art. As noted in the paper, internationally recognised artists from Soteria are credited by name, whereas the users from Kokoro-karada-art are anonymised to respect privacy. The main body of the paper provides detailed descriptions of each piece, including materials and themes.

Figure 1. Untitled artwork by Sasaki K.

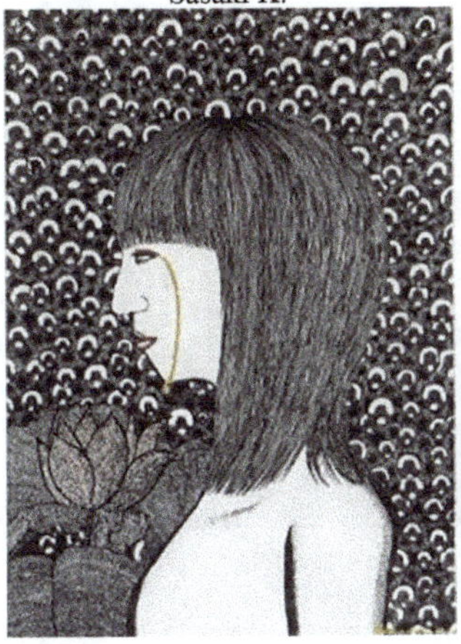

Figure 2. Untitled artwork by Sasaki K.

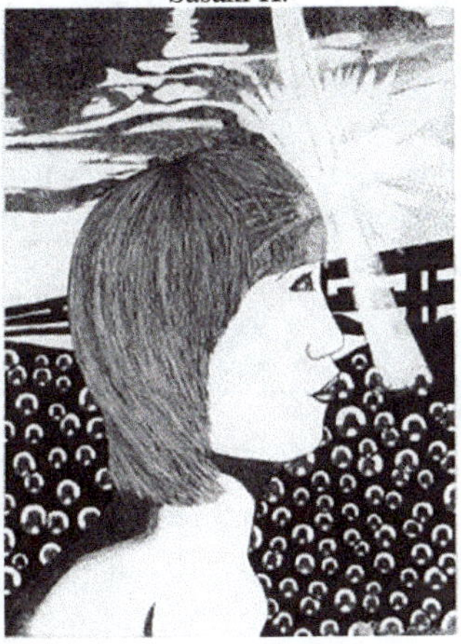

Figure 3. Untitled artwork by Sasaki K.

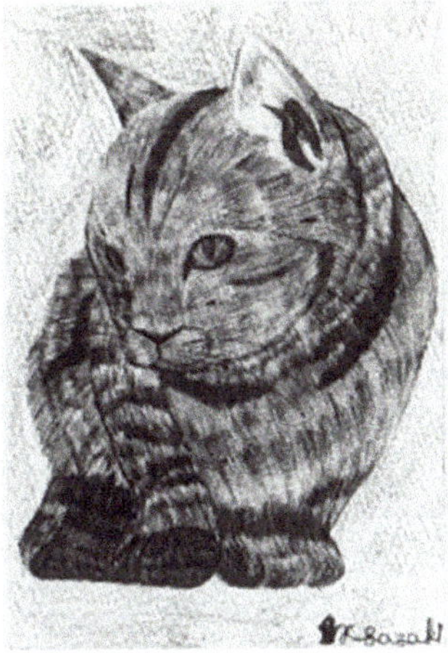

Figure 4. Untitled artwork by Sato M.

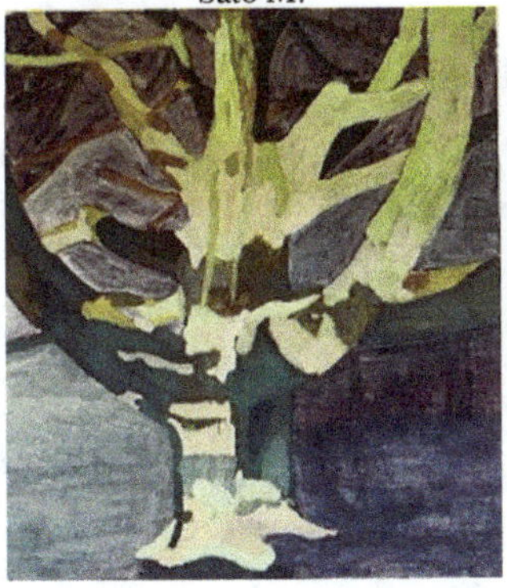

Figure 5. Untitled artwork by Sato M.

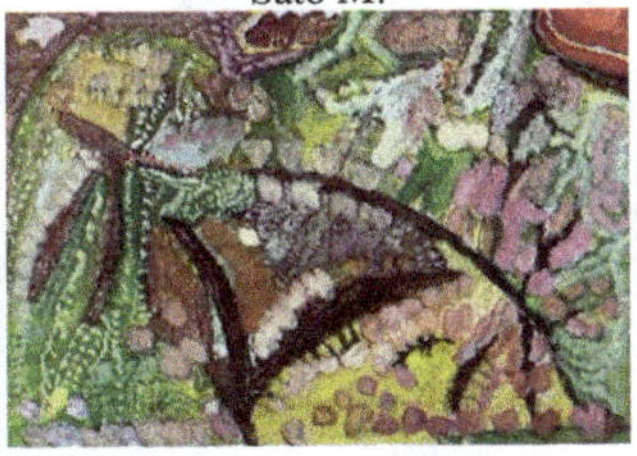

Figure 6. Untitled artwork by Sato M.

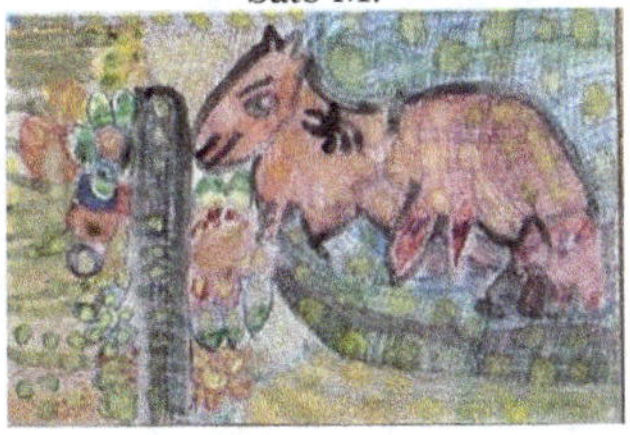

Figure 7. Untitled artwork by A.

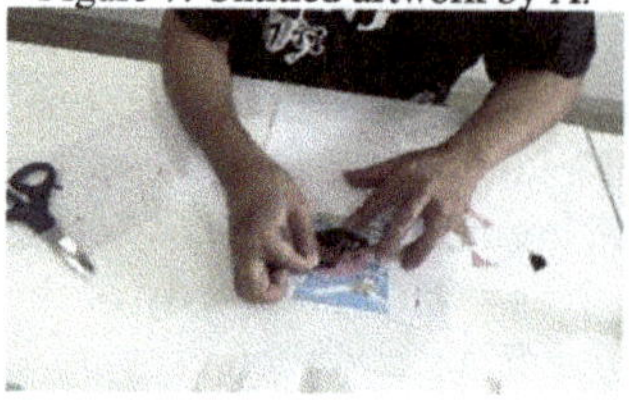

Figure 8. Untitled artwork by A.

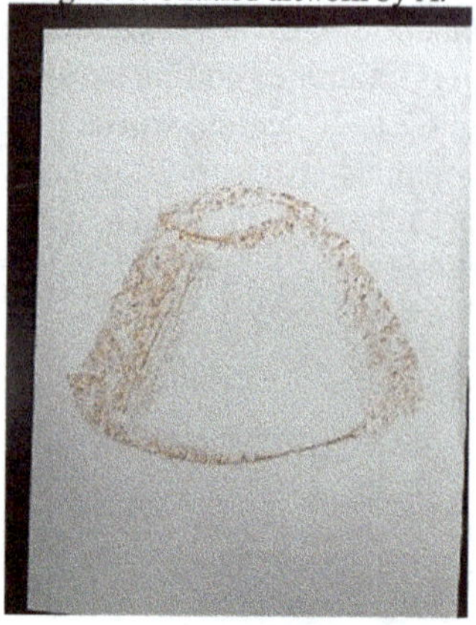

Figure 9. Untitled artwork by A.

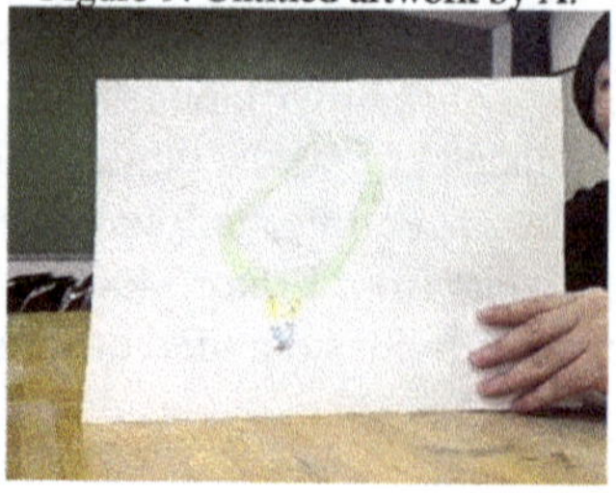

Figure 10. Untitled artwork by B.

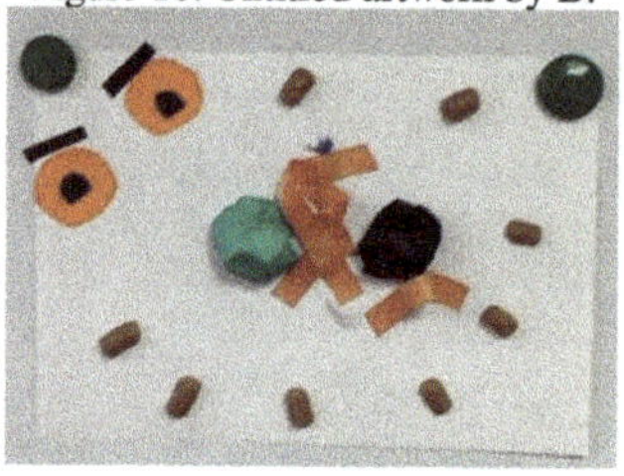

Figure 11. Untitled artwork by B.

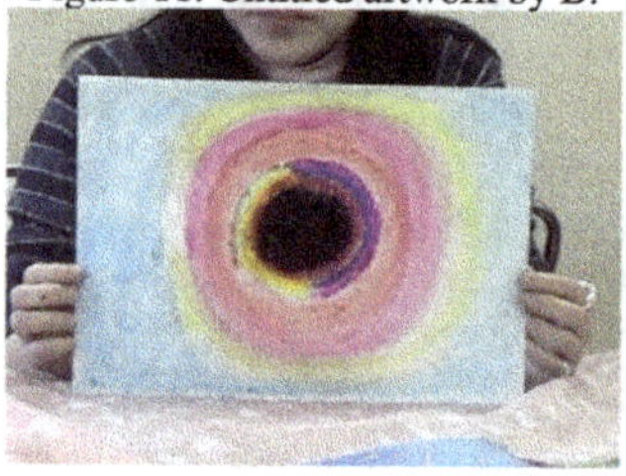

Figure 12. Untitled artwork by B.

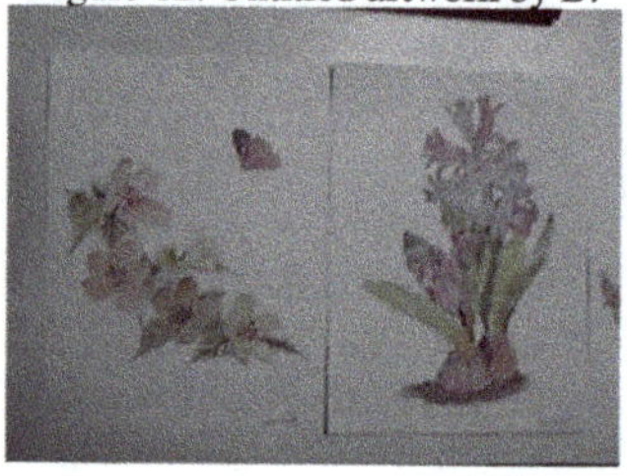

APPENDIX II

In this appendix, the full set of interview questions posed to the facilitators and selected users of the two Japanese art therapy centres is provided. A curated selection of their responses, translated into English, is also included to highlight the lived experiences and reflections that inform this study.

Questions for the tutors:

1. How do you think music or art therapy can help people find out who they are?
2. How many people work at the Centre?
3. Why is the activity mainly collective or individual?
4. What tools are used? Have they ever used tools that are usually thought of as “non-Western” or “Eastern”?
5. How do users start enrolling in the centre? Is it voluntary or is it based on medical advice?

1. 音楽療法・アートセラピーは、ユーザーが個人のアイデンティティを定義するのにどのように役立つと思いますか。
2. センターで働いている人の何人がいますか。
3. 活動は主に個人ですか、それとも集団ですか。それはなぜですか。
4. どんな音楽や楽器・芸術的手法を使っていますか。センターで「西洋」か「東洋」の楽器・芸術的手法を使った経験はありますか。
5. ユーザーはどのようにセンターに参加し始めていますか?自発的にまたは医師のアドバイスを受けてからですか。

Questions for each user:

1. How old are you?
2. What gender are you? “Male”, “female”, “intersex” or “prefer not to specify”
3. What is the nature of your discomfort or disability? How did you feel when you arrived at the Centre?
4. What musical instrument/genre do you prefer? What techniques, subjects or colours do you prefer in art?
5. How often do you go to the Centre?
6. How long have you been going there?
7. Are there any changes or improvements?
8. What have been the changes in the creative process?
9. What were the changes in the way we express ourselves and relate to others?
10. Were there any changes in relation to the pathological condition?

11. Can you describe some of your artistic creations that you think best represent your style?

1. 年齢・年齢層
2. 性別:「男性」、「女性」、「他」、「特定しないことを希望する」
3. 不快感または障害の種類
4. ユーザーはどの楽器や音楽ジャンルを好みますか。ユーザーが好む代表的な芸術技法/主題/色は何ですか。
5. 利用頻度
6. 利用期間
7. 変更、改善はありましたか。
8. 芸術的にどんな変化がありますか。
9. 人との関係または自己表現の変化はありましたか。
10. 病状に対する変化はありましたか。
11. 芸術作品の中で、特にあなたのスタイルを象徴するものについて説明していただけますか。

NPO Tokyo Soteria Art Circle

Sasaki K.

- 最近は、最初にコンセプトを決めてから、制作を開始するようにしている。
- 制作中は、時には、苦行、時には、楽しい。
- テーマは、女性と猫。他人の判断を恐れるから自分の心の内側に秘めている女性の感覚を表現する。
- 制作後は、完成した喜びと燃え尽きた感がある。
- I recently decide on a concept first, then start creating.
- The process of creation is sometimes painful, and sometimes fun.
- The theme is women and cats. I want to express the feminine feelings hidden inside my heart due to fear of the judgement of others.
- Upon completion of the work, a sense of elation mixed with fatigue is often experienced.

Sato M.

- 20代の時に生け花を習っていた。最初は、趣味程度でしたが、28歳の時に生け花の師範になりたいと思っていた。29歳の時に師匠から特訓を受け、30歳の時に免状を取得した。今でも生け花が好きで、自宅でも花を生けている。絵画の制作では、花をモチーフにすることが多い。

- 制作中は、アドバイスをもらえるので、それが役に立っている。
- 自分なりに工夫して使っている。
- 最初は、絵が上手に描けるようになれば良いと思っていたが、2年間、アートサークルに通い、主治医の先生から、「アートサークルへは、90歳くらいまで通えるよ」と言われ、楽しんで制作を続けたいと思っている。
- I learned flower arranging in my 20s. It started as a hobby, but by 28 I was set on becoming an Ikebana master. At 29, I received intensive training from a master, and at 30, I obtained my license. I am still passionate about flower arranging and enjoy creating floral arrangements at home. When I create paintings, I often use flowers as a motif.
- I seek guidance from others during my creative process, which I find beneficial.
- I conceptualise and execute my designs my own way.
- Initially, my goal was simply to become proficient in painting, but after two years of attending the atelier, my doctor told me, "You can continue attending the atelier until you're about 90 years old", which has motivated me to continue creating while enjoying it.

Kokoro Karada Art

A. セラピー当初は話もできず、椅子に座ったままーっとしていました。意欲がなく、ただこの場所に来ているだけの時間が何日も続きました。半年経つ頃から、少しずつ言葉が出るようになり、絵が描けるようになりました。彼は私に「これは私には難しすぎる」とか「分からない」とか「手伝ってほしい」などと言い始めました。自分で説明書を読んでペーパークラフトができるようになりました。徐々に会話が増え、よく笑い、冗談を言うようになりました。そのうち作業所に通うことが決まり、私とのセッションは終了しましたが、お母さまはその後も近況報告をしてくださいました。今では作業所で収入を得るまでになったそうです。家族の介助、本人の努力、医療、そしてアートセラピー、当時は回復が難しいと言われていましたが、ここまで回復されたことは本当に素晴らしく、私にとってこの経験はとっても嬉しいことでした。

At the start of the therapy, he was unable to speak and just sat in a chair, lost in thought. He had no motivation, and many days he continued to just come to this place. After six months, he started to speak up and was drawing pictures. He started to tell me things like: "This is too difficult for me" or "I don't understand", "Can you help me?". He could read instructions and make paper crafts independently. He started talking more, laughing and joking a lot. Eventually, he decided to attend a workshop, and my sessions with him came to an end. However, his mother continued to give me updates on his situation. He now earns an income from the workshop. His recovery was challenging, but he overcame it thanks to his family, his own efforts, medical care and art therapy. I am very happy that he has made it this far and this experience has made me very happy.

B. 3年ほど仕事を休職、辛い日々を送っている女性を紹介されました。彼女の不調のほとんどは、うつ病や対人恐怖症に関連した症状を反映していました。セッションの予約をしてもセラピーの場所までたどり着けないことが何度もありました。それでもあきらめずに通って来られました。そのころ食事は砂を食べているようだと言われていました。彼女のアートセラピーの経験は3つの段階に分けられます。アートセラピーを開始「苦しくて、アリ地獄に引きずり込まれるような感覚。もがいてもどんどん砂の中に埋もれていく感じ。何とか今の状況から脱する方法はないものか」。アートセラピー途中「アートセラピーは私に合っていると思う。アートセラピーは私の心の中を代弁してくれる」。アートセラピー後「スッキリとした。楽しい。アートセラピーを続けたい。アートセラピーに出会ってよかった」。

セッションでは、その感覚を絵に描いたり、踊ったり、泣いたり、笑ったり、こころの切り替え方を勉強したり。彼女にとって、それはドラマティックな時間だっただろうと思います。そのうちセッションの間隔が開いてきました。回復の兆しです。おしゃれになったり買い物をしたり。やがて職場にも復帰しました。時々しんどいことはあるけれど乗り越えました。そして好きな人に出会って結婚しました。カウンセリングだけでは得られなかったセッションの効果だと思います。

I met a woman who had been out of work for about three years and was struggling. Most of her ailments reflected symptoms related to depression and interpersonal phobia. She frequently failed to attend therapy sessions, despite having booked them. But she didn't give up. She kept coming. She described the sensation of eating as akin to eating sand. Her experience with art therapy can be divided into three stages. Before: "It's painful, and I feel like I'm being dragged into an antlion pit. No matter how hard I struggle, I feel like I'm getting buried deeper and deeper in the sand. Is there any way to escape this situation?". During: "I think art therapy suits me. Art therapy speaks for what's inside my heart." After: "I feel refreshed. It's fun. I want to continue art therapy. I'm glad I discovered art therapy."

During the sessions, she drew pictures of those sensations, danced, cried, laughed, and learned how to change her mindset. This was undoubtedly a very dramatic time for her. Eventually, the time between sessions became longer. This was undoubtedly a sign of recovery. She started dressing up and going shopping. She returned to work. She faced challenges, but she overcame them. Then she found love and got married. I achieved results through art therapy that I would not have been able to achieve with counselling alone.

Chapter 13
Bibliotherapy and Heterolingualism in Nagori:
Body and Language Interactions

Anna Bourges-Celaries
http://orcid.org/0009-0003-8615-7550
University of Montreal, Canada

ABSTRACT

This article explores the potential therapeutic effects of heterolingual literature in the context of bibliotherapy closely linked to cognitive behavourial therapy, through a close reading of Sekiguchi Ryōko's exophonic essay Nagori (2018). According to Sekiguchi, French people are as sensitive as Japanese people to the unique sensation of nagori, but lack a word to express it. Althought this essay is mainly written in French, Sekiguchi decided to use the Japanese word "nagori" as the title of her book, along with many other Japanese words within the text. This literary practice is called heterolingualism, and I argue that it impacts the body and the mind of the readers. Studies in neurosciences have called attention to the fact that there are strong relationships between word and face processing. The readers' interactions with a written text mirrors the dynamics between body and language that heterolingualism enhances as it provides more scope for cultural and emotional awareness.

INTRODUCTION

This article explores the potential therapeutic effects embedded in heterolingual literature, particularly in the context of bibliotherapy inspired by cognitive

DOI: 10.4018/979-8-3373-3521-6.ch013

behavourial therapy, through a close reading of Sekiguchi Ryōko's exophonic essay *Nagori* (2018). Bibliotherapy has been known as such since the beginning of the last century, as the term "bibliotherapy" was coined in 1916 in an article in *The Atlantic Monthly* by Samuel McChord Crothers (1857-1927), and has been used ever since. Bibliotherapy, book therapy or poetry therapy—these terms can be used interchangeably according to Mari Alschuler (2006)—is a creative and therapeutic approach using literature of all forms to help solve or cope with mental or physical illnesses. The etymology of the word "bibliotherapy" comes from the Greek: *biblion* (βιβλίον) meaning "book", "letter"; and *thérapeìa* (θεραπεία) meaning "cure" or "treatment". Bibliotherapy is often applied based on Cognitive Behavioural Therapy, also commonly known as CBT, and group therapy (Alschuler 2006, p. 253).

It appears that the experience of emotions is not purely personal but influenced by psychological and societal patterns. Indeed, two of the founders of CBT, Aaron Beck (1921-2021) and Albert Ellis (1913-2007), were inspired by the philosophy of Stoicism when establishing the model on which CBT is based, as Jules Evans writes in his book *Philosophy for Life And Other Dangerous Situations* (2012).

> *Albert Ellis told me, for example, that he had been particularly impressed by a saying of the Stoic philosopher Epictetus: 'Men are disturbed not by things, but by their opinions about them.' This sentence inspired Ellis's 'ABC' model of the emotions, which is at the heart of CBT [...]. (p. 4)*

This led Kelda Green to explore the connection between ancient Greek philosophy and CTB[1] in her book, *Rethinking Therapeutic Reading* (2020), revealing that bibliotherapy and literary texts are linked on a deep level. Green also establishes a model of therapy based entirely on bibliotherapy. Studies such as Kelda Green's underline the potent healing ability that literary reading holds and support this speculative exploratory work in the interdisciplinary field of psychology and literature.

My previous research on exophonic writings led me to work with heterolingualism, since exophony is intrinsincally linked to heterolingualism. Indeed, exophony is a term used to describe writers who do not write in their native language. Heterolingualism is a concept developed by Rainier Grutman, while working on French Canadian Literature. He defines it as: "the presence in a text of foreign idioms, in whatever form, as well as varieties (social, regional or chronological) of the main language[2,3]" (2019, p. 60) Exophonic writings often form, if not always, a literary space where heterolingualism is at play, which prompted me to observe that it could also be used as a methodological tool since it enhances cultural transfers due to the impact on the brain when exposed to a different language through reading (Bourges-Celaries, 2024b). Indeed, different results from studies in neuroscience support the claim that the region of the brain that processes words and script systems is close and somehow linked with the part that recognises faces (Behrmann & Plaut, 2014; Yang et al, 2022). This evidence led me to consider the way the written word, affect, and emotions are linked; an idea supported by the fact that "emotional words represent highly symbolic emotional stimuli that acquire personal significance" (Straube et al, 2011, p. 67). There is also evidence of the impact words have on emotions' representation (Lee & Satpute, 2024).

In this article, I propose that texts which are both exophonic and heterolingual can serve as powerful tools for bibliotherapy, particularly in alleviating suffering related to emotional challenges such as alexithymia. Medically trained experts may notice some limitations in this approach; therefore, I kindly ask readers for their indulgence and encourage them to retain any elements they find relevant, as this study represents a preliminary theoretical step towards using heterolingual writings for curative purposes. Drawing on recent studies about effective therapeutic methods for alexithymia, this article will focus on this condition as a potential target for healing through bibliotherapy. Indeed, alexithymia is "understood as a multi-faceted construct that primarily describes difficulties in (a) identifying emotions, (b) finding appropriate words to describe emotions and (c) an externally oriented thinking style" (Mazza et al, 2026, p. 3). Alexithymia is often associated with physical illnesses—such as brain injuries—as well as developmental disorders—such as the autism spectrum disorder—and mental health conditions, including traumatic experience or anorexia nervosa for example.

I argue that the dynamic between heterolingualism and bibliotherapy, and its possible implementation as a therapy, can be explored by analysing an excerpt from the essay *Nagori* (2018) by Japanese author Sekiguchi Ryōko (1970-). Sekiguchi is known for writing both in her native Japanese and in French. *Nagori* is written in French and is, therefore, an exophonic text, but also a heterolingual one, making it a solid sample to consider the curative effect of heterolingual literature.

First, I will show how neuroscience corroborates the interplay between heterolingual writings and bibliotherapy, and its potential impact on alexithymia. Second, I will demonstrate how heterolingualism can be used to serve the purpose of CBT, that is modifying thought patterns, which illustrates the effect heterolingualism holds for people suffering from alexithymia. Third, I will review the limitations and advice regarding this project that came to light during this study.

LITERATURE, LANGUAGES AND BIBLIOTHERAPY

Exophony, Heterolingualism and Alexithymia

There are many theories and terms attached to the literary practice of writing in a language that is not one's native tongue, such as translingualism, multilingualism, or migrant literature, to name but the most familiar ones. The term "exophony" is also used occasionally, but is not as neatly defined as other related concepts are. The word "exophony" was first used by the exophonic Japanese writer Tawada Yōko in her essay『エクソフォニー・母語の外へ出る旅』[*Exophony: Voyages Outside the Mother Tongue*], an essay about exophony. She had heard Robert Stockhammer use this word to describe the work of authors changing languages to write while attending a conference held in Dakar in 2002 (Tawada, 2003, p. 3). Tawada writes both in German and Japanese and was invited to Dakar to discuss her experience as an author who writes in German, even though German is not her native language. Her participation in this conference led Tawada to write an essay about exophony in 2003. In this essay, Tawada wrote: "Until this day, I had often heard words such as 'migrant literature' or 'creole literature', 'exophony' has a broader meaning and refers to the general state of having left one's mother tongue.[4]" (p. 3) This observation made by Tawada shows that exophony as a concept broadens this literary practice beyond the limits of national borders by excluding terms such as "migrant" and "creole". Indeed, following that same conference in Dakar, another book was published in 2007: a collective monograph titled *Exophonie: Anderssprachigkeit (in) der Literatur* [Exophony: Linguistic Otherness of/in Literature]. This collective monograph remains to this day one of the main references regarding exophony. In its introduction, the editors Susan Arndt, Dirk Naguschewski, and Robert Stockhammer explore the etymology of "exophony": it comes from the Greek with "exo" meaning "outside, outer, external", and "phony" that derives from "phōnē" which means "voice".

Although the term "exophony" is either used as an analytical tool applied to the interpretation of texts defined as *multilingual* or *translingual*, or as a barely defined theory, exophonic writings bear a particular dimension distinguishing them from multilingual and translingual texts: choice. Indeed, during my doctoral research on exophony, I observed that some writers—who were not subjected to exile, colonialism, or their consequences—often adopt a unique position as writers. I thus developed the following definition: exophony is the act of choosing to write in a language that is not one's native language, meaning a language that the writer learns as a young adult or adult. This choice is not the result of any kind of external pressure, such as exile, war, or colonialism (Bourges-Celaries, 2024a). Sekiguchi Ryōko, the author of *Nagori*, falls into the exophonic category as she was born in 1970 in Tōkyō, where she grew up. She studied both in Japan and France and moved of her own accord to France almost 30 years ago. She started writing in French in 2003. *Nagori*, published in 2018, is an essay mostly about seasons and foods, and the way they affect us. Since *Nagori* was written in French, Sekiguchi's literary practice is a perfect example of exophony, as she was under no pressure to leave Japan to move to France, nor was she forced or coerced in any way to write in French.

In *Nagori*, Sekiguchi transcribes Japanese words into Latin alphabet. It facilitates the process of sharing Japanese words and concepts with her French-speaking readers, as it directly supports the cultural transfer between Japanese language/culture and French language/culture. According to Michel Espagne and Michael Werner, implementing a cultural transfer means "linking two autonomous, asymmetrical systems" (1988, p. 5). Therefore, the fact that the author also chose to give a Japanese title to this essay she wrote in French confirms her willingness to establish a connection between the French language/culture and the Japanese language/culture. Indeed, in an interview, Sekiguchi stated that she wanted to give to French-speaking people a word to name that singular feeling that is *nagori* (Hirsch, 2018), thus making her use of heterolingualism a tool for sharing. Sekiguchi defines "nagori" in the essay as: "the nostalgia of the season that has just left us". She explains that this word can be used to talk about something from the past that is somehow still lingering in the present. She gives examples such as a child who reminds their family of their deceased parents, or how some flowers sometimes remain on a tree long after the end of the season (p. 29).

Although it is clear that through the use of heterolingualism, exophonic writers show a willingness to share, and even pass on, some cultural and linguistic aspects by incorporating words of their native language into the text they choose to write in a different language, it should be noted that the aim of this study is not to observe the effect of Japanese words and culture on non-Japanese-speaking people per se. The nature and influence of Japanese culture will be considered as one element of this study, but the goal is to investigate whether the use of unfamiliar and unknown foreign words can work as an external stimulus and help people who suffer from alexithymic-based difficulties to gain a better grasp of their own emotions by bypassing culturally and socially charged terms that influence our perceptions of emotions. The primary causes of alexithymia may be language impairment and difficulty with interoception—the ability to be aware of internal sensations in the body (Mazza et al, 2026, p. 7)—which explains why alexithymia is not a diagnosis but a subclinical construct that can be experienced by very diverse populations and at different levels. Therefore, there are as many obstacles as there are possibilities when it comes to the use of bibliotherapy for alexithymic-based symptoms.

As expected, foreign words cannot be used as terms from the natural semantic metalanguage (NSM) developed by Anna Wierzbicka and Cliff Goddard. NSM is "a mini-language which corresponds to the intersection—the common core—of all languages. This intersection of all languages has been discovered empirically, through extensive cross-linguistic studies undertaken by many scholars over many years." (Wierzbicka, 2009, p. 4). Words from any language are essentially the opposite of universal. Indeed, NSM opposes the idea that words and their concepts are universal, for "Emotion terms are always language- and culture-specific and therefore carry with them a particular linguistic and cultural slant." (p. 7) In the case of *Nagori*, whether Japanese words are understood and welcomed wholly as Japanese by French-speaking readers, and the impact they have, is a subject for another study that would further explore the topic of this article. One could argue that this objective might be attained by using made-up words—or pseudowords that "are units of speech that seem to be a word in a language but are not part of the standard vocabulary of [the native language of the treated patient]" (Nwokah & Graves, 2009, p. 436)—but in order to propose a substantial and long-lasting method of therapy, relying on literature that already exists is more realistic—unless one is also a writer willing to experiment with made-up words.

Bibliottherapy, CBT and Emotions

Books and literature, especially self-help books, have a long history in healing. In ancient Egypt, teachings and maxims were written down. Called *sebayt* (meaning *instructions*), these texts were collections of advice on how to behave properly in society or how to address more personal issues (Chadefaud, 1993, p. 53). From ancient Egypt to the present day, the written word has always been a resource for navigating life. Many attribute the term "self-help" to Samuel Smiles (1812-1904), a British author who published *Self-Help* in 1859, a book about self-improvement that became very popular after its publication[5]. Bibliotherapy and the idea that people can actually help themselves through reading appropriate books (usually self-help books or morally accepted writings such as religious texts) gained momentum, and in 1980, the American psychiatrist David Burns wrote a self-development book called *Feeling Good*. In 2020, he updated it, changing its title to *Feeling Great*. These two books are often used in bibliotherapy with English-speaking people (Correll et al, 2024; Naylor et al, 2010). The fact that Burns updated his book forty years after its first publication shows that bibliotherapy is a therapeutic method gaining increasing interest. As the full titles of *Feeling Good* and *Feeling Great* show ("The New Mood Therapy" and "The Revolutionary New Treatment for Depression and Anxiety"), bibliotherapy was initially conceived mostly as a drug-free treatment for mild depression (Moldovan et al, 2013). Recent studies have conducted experiments using bibliotherapy with patients with more serious issues, such as psychopathic disorder and schizophrenia (Kasperek-Zimowska et al, 2021; Rafiei et al, 2023). However, these studies used literature such as poetry, diaries, biographies. The results were positive and invite further investigation into the curative effect literature holds.

Indeed, most heterolingual books address the feeling of not belonging to the community these writers live in, as studies in translation have underscored (Gauvin, 2009; Suchet, 2014). Although the causes differ, alexithymic invididuals may find resonance in heterolingual writings, as they struggle to identify and regulate their emotions due to an inability to express what they feel through words—similar to the experience of lacking the right words in a non-native language. Moreover, it has been observed that adult "Participants showed evidence of learning after just two exposures, especially for words learned in emotional contexts." (Dong et al, 2025, p. 2177-2178) Undertaking therapy is a highly emotional context, which sets up appropriate conditions for learning new words to identify and express emotions. Although not written for therapeutic purposes, such texts may prove highly valuable to individuals seeking therapy by providing an opportunity to reflect on these issues outside the conventional clinical setting, which can sometimes feel intimidating.

There are methods of therapy that integrate elements of bibliotherapy, such as poetry therapy, which "can incorporate journal therapy, therapeutic reading (bibliotherapy), and narrative therapy." (Alfrey et al, 2021, p. 2). Poetry therapy ranks amongst the category of arts therapies because it includes a creative dimension that bibliotherapy alone does not provide. Regarding alexithymia, it has been observed that integrative therapies yield the best results: "[...] a large effect size was observed for integrative therapies, indicating that integrative therapies were more effective at reducing levels of alexithymia than unimodal therapies." (Mazza et al, 2026, p. 15) This evidence supports the necessity of applying bibliotherapy alongside CBT, which can modify thought patterns—relying on the balanced approach such an integrative therapy harbours.

Therefore, using CBT and bibliotherapy as elements of an integrative therapy is more effective than using either one separately. The aforementioned therapeutic method developed by Kelda Green in bibliotherapy includes a creative aspect, as participants were asked to keep a journal and write letters to fictional characters from the book they were assigned to read. There are several creative approaches to CBT, and the arts are often used as tools within CBT (Wang & Xiao, 2021; Yi et al, 2024). However, in the case of alexithymia, CBT and arts therapies are usually not combined. A tailored integrative therapy—including bibliotherapy, CBT and active creative practices following Green's method—can also explore the interplay between CBT and arts therapies for aleximythic individuals, especially since arts therapies have yielded successful results regarding alexithymia (Cirillo et al, 2025; Heiman et al, 2013; Meijer-Degen & Lansen, 2006). Thanks to art therapy (theatre-based activities in this instance), "measurable movement in domains linked to emotional recognition and verbalization" (Cirillo et al, 2025, p. 12) have been observed when treating alexithymia in adolescent patients with severe anorexia nervosa. Art therapies are empowering as they require patients to use their own capacities (Meijer-Degen & Lansen, 2006, p. 172).

In the case of exophonic and heterolingual texts, readers also have to be active as they learn and adapt to new words. To grasp the performative effect heterolingualism can have through the use of literature in bibliotherapy, the work of the neuroscientist and psychologist Lisa Feldman Barrett—an expert in the psychology of emotion who developed a theory in neuroconstructivism, a theoretical framework focusing on the construction of representations in the brain—is crucial. According to the theory of constructed emotion: "emotions are constructions of the world, not reactions to it." (2017, p. 16) This means that emotions are sensory events-based representations; we build representations of them based on what we experimence from an event, which is therefore interpreted in accordance with beliefs and values from our culture and personal history. Most events are not fundamentally good or bad, nor do they inherently possess characteristics that will always make us feel a specific emotion. Therefore, our brains build representations of impending events based on previous experiences, as Barrett clearly states.

> *[...] the brain constructs meaning by correctly anticipating (predicting and adjusting to) incoming sensations. Sensations are categorized so that they are (i) actionable in a situated way and therefore (ii) meaningful, based on past experience. When past experiences of emotion (e.g. happiness) are used to categorize the predicted sensory array and guide action, then one experiences or perceives that emotion (happiness). (p. 9)*

If emotions are constructed representations, one wonders what happens when people are confronted with an entirely novel event/item. This raises many questions, such as how readers would adopt a foreign word to express their emotions, and why they would do so. Regarding the relationship between emotions and words, cultural evolutionary theories describe two aspects that activate this dynamic: proximate mechanisms and ultimate explanations.

> *Ultimate explanations focus on why a cultural trait is favored. A proximal mechanism focuses on what leads people to adopt a cultural trait. [...] Past cultural evolutionary work has suggested ultimate explanations of why humans have emotion words in the first place, and proximate explanations of how cultures develop such diverse emotion languages. (Jackson & Lindquist, in press, p. 12)*

Proximate causes support the adoption of new words, and according to Joshua Conrad Jackson and Kristen Lindquist, there are three potential mechanisms "through which speakers may come to develop words that name emotions" (p. 13): attractors, social learning strategies, and features of the structure of languages themselves (p. 14). Attractors can function as proximate mechanisms that draw people to adopt a foreign word. Here is an example discussed by Jackson and Lindquist regarding the adoption of foreign words in a given language:

> *Emotion scientists once referred to the German word schadenfreude, pleasure at another's pain, as an emotion category with no English equivalent. However, English-language speakers were happy to adopt schadenfreude into their vocabulary [...]. Why has this borrowed word become so popular amongst English speakers? One possibility is because schadenfreude captures a set of feelings and*

regularly encountered circumstances that English speakers could immediately relate to, even if English did not itself originally compress those experiences into a single word. For English speakers, schadenfreude was an experiential category in search of a word, and the German language provided one. In this example, the word schadenfreude is an "attractor," a destination that pulls culture towards it in the same way that gravity pulls objects towards earth. (p. 14)

As mentioned, there are various conditions that may cause alexithymia, and some people experiencing alexithymic symptoms may benefit from this attractor mechanism, which can help them gravitate towards foreign words that may capture how they feel.

IMPLEMENTING HETEROLINGUAL BIBLIOTHERAPY

Words and Emotions

Almost a hundred years ago, renowned psychology professor William Hunt (1903-1986) had already hinted at the importance of words regarding emotions, noting the subjective nature of the latter and stating that "[...] the only universal element in any emotional situation is the use by all the subjects of a common term of report, *i.e.* 'fear'." (1941, p. 266) The use of an emotional term such as fear is influenced by a categorisation process that functions alongside the aforementioned constructed representations.

The events that people call ''anger,'' ''sadness,'' ''fear,'' and so on, result when core affect is conceptualized using knowledge of emotion (effectively, what a person knows about the category of anger, sadness, or fear, etc.). In an instant, conceptualization proceeds efficiently and automatically, transforming internal sensory information from the body into psychologically meaningful state by combining it with external sensory information about the world and situation-specific knowledge of emotion learned from prior experience. The result is an intensional state that is at once affective and conceptual. (Lindquist & Barrett, 2008, p. 898)

Because the emotional states associated with the term *fear*, for example, are various, measures such as the NSM have been developed to understand the conceptual unity of human categorisation of emotions (Wierzbicka, 2009, p. 12). It appears that although all people can experience fear regardless of their cultures and languages, what might be called *fear* by some might be labeled *surprise* by others, since—from an English-speaking point of view—there are languages that do not have two clearly distinct categories for *fear* and *surprise* (p. 7). Therefore, words play an important role in the way we construct emotions, for they help build representations of emotional experiences. Hence Sekiguchi Ryōko's statement in *Nagori*: "Sensibility springs from words: one cannot feel what has no name[6]." (p. 23) Although numerous avenues remain to explore regarding the relationship between words and emotions, science and the arts agree on how essential words are for expressing and experiencing emotions. Indeed, it has been proven that the human brain reacts to words evoking the idea of pain, even when one is not talking about actual pain but imagining it.

> *Our study provides evidence that the processing of pain-related words leads to activations within regions of the pain matrix. [...] During the imagination task, the specificity of pain-related words is reflected in a central nervous activation of regions associated with the cognitive dimension of pain [...]. (Richter et al, 2010, p. 204)*

This observation is supported by the fact that it has been established that there is "a close connection between regions of the brain that process lexical semantics and regions that are activated during emotion perception." (Jackson & Lindquist, in press, p. 25) The emotion perception process appears to rely on words and is even potentially activated during imagination tasks. As previously mentioned, not only are words linked to faces and have a direct impact on our perception of the environment, but they also shape the entire human experience of feeling: "[...] the language of emotions can causally affect how people recognize emotions, conceptualize emotions, and even experience emotions. This evidence suggests that emotion language changes the structure of thought, as well as communication." (p. 30) The enabling potential of words to change the structure of thought and communication is exactly the topic this article explores and endeavours to do so by reviewing the exophonic heterolingual aspect of *Nagori*.

The Case of *Nagori*

Exposure to new words can help individuals with alexithymic symptoms to express the unnamed yet experienced, thereby creating new positive experiences. Moreover, discovering foreign words and concepts might help broaden one's perception of life. Heterolingual texts can provide new words for people to regain their past. In addition, thanks to the autobiographical aspects of *Nagori*, a feeling of closeness is established, which might also facilitate entering the phase of opening up. In *Nagori*, Sekiguchi Ryōko introduces key elements to discuss foods from her familiar Japanese point of view in a clear and simple way, making it accessible to French-speaking readers.

> *[...] there are three different words to describe how food changes through seasonality: hashiri, sakari and nagori. They respectively refer to the equivalent of*

'spring', 'peak season', and the last one, nagori, refers to the late season, 'the nostalgia of the season that has just left us'.[7] *(p. 27-28)*

The way the author opens up about Japanese culture is straightforward: first, Japanese words are introduced and immediately translated. Second, Sekiguchi further contextualises for readers to fully grasp what *hashiri*, *sakari*, and *nagori* mean. She explains that *hashiri* also refers to the "opening of the season[8]" (p. 28), and that the word *hashiri* is "the verbal noun from the verb *hashiru*, 'to run', which refers both to the act of running and to something rolling, but also to the idea of 'precursor' […][9]" (p. 28). As for *sakari*, Sekiguchi writes: "*Sakari* means 'acme', 'apogee', or refers to the time when animals are in heat.[10]" (p. 28) As covered in the introduction, *nagori* is a more complex phenomenon, and the author gives a thorough explanation of its meaning, providing many examples to guide readers.

As for nagori, it holds a broader acceptation. First and foremost, it means the trace, the presence or the atmosphere of something from the past, something that is no more. […] Nagori can also be used to talk about the damage or consequences of an event, such as the nagori of an earthquake or of an illness. […] There are many idiomatic phrases using 'nagori'. First, some are about a phenomenon that lingers against all odds long after its time has passed, like nagori no yuki, 'nagori's snow': the snow that does not melt, or keeps on falling even when it's spring already […]. Second, those phrases can also express nostalgia or regret that is found in an item or a landscape. For example, the phrase nagori no sora, 'nagori's sky', is not about how the sun sets late in summer and the sky remains accordingly bright late in the evening, but about the way the sky appears when leaving someone with regret, or about the sky we contemplate on New Year's Eve while thinking of the year that is about to end.[11] *(p. 28-30)*

This information appears at the beginning of the book[12]. Once *hashiri*, *sakari* and *nagori* are translated and contextualised, they are used throughout the book as any other word.

When reading foreign words from a language one does not understand, there are no prior experiences associated with these specific terms that can guide the reader towards any known emotion. The primary influences on how one receives words from an unfamiliar language is therefore cultural bias and labels attached to that language, since it has been established that words expressing emotions are always culture- and language-specific. Japan's history of crafting a unique image of itself is long-standing, and relations between France and Japan began in 1858, the year of the first Franco-Japanese treaty. The term *Japonisme*—the fascination for Japanese objects and arts—is a French word coined by the critic and art collector Philippe Burty in 1872 (Ono, 2001, p. 1). During the period of *Japonisme*, Japan was perceived in France as "a new continent of aesthetics[13]" (Thirion, 1961, p. 130), and consequently as "a reconciliation between entering modernity and carrying on tradition[14]" (Rafoni, 2008). This highly dynamic and positive image of Japan may vary slightly in other French-speaking countries. Nonetheless, for French readers who do not speak Japanese but are influenced by this image, *Nagori* holds promising potential. Indeed, while using a language that might evoke negative associations related to a country and its culture would likely hinder the therapeutic process of regaining one's past through neutral words, positive cultural labels attached to certain languages might, conversely, motivate patients to engage with exophonic heterolingual bibliotherapy.

As presented earlier, according to Feldman Barrett's theory of constructed emotion, emotions are events-based representations. Therefore, the way emotions are constructed depends on how individuals define concepts such as happiness, which in turn is shaped by the previous events and sensations associated with that emotion. Words contribute directly to this process. In writings such as *Nagori*, confusion is minimised because *hashiri*, *sakari*, and *nagori* have been translated and contextualised for French-speaking readers, providing a framework for the emotional construction process. Readers still face the challenge of encountering novel and foreign words, which disrupt their existing emotional representations; however, this challenge also presents an opportunity to expand one's understanding of self and others. Introducing new words and concepts may alter thought patterns. The previously mentioned proximate mechanism of an attractor factor can supply the brain with a new tool, free from the emotional baggage words that native language words might carry since. Since emotions are constructed representations and words play a performative role in how we experience and express them, this process is significant.

Because of their novelty and the positive image of Japan in France, the words *hashiri*, *sakari*, and *nagori*, as well as the concepts related to time and seasonality that they convey, stimulate the imagination of readers. Moreover, the themes of seasons and the life cycle of foods are inevitably linked to the human life cycle, as Sekiguchi clearly states in her book: "We all live the same season, along with the birds, the animals, the fish and the plants. Those who are alive meet there. But they are not all young at the same time, just like us human beings. Because of this, *nagori*'s time is different for everyone.[15]" (2018, p. 67-68) *Hashiri*, *sakari* and *nagori* are words that naturally provoke reflection on human life and its cycles. These terms function as exophonic heterolingual anchors facilitating cultural transfer, which can support individuals seeking ways to process and express their emotions. A close-reading of key excerpts of *Nagori* will contribute to our understanding of the impact foreign words can have on emotional representations and their potential to alleviate alexithymic symptoms.

"People like vegetables in hashiri also for their bitterness, as if the energy buried in the earth, an almost metallic energy that remained dormant, finally emerged, concentrated, in the buds.[16]" (p. 98)

"[...] we never really are in just one season, except at the peak point that is sakari, and that only lasts a moment, like an athlete's jump.[17]" (p. 98)

"The start of a season is always the nagori of the previous one [...].[18]" (p. 98)

These examples are taken from a paragraph where Sekiguchi explains that vegetables have a uniquely bitter taste when they are still young and not fully ripe. This bitterness heralds both the awakening of spring and "winter's *nagori*" (p. 98). Due to Sekiguchi Ryōko's heterolingual practice, the Japanese words are integrated into the French text and perform semantic functions that no French equivalent could fulfill, blending seamlessly with the French language.

When comparing second language acquisition, it has been observed that "congruence between the orthographic structures of L1 and L2 facilitates the acquisition of a novel surface word form *per se*" (Fu et al, 2025, p. 12) Therefore, Sekiguchi's heterolingual practice and transcription of kanji into the Latin alphabet contribute to the fluidity of reading her essay. Moreover, the terms *hashiri*, *sakari*, and *nagori* evoke processes, which grants them semantic flexibility and allows for colexifications—the phenomenon where one word has multiple related meanings in a language. A recent study using an artificial language explored the cross-linguistic tendency for colexification of similar concepts. This study claims that "Speakers readily colexify similar concepts, unless distinguishing them is necessary for successful communication, in which case they do not." (Karjus et al, 2021, p. 23) Communicative needs thus play a pivotal in shaping how individuals adopt and use both novel and established lexical items. The artificial language employed in the study does not ressemble English but consists of artificial words—such as *fuwo* or *qohe*—allowing for an analogy to be drawn between this artificial system and an actual foreign language. This analogy suggests the potential for individuals with alexithymia-related difficulties, whose communicative needs remain unmet by their first language, to adopt and employ unfamiliar foreign words as tools for self-expression.

The aforementioned translation and contextualisation of the Japanese terms are supported by the author's prose, which establishes a conceptual framework aligned with the themes of her essay. Through a masterful deployment of syntactic structures and carefully selected lexical fields, the author intimates that the appeal of the vegetables in *hashiri* lies in their singular evocation of youthfulness, or even life itself, using expressions such as *dormant energy emerging*. Sekiguchi characterises the buds as imbued with vitality that could be assimilated through the consumption of these vegetables. This evocation of youth, dynamism, and latent potentiality is encapsulated in the term *hashiri* which is intricately woven in the text's fabric through the author's framing of *Nagori*. Although, *hashiri* is unfamiliar to most Francophone readers, its heterolingual presentation enables it to convey that sensation of youthful vitality, readily associated with the fundamental affect of well-being.

A more detailed close reading of Sekiguchi's prose reveals that *hashiri* is metaphorically represented as a seed germinating beneath the soil's surface. The author achieves this by juxtaposing succinct verbal phrases— such as "finally emerged", and "concentrated"—which mirror the stages of *hashiri*'s energetic growth, and by constructing extended sentences that evoke the imagery of roots. The vegetables' "almost metallic" and somewhat bitter taste is attributed to the earth's sharp energy they embody; however, this emergent energy may be harnessed through CBT and/or creative practices. Following Kelda Green's method, participants might be invited to elaborate on the ideas and sensations elicited by *hashiri* during group sessions with peers facing analogous challenges or, where interpersonal interactions proves difficult, through solitary creative practices such as journaling. Such exercises may facilitate the association of *hashiri* with previously unidentifiable emotions. Using the text's specific lexical items, particularly unfamiliar terms, as prompts can assist participants in identifying the emotional states evoked by the reading. The lexical field surrounding *hashiri* conjures notions of strength ("almost metallic", "concentrated") alongside those of potentiality ("energy", "dormant", and "buds"). These familiar yet evocative words enable readers to reconsider emotional concepts beyond the confines of their native language's lexicon.

For those responsive to bibliotherapy and willing to engage with linguistic stimuli, guidance towards a particular term may prove beneficial. The term *sakari* may resonate more profoundly with certain individuals. Within the text, *sakari* signifies strength and momentum, tempered by the caveat that, like opportunity, it is ephemeral and demands readiness to seize. The excerpt illustrating *sakari* is notably more concise than that for *hashiri*, its brevity reflecting the alertness required to apprehend *sakari* and its attendant affective nuances. Sekiguchi's diction captures the exhilaration embodied by *sakari*, eschewing connotations of stress or fatigue. She describes *sakari* as a "peak point", connoting achievement, success, and intensity. The simile of "like an athlete's jump" serves to anchor this concept in embodied experience, potentially facilitating participants' reappraisal of past events and the verbal encapsulation of previously unnamed emotions.

The titular term *nagori* offers yet another avenue for participants to engage with their affective landscape through bibliotherapy. Associated with the nostalgia, *nagori* conveys a bittersweet affect, signifying both an ending and a beginning. It thus embodies the therapeutic potential for renewal. In *Nostalgie* (2015), Barbara Cassin describes nostalgia as "the pain of return" (p. 17), analysing Homer's *Odyssey* through the lens of "[the] link between nostalgia and native soil or patriotism, in order to bring out of nostalgia a different story that would guide us to the threshold of a broader and more welcoming way of thinking, a vision freed from all forms of belonging[19]" (p. 23). This notion of recognition resonates deeply with alexithymia, understood as the difficulty in identifying, recognising, and articulating one own's emotions. Cassin's close reading of the *Odyssey* associates nostalgia with recognition—being known and acknowledged by others. Ulysses, who undergoes profound transformation during his absence from Ithaca, is initially recognised only by his dog. Barbara Cassin thus highlights that the anguish inherent in nostalgia derives from the uncertainty of whether return is ever truly possible, as Ulysses "keeps never coming back. The question posed by the *Odyssey* is whether Ulysses, the sole survivor who has not yet returned home, is 'returnable'— *nostimos* in [ancient] Greek [...][20]" (p. 26). In the context of alexithymia, the notion of being *returnable* may be rephrased as being *knowable*. Indeed, for individuals whose alexithymic symptoms arise from a traumatic experience for instance, the process of identifying and expressing emotions are essential for their well-being, as these processes enable them to live with and manage their emotions—both positive and negative—and foster mutual understanding with others. Thus, *returning* is necessary for emotional well-being: returning as revisiting old wounds, or returning as confronting and overcoming one's own difficulties to prevent the perpetuation of maladaptive behaviours that undermine well-being. The objective of any therapeutic intervention is therefore to facilitate a *return*, but a transformed one; this implies that the individuals should not repeat the patterns that originally provoked anxiety—often manifested somatically in alexithymia.

It is thus a legitimate question to ask oneself: Am I *returnable*, as Cassin puts it, or am I destined to avoid feeling and confronting my emotions altogether? Barbara Cassin observes that nostalgia is not solely linked to a place, an event, or a specific moment in time; it may also be connected to language. She notes: "The only direct and immediate recognition is that of his dog Argos who, lying on a pile of manure, full of lice, raises his head and ears; he 'feels' Ulysses, he 'recognises' him.[21]" (p. 40) In French, the verbs "to feel" and "to smell" are expressed by the same word, *sentir*. Cassin's observation draws not only on this linguistic particularity of French but also on the original ancient Greek of the *Odyssey*, where Homer employs the term "*noein*: the same verb refers to divine intuition" (p. 40). Through French, Cassin reveals how this divine intuition is momentarily embodied in Ulysses' dog, and how nostalgia and *nagori* are transmitted and transformed through bodies and words.

The impact words have is commensurate with their symbolic emotional stimulus. Consequently, new words can acquire symbolic emotional potential by fostering familiarity during therapy. Creative practices, such as journaling with writing prompts, can nurture this process, while reading also contributes through its lexical fields, stylistic devices and syntactic structures as previously discussed. Indeed, it has been demonstrated that "both negative and positive words caused increased activation in the amygdala" (Straube et al, 2011, p. 71) Curated negative and positive words, employed through bibliotherapy, can thus enhance emotional responsiveness and facilitate novel modes of emotional identification.

PERSPECTIVE ON PRACTICING BIBLIOTHERAPY: LIMITATIONS AND RECOMMENDATIONS

As demonstrated in the first part of this article, bibliotherapy has long been employed in Cognitive Behavioural Therapy (CBT). Although CBT is widely regarded as the most effective treatment for alixithymia, recent studies have revealed a "significant heterogeneity" in the outcomes of CBT-based interventions (Mazza et al, 2026, p. 15). This variability is partly attributable to methodologies limitations, notably that "many studies do not compare CBT to another active control group: A large proportion of studies into CBT utilise a waitlist control." (p. 19) Consequently, the inclusion of an active control group is essential in any experimental design evaluating the therapeutic efficacy of heterolingual bibliotherapy.

CBT is an issue-oriented approach that assists individuals in identifying maladaptive thought patterns and understanding how these patterns distort their self-perceptions and their interpretation of situations. Its primary aim is to facilitate cognitive restructuring and behavioural change. CBT employs practical techniques such as journaling, breathing exercises, or role-playing; reading is also recognised as a therapeutic tool within this framework. It is crucial to emphasise that therapists intending to integrate literature and heterolingualism as CBT modalities must possess a comprehensive knowledge of literary theories and practices to effectively guide patients. As Rafiei et al (2003, p. 268) note, "[…] what is essential is a well-written bibliotherapy program and books that cater to the needs and tastes of clients and the active presence of the bibliotherapist." Alternatively, therapists lacking this expertise should collaborate closely with literary specialists to ensure appropriate book selection.

Conversely, literary experts specialising in exophonic heterolingual writings must work alongside trained psychologists. A common pitfall is the inclination to select texts that closely mirror the patients' life experiences. However, studies indicate that "matching the story to the client's life risks oversimplifying the process and reducing the range of discussion." (Detrixhe, 2010, p. 66) In some instances, engaging with literature that directly reflects one's difficulties adversely affect well-being. For example, "[…] reading about someone else who has an eating disorder may be experienced as harmful rather than helpful with respect to mood, self-esteem, body-directed feelings, and diet and exercise habits by respondents both with and without personal eating-disorder experience." (Troscianko, 2018, p. 13) Therefore, selecting fiction and non-fiction works, that allow for interpretative openness appears to be the most prudent approach, supporting a literary and creative methodology particularly suited to alexithymia.

An additional critical consideration regarding heterolingual bibliotherapy concerns the choice of target-language—the language used to establish new word-emotion associations (Japanese, in the case of the essay *Nagori*). There are two principal implementation strategies. The first involves employing a language entirely unfamiliar to the patient. Prior exposure to the foreign lexemes featured in the selected texts might diminish their efficacy as novel emotional carriers. Heterolingualism can exert a profound impact on patients, as neuroplasticity enables all brains—regardless of age—to reorganise in response to environmental stimuli, including foreign words used to approach challenging emotional topics from new perspectives. The second strategy involves using a foreign language with which the patient is familiar and emotionally connected. If therapists identify a positive affective bond between the patient and a particular language or culture, this may facilitate the cognitive reframing CBT seeks to achieve. While the emotional impact of foreign words may be equally potent in this context, such interventions require careful tailoring to individual needs to avoid inadvertently evoking negative associations stemming from prior experiences potentially unknown to the therapist.

Cultural Perspectives and Limitations

Cultural bias must also be addressed when prescribing bibliotherapy. Harré (2003, p. 151-152) observes that "Social representations exist in formal and syntactic structures of spoken and written languages, as well as in the semantic organisation of their lexicons[22]." Consequently, a person's first language can influence the reception of newly encountered words in complex ways. It can occur in many ways. For instance, the Japanese word *nagori*, when pronounced with a French accent, differs from its original pronunciation. The final syllable, pronounced [ʁi] in French, homophonously ressembles the French word *riz* ("rice"), potentially evoking disparate associations depending on the individual. Some may perceive this as a meaningful link to food, resonating with the essay's thematic focus, thereby reinforcing cohesion between vocabulary and theme. Others may find the association distracting, hindering their ability to connect the nostalgic sentiment of *nagori* with the mundane culinary reference.

Cultural bias may further impede the therapeutic efficacy of heterolingual bibliotherapy due to the sociocultural connotations attached to certain languages or countries. As noted earlier in this article, Japan and its culture enjoy a generally positive image in France, which may facilitate engagement with heterolingual texts that include Japanese terms. Indeed, Japan is a well-known and popular country: millions of people visit Japan every year[23], and many globally recognised brands are Japanese. Moreover, Japan has cultivated a carefully constructed image of its culture, language, and identity partially supported by *nihonjinron* (日本人論) discourses, as Iwabuchi Kōichi discusses in his book about Japan and globalisation.

> *Japan's obsession with the uniqueness of its own culture has been widely observed in the popularity of Nihonjinron discourses, which explain distinctive features of Japanese people and Japanese culture in essentialist terms. Those Japanese cultural practices and materials that have been internationally exhibited or represented in the global forum have been predominantly officially sanctioned items of "traditional" culture which have little to do with contemporary Japanese urban culture. (2002, p. 6-7)*

The term 日本人 (*nihonjin*) means "Japanese people", and 論 (*ron*) means "discussion, study, treatise". *Nihonjinron* refers to debates about Japan and Japanese identity conducted by Japanese people themselves. The ideological currents underpinning this movement are often nationalistic, producing literature that does not critically examine Japanese culture and society but rather perpetuates a consistent idealised image to maintain "the idea [...] underlying all the *Nihonjin-ron*, of Japanese immutability, remains intact[24]" (Pigeot, 1983, p. 21).

Iwabuchi further explains that Japan has a long history of exercising "transnational cultural power", beginning with the indigenisation—"Japanisation"—of cultural elements from closely related ethnic groups. For example:

> *A glance at transformations in the meaning of the term Japanization, which articulates Japanese transnational cultural power, reveals the shift in Japanese cultural orientation. In prewar Japan, Japanization was articulated in the term kōminka, which means "the assimilation of ethnic others (such as Ainu, Okinawans, Taiwanese, and Koreans) into Japanese imperial citizenship under the Emperor's benevolence." Japanization also referred to the indigenization and domestication of foreign (Western) culture. (p. 9)*

The indigenisation of Western cultural aspects operates alongside the Western Orientalism of Japan, as well as the related phenomena of *Japonisme* and self-Orientalism at work in Japan (Iwabuchi, 2002; Nishihara, 2005). Many Japanese artists incorporated Orientalist perspectives into their work; a notable example is the writer Tanizaki Junichirō (1886-1965) who "orientalizes Japan itself when he expresses the charm and beauty of the country from the perspective of a Westerner (Self-Orientalism, Japan as the object)." (Nishihara, 2005, p. 246)

Although Japan's case may appear unique when how a country's image and cultural identity influence readers' reception of heterolingual texts containing foreign words, the essential point remains how such images and the messages it conveys shape the reception of the heterolingual dimension. Indeed, beliefs actively contribute to identify information, as one's "environment is made of the reality of everyday objects but also of a set of imaginary and symbolic representations[25]" (Stoloff, 2020, p. 117).

Therefore, it is crucial to consider patients' experiences and perspectives in order to select appropriate heterolingual texts. Based on the languages and cultures familiar to the bibliotherapist or clinical study coordinators, a curated collection of heterolingual books can be assembled. Participants should then complete a survey assessing their familiarity with specific languages, cultures, and countries, enabling the bibliotherapist to identify which texts may be most beneficial.

Another dimension of cultural bias relevant to the essay *Nagori*—and a reminder of the importance of thorough knowledge of the target culture and language for implementing exophonic heterolingual bibliotherapy—concerns Sekiguchi's explaination of specific countries' customs, such as the enjoyment of foods in *hashiri*, *sakari* or *nagori*, which vary according to climate, preservation methods, and current gastronomic trends[26]. Thus, individual preferences for foods associated with *hashiri*, *sakari,* or *nagori* are culturally influenced. Cultural bias also shapes the symbolic meanings and representations attributed to foods.

Additionally, many reports indicate that bibliotherapy within CBT is often delivered in one-on-one sessions, supplemented by brief telephone calls to monitor patients' reactions to prescribed reading materials and to support their self-directed therapeutic process (Correll et al, 2024; Gualano et al, 2017; Moldovan et al, 2013). Bibliotherapy has also been widely employed in group settings. For example, in studies previously mentioned involving patients with schizophrenia and psychopathy, bibliotherapy was integrated into CBT group sessions, an alternative implementation method. Group sessions provide opportunities for patients with similar challenges or language skills to gather and support each other, fostering a sense of community that may enhance well-being. It has been observed that "the potential of the group to help individual participants" is significant (Kasperek-Zimowska et al, 2021, p. 285). Indeed, group activities can yield notable improvements in addressing individual issues such as irresponsibility, as demonstrated in a study on psychopathic disorder: "Since reading aloud was a group activity and each person was responsible for reading part of the material aloud, this increased the sense of responsibility in both the control and experimental groups" (Rafiei et al, 2023, p. 268). It has also been observed that group sessions contributed to patients' well-being, as they reported "feel[ing] good because they were together" (2023, p. 268). Another important observations, made by Beata J. Kasperek-Zimowska and colleagues in their work with patients suffering from schizophrenia, highlighted the significance of interpersonal dynamics within the group, which were both meaningful to patients and instrumental in enhancing therapeutic efficacy.

> *A patient attending this form of treatment benefits from the influence of various forms of interaction, beginning with the therapeutic community, through group psychotherapy and ending with individual psychotherapy. The therapeutic community allows for the definition of rights and obligations, roles in the community*

and the scope of influence on the group. Social skills training provides an opportunity to improve or learn such capabilities as establishing and maintaining contact with others, managing an illness (e.g. how to identify and react to a relapse) […]. (2021, p. 285)

The therapeutic potential of heterolingual texts may similarly be optimised by grouping patients according to linguistic competencies and shared language communities—that is, forming groups composed of individuals assigned heterolingual texts utilising the same target language. Such linguistic affinity could facilitate emotional processing by fostering a shared cultural and linguistic interest. Participants with a common linguistic background may engage more deeply with the words of the target language, enriching their discussions of the heterolingual texts they have read. This dynamic has the potential to amplify the positive effects typically observed in group therapy settings and to foster the formation of supportive interpersonal bonds, thereby enhancing participants' capacity to articulate their thoughts and emotions.

While the creation of linguistic communities appears highly beneficial, it is important to emphasise that group bibliotherapy should complement, rather than replace, individual therapy.

CONCLUSION

Heterolingualism, when mediated through carefully selected literature, appears to hold significant potential for therapeutic and transformative effects on individuals. By fostering enhanced interactions between body and mind, new foundations for well-being may be established through language. The use of exophonic heterolingual literature for bibliotherapeutic purposes represents a promising avenue warranting further exploration.

Interdisciplinary approaches such as this not only stand to advance both literary, psychological, and neuropsychological research but also offer the prospect of novel therapeutic modalities and research topics by bridging disciplines that rarely work intersect. Bibliotherapists—or collaborative teams comprising therapists and literary experts—must carefully select texts that align with the specific needs, backgrounds, and preferences of their patients.

It is important to recognise that cultural differences and biases are not confined solely to foreign cultures but are also inherent within one's own culture and language, as individuals invariably rely on internalised representations to construct and interpret their emotions. Accordingly, cultural and linguistic diversity should be regarded not as obstacles to be circumvented but as potential keys to fostering well-being, particularly engagement with exophonic heterolingual texts.

REFERENCES

Alfrey, A., Field, V., Xenophontes, I., & Holttum, S. (2021). Identifying the mechanisms of poetry therapy and associated effects on participants: A synthesised review of empirical literature. *The Arts in Psychotherapy, 75*. Advance online publication. DOI: 10.1016/j.aip.2021.101832

Alschuler, M. (2006). Poetry, the Healing Pen. In Brooke, S. (Ed.), *Creative Therapies Manual* (pp. 253–262). Charles C Thomas Publisher Ltd.

Arndt, S., Naguschewski, D., & Stockhammer, R. (Eds.). (2007). *Exophonie: Anderssprachigkeit (in) der Literatur*. Kulturverlag Kadmos.

Barrett, L. F. (2017). The theory of constructed emotion: An active inference account of interoception and categorization. *Social Cognitive and Affective Neuroscience, 12*(1), 1–23. PMID: 27798257

Behrmann, M., & Plaut, D. C. (2014). Bilateral Hemispheric Processing of Words and Faces: Evidence from Word Impairments in Prosopagnosia and Face Impairments in Pure Alexia. *Cerebral Cortex (New York, N.Y.), 24*(4), 1102–1118. DOI: 10.1093/cercor/bhs390 PMID: 23250954

Bourges-Celaries, A. (2024a). *L'exophonie chez les autrices Shimazaki Aki, Tawada Yōko et Sekiguchi Ryōko* [Exophony in the works of authors Shimazaki Aki, Tawada Yōko, and Sekiguchi Ryōko] [Doctoral dissertation, University of Montréal]. Papyrus. DOI: 10.71781/14100

Bourges-Celaries, A. (2024b). Des espaces japonais du français. In M. O. M., Hertrampf & D., Mistreanu (Eds), *Langue(s) et espaces dans les xénographies féminines en français*. 55–68. AVM Verlag.

Cassin, B. (2015). *La nostalgie* [Nostalgia]. Pluriel.

Chadefaud, C. (1993). *L'écrit dans l'Égypte ancienne* [*Writing in ancient Egypt*]. Hachette.

Cirillo, F., Spina, G., Irrera, M., Bozzola, E., Mascolo, C., Gargiullo, L., Burla, V., Roversi, M., Carlevaris, C. M., Dusi, S., Pretelli, I., & Marchili, M. R. (2025). The Impact of Expressive Arts Therapy on Alexithymia Levels in Adolescent Inpatients with Severe Anorexia Nervosa. *Children (Basel, Switzerland), 12*(10). PMID: 41153576

Correll, A. B., Correll, T. L., & Correll, M. C. (2024). Literary Prescriptions: Applying Bibliotherapy in a Psychotherapeutic Context. *Innovations in Clinical Neuroscience*, *21*(7-9), 15–21. PMID: 39329026

Crothers, S. M. (1916, September). Literary Clinic. *Atlantic Monthly*.

Detrixhe, J. J. (2010). Souls in Jeopardy: Questions and Innovations for Bibliotherapy With Fiction. *The Journal of Humanistic Counseling, Education and Development*, *49*, 58–72. DOI: 10.1002/j.2161-1939.2010.tb00087.x

Dong, Y., Mak, M. H., Hepach, R., & Nation, K. (2025). Learning new words via reading: The influence of emotional narrative context on learning novel adjectives. *Quarterly Journal of Experimental Psychology*, *78*(10), 2167–2180. DOI: 10.1177/17470218241308221 PMID: 39641281

Espagne, M., & Werner, M. (Eds.). (1988). *Transferts. Les relations franco-allemandes dans l'espace francoallemand*. Éditions Recherche sur les civilisations.

Evans, J. (2012). *Philosophy for Life And Other Dangerous Situations*. Ebury Publishing.

Fu, Y., Yang, J., Bermúdez-Margaretto, B., Wang, H., Cordón, D. E. J., & Domínguez, A. (2025). From eye to cortex: Tracing the neurocognitive dynamics of bilingual novel word acquisition. *Brain and Language*, *270*. Advance online publication. DOI: 10.1016/j.bandl.2025.105632 PMID: 40865422

Gauvin, L. (Ed.). (2009). *L'écrivain francophone à la croisée des langues: Entretiens*. Karthala., DOI: 10.3917/kart.undef.2009.02

Green, K. (2020). *Rethinking Therapeutic Reading: Lessons from Senecca, Montaigne, Wordsworth and George Eliot*. Anthem Press.

Grutman, R. (2019). *Des langues qui résonnent: L'hétérolinguisme au XIX*e *siècle québécois* [*Languages that resonate: Heterolingualism in 19*th *Century Quebec*]. Classiques Garnier.

Gualano, M. R., Bert, F., Martorana, M., Voglino, G., Andriolo, V., Thomas, R., Gramaglia, C., Zeppegno, P., & Siliquini, R. (2017). The long-term effects of bibliotherapy in depression treatment: Systematic eview of randomized clinical trials. *Clinical Psychology Review*, *58*, 49–58. DOI: 10.1016/j.cpr.2017.09.006 PMID: 28993103

Harré, R. (2003). Grammaire et lexiques, vecteurs des représentations sociales. [Grammar and lexicons, media of social representations] In Jodelet, D. (Ed.), *Les représentations sociales* [*Social representations*]. (pp. 149–169). Presses Universitaires de France. DOI: 10.3917/puf.jodel.2003.01.0149

Heiman, M., Strnad, D., Weiland, W., & Wise, T. N. (1994). Art Therapy and Alexithymia. *Art Therapy: Journal of the American Art Therapy Association, 11*(2), 143–146. DOI: 10.1080/07421656.1994.10759067

Hirsch, J.-P. (26th October 2018). *Ryoko Sekiguchi Nagori* [Video]. YouTube. https://www.youtube.com/watch?v=4WT2K9jJadM

Hunt, W. A. (1941). Recent Developments in the Field of Emotions. *Psychological Bulletin, 38*(5), 249–276. DOI: 10.1037/h0054615

Iwabuchi, K. (2002). *Recentering Globalization: Popular Culture and Japanese Transnationalism*. Duke University Press.

Jackson, J. C., & Lindquist, K. (in press). Origins and Consequences of Cultural Variation in Emotion Vocabulary. In Yik, M. (Ed.), *The Oxford Handbook of Emotion and Culture*. Oxford University Press.

Karjus, A., Blythe, R. A., Kirby, S., Wang, T., & Smith, K. (2021). Conceptual Similarity and Communicative Need Shape Colexification: An Experimental Study. *Cognitive Science, 45*. Advance online publication. DOI: 10.1111/cogs.13035 PMID: 34491584

Kasperek-Zimowska, B. J., Bednarek, A., Giguere, M., Orłowski, W., & Sawicka, M. (2021). The specificity of the use of bibliotherapy as an element of psychiatric rehabilitation in a group of patients suffering from schizophrenia. *Advances in Psychiatry and Neurology/Postępy Psychiatrii i Neurologii, 30*(4), 278–286. DOI: 10.5114/ppn.2021.111946

Lee, K. M., & Satpute, A. B. (2024). More than labels: Neural representations of emotion words are widely distributed across the brain. *Social Cognitive and Affective Neuroscience, 19*(1), 1–11. DOI: 10.1093/scan/nsae043 PMID: 38903026

Lindquist, K. A., & Barrett, L. F. (2008). Constructing Emotion: The Experience of Fear as a Conceptual Act. *Psychological Science, 19*(9), 898–903. DOI: 10.1111/j.1467-9280.2008.02174.x PMID: 18947355

Mazza, A., Davis, P., Johnson, L., Larkin, F., & Cole, S. N. (2026). Identifying therapies to effectively reduce alexithymia: A systematic review and meta-analysis. *Journal of Affective Disorders, 400*, 1–13. DOI: 10.1016/j.jad.2026.121167 PMID: 41525940

Meijer-Degen, F., & Lansen, J. (2006). Alexithymia—A challenge to art therapy: The story of Rita. *The Arts in Psychotherapy*, *33*(3), 167–179. DOI: 10.1016/j.aip.2005.10.002

Moldovan, R., Cobeanu, O., & David, D. (2013). Cognitive bibliotherapy for mild depressive symptomatology: Randomized clinical trial of efficacy and mechanisms of change. *Clinical Psychology & Psychotherapy*, *20*(6), 482–493. DOI: 10.1002/cpp.1814 PMID: 22941790

Naylor, E. V., Antonuccio, D. O., Litt, M., Johnson, G. E., Spogen, D. R., Williams, R., McCarthy, C., Lu, M. M., Fiore, D. C., & Higgins, D. L. (2010). Bibliotherapy as a Treatment for Depression in Primary Care. *Journal of Clinical Psychology in Medical Settings*, *17*, 258–271. DOI: 10.1007/s10880-010-9207-2 PMID: 20803165

Nishihara, D. (2005). Said, Orientalism, and Japan. *Alif: Journal of Comparative Poetics*, *25*, 241–253.

Nwokah, E. E., & Graves, K. N. (2009). Word Play: The Creation and Function of Novel Words in the Pretend Play of Two Siblings. *American Journal of Play*, *1*(4), 429–450.

Ono, A. (2001). *Japonisme in Britain: A Source of Inspiration: J. McN. Whistler, Mortimer Menpes, George Henry, E. A. Hornel and Nineteenth Century Japan* [Doctoral dissertation, University of Glasgow]. Enlighten Team.

Pigeot, J. (1983). Les Japonais peints par eux-mêmes: Esquisse d'un autoportrait [The Japanese painted by themselves: Sketch of a self-portrait]. *Le Debat*, *1*(23), 19–33. DOI: 10.3917/deba.023.0019

Rafiei, A., Noruzi, A., & Ferdousi, T. (2023). Cognitive bibliotherapy for delinquent adolescents with psychopathic disorder: A quasi-experimental study. *Journal of Poetry Therapy*, *36*(4), 259–272. DOI: 10.1080/08893675.2023.2179437

Richter, M., Eck, J., Straube, T., Miltner, W. H. R., & Weiss, T. (2010). Do words hurt? Brain activation during the processing of pain-related words. *Pain*, *148*(2), 198–205. DOI: 10.1016/j.pain.2009.08.009 PMID: 19846255

Sekiguchi, R. (2023). *Nagori*. P.O.L. (Original work published 2018)

Stoloff, J-C. (2020). Identifier, s'identifier, croire [Identifying, self-identifying, believing]. *Le présent de la psychanalyse*, *4*(2), 115–129.

Straube, T., Sauer, A., & Miltner, W. H. R. (2011). Brain activation during direct and indirect processing of positive and negative words. *Behavioural Brain Research*, *222*, 66–72. DOI: 10.1016/j.bbr.2011.03.037 PMID: 21440008

Suchet, M. (2014). *L'Imaginaire hétérolingue* [*The Heterolingual Imagination*]. Classiques Garnier.

Tawada, Y. (2003). エクソフォニー・母語の外へ出る旅 [*Exophony: Voyages Outside the Mother Tongue*]. Iwanami Shoten.

Thirion, Y. (1961). Le japonisme en France dans la seconde moitié du XIXe siècle à la faveur de la diffusion de l'estampe japonaise [Japonisme in France in the second half of the 19th century thanks to the spread of Japanese prints]. *Cahiers de l'Association internationale des études françaises, 13*, 117–130. DOI: 10.3406/caief.1961.2193

Troscianko, E. T. (2018). Literary reading and eating disorders: Survey evidence of therapeutic help and harm. *Journal of Eating Disorders, 6*. Advance online publication. DOI: 10.1186/s40337-018-0191-5 PMID: 29692896

Wang, C., & Xiao, R. (2021). Music and art therapy combined with cognitive behavioral therapy to treat adolescent anorexia patients. *American Journal of Translational Research, 13*(6), 6534–6542. PMID: 34306394

Wierzbicka, A. (2009). Language and Metalanguage: Key Issues in Emotion Research. *Emotion Review, 1*(1), 3–14. DOI: 10.1177/1754073908097175

Yang, Q., Cao, X., & Jiang, X. (2022). The Role of Multilingual Script Systems in Face Processing. In Jiang, X. (Ed.), *Multilingualism–Interdisciplinary Topics* (pp. 85–100). IntechOpen.

Yi, C., Naixin, L., Onosahwo Iyendo, T., & Apuke, O. D. (2024). Cognitive behavior, art, and music therapies intervention for treating the depression of children: A randomized control trial. *Psychiatry Research, 333*. Advance online publication. DOI: 10.1016/j.psychres.2024.115716 PMID: 38244284

APPENDIX

Translation Notes

1. See Chapter 1 "Senecan Tragedy and Stoic philosophy" pp. 9-26.
2. « […] la présence dans un texte d'idiomes étrangers, sous quelque forme que ce soit, aussi bien que de variétés (sociales, régionales ou chronologiques) de la langue principale. »
3. Unless otherwise stated, all translations are mine. In the interests of accuracy, the original citations are displayed in the footnotes.
4. 「これまでも「移民文学」とか「クレオール文学」というような言葉はよく聞いたが、「エクソフォニー」はもっと広い意味で、母語の外に出た状態一般を指す。」
5. See the website of the Oxford University Press: https://global.oup.com/academic/product/self-help-9780199552450?cc=fr&lang=en&#
6. « La sensibilité naît des mots: on ne saurait sentir ce qui n'a pas de nom. »
7. « […] il existe trois termes différents pour décrire l'état de saisonnalité d'un aliment: *hashiri*, *sakari* et *nagori*. Ils désignent l'équivalent de "primeur", de "pleine saison", et le dernier, *nagori*, de l'arrière-saison, "la nostalgie de la saison qui vient de nous quitter". »
8. « l'ouverture de la saison »
9. « la forme substantive du verbe *hashiru*, "courir", désigne à la fois l'acte de courir et quelque chose qui glisse, mais aussi bien ce qui est "précurseur" »
10. « *Sakari* signifie "l'acmé", "le comble", ou les animaux en rut. »
11. « *Nagori*, quant à lui, possède une acception beaucoup plus large. Il signifie avant tout la trace, la présence, l'atmosphère d'une chose passée, d'une chose qui n'est plus. […] *Nagori* se dit aussi des conséquences, des dégâts ou des suites d'un événement, comme le *nagori* d'un tremblement de terre ou d'une maladie. […] Les expressions idiomatiques avec *nagori* abondent. D'une part, il peut s'agir d'un phénomène qui persiste au-delà de son temps, contre toute attente, comme *nagori no yuki*, "la neige de *nagori*", à savoir: la neige qui persiste après l'arrivée du printemps ou la neige qui tombe au printemps […]. D'autre part, il peut s'agir d'une nostalgie ou d'un regret, reflété sur un objet ou sur un paysage. En l'occurrence, l'expression *nagori no sora*, "ciel de *nagori*", ne désigne pas le ciel d'été qui reste longtemps clair, mais le ciel tel qu'on le voit lorsque l'on quitte quelqu'un à regret, ou le ciel de la nuit du réveillon, que l'on contemple avec le sentiment de l'année qui s'achève. »

12. I am referring to the 2020 edition of *Nagori*, making these explanations appear from page 27 to page 30. The essay in itself is approximately a hundred and thirty pages long.
13. « un contient esthétique nouveau »
14. « la conciliation de l'entrée dans la modernité et de continuation de la tradition »
15. « Nous vivons tous la même saison, avec les oiseaux, les animaux, les poissons et les végétaux. Ceux qui sont en vie s'y rencontrent. Seulement, le temps de la jeunesse des uns n'est pas celui des autres, tout comme pour les humains. De ce fait, le temps de *nagori* est différent pour chacun. »
16. « On apprécie les légumes de *hashiri* y compris pour cette amertume, comme si l'énergie enfouie sous la terre, énergie presque métallique demeurée en sommeil, surgissait alors, concentrée, dans les bourgeons. »
17. « [...] on n'est jamais tout à fait dans une seule saison, sauf en ce point d'acmé qu'est le *sakari*, qui ne dure qu'un instant, comme le saut d'un athlète. »
18. « Le début d'une saison est toujours le *nagori* de la saison précédente [...]. »
19. « Le lien entre la nostalgie et le sol natal ou le patriotisme, pour faire de la nostalgie une toute autre aventure nous conduisant au seuil d'une pensée plus large, plus accueillante, d'une vision du monde délivrée de toutes les appartenances. »
20. « [...] n'a pas cessé de ne pas revenir. La question de l'*Odyssée* est de savoir si Ulysse, le seul des survivants à ne pas être rentré chez lui, est "revenable", *nostimos* en grec [...]. »
21. « La seule reconnaissance directe et immédiate est celle de son chien Argos, couché sur le tas de fumier, plein de poux, qui lève la tête et les oreilles. Il "sent" Ulysse, il le "reconnaît". »
22. « Les représentations sociales existent dans les structures formelles, syntaxiques des langues parlées et écrites aussi bien que dans l'organisation sémantique de leurs lexiques. »
23. Between January 2025 and April 2025, almost 15, 000, 000 people visited Japan (Source: https://www.tourism.jp/en/tourism-database/stats/inbound/).
24. « que reste intacte l'idée [...] sous-jacente à l'ensemble des *Nihonjin-ron*, de l'immutabilité japonaise. »
25. « [...] environnement est tissé à la fois par la réalité de ces objets, mais aussi par tout un ensemble de représentations imaginaires et symboliques. »
26. See Chapter 7 « Nouvelles rencontres, nouveaux départs » pp. 89-111.

Chapter 14
Well-Being With Arts for Peace of Mind:
Creativity and Movement as Integrative Therapeutic Strategy

Charlène Clonts
http://orcid.org/0000-0003-4228-4868
Kyushu University, Japan

ABSTRACT

The chapter investigates the transformative potential of art-based movement – esp. Art-Yoga – as integrative strategies for mental health. Drawing on interdisciplinary research across psychology, philosophy, neuroscience, and the arts, it argues for a holistic paradigm that embraces embodied cognition, emotional regulation, and creative expression. The Well-Being with Arts project, Japan, was extended to Turkey: it serves as a case study demonstrating the therapeutic efficacy of combining yoga, dance, music, and poetry. Empirical findings reveal significant reductions in stress, anxiety, and fatigue, alongside increases in vitality, pride, and emotional clarity. The chapter situates these outcomes within broader cultural and philosophical contexts, including ancient yogic wisdom and enactive cognitive science, proposing that mindful artistic engagement fosters resilience, relational intelligence, and a deeper sense of self. It promotes the integration of arts and movement into mental healthcare as a culturally sensitive, inclusive, and sustainable approach to well-being.

INTRODUCTION

The contemporary landscape of mental health and well-being is increasingly shaped by a renewed interest in the dynamic interplay between body and mind.

DOI: 10.4018/979-8-3373-3521-6.ch014

Within this context, the present chapter examines how creativity and movement—particularly through art-based practices, such as the Art-Yoga whose effects have been investigated at Kyushu University, Japan (Clonts et al. 2026)—can serve as integrative modalities for cultivating peace of mind and psychological resilience. In the digital age, where cognitive overload, social fragmentation, and disembodiment increasingly characterize daily life, the integration of body, mind, creativity, and emotion has emerged as a vital axis for promoting mental health and well-being. Moreover, a growing body of interdisciplinary research underscores the therapeutic and developmental potential of embodied and creative practices, revealing their capacity to foster emotional regulation, cognitive flexibility, and holistic self-awareness.

Theoretical and empirical advances across disciplines have undeniably converged to affirm that the body is not merely a passive recipient of mental states but an active agent in shaping emotional, cognitive, and social experience. Recent studies have operationalized the mind-body connection through constructs such as interoceptive attention, sensation-emotion articulation, and body-mind values. For instance, Van Bael et al. (2023) developed the Body-Mind Connection Questionnaire (BMCQ), demonstrating that individuals who are more attuned to their internal bodily states and capable of articulating these sensations in emotional contexts exhibit greater psychological resilience and self-regulation. Similarly, Rodriguez-Jiménez et al. (2022) found that embodied practices like Hatha-Yoga and Dance Movement Therapy significantly reduced stress, and enhanced self-knowledge and kinaesthetic empathy among educators, suggesting that body-based interventions can be powerful tools for emotional and rational development.

Defined in this chapter in a broad way, not only as visual arts but also as literature, staged and in-situ performance, dance, music and "Ways", the arts have been long recognized in the fields dealing with mental health for their expressive and symbolic capacities. They are now being validated through neuroscientific research as mechanisms for emotional healing. Indeed, Barnett and Vasiu (2024) reviewed neuroimaging studies showing that engagement with creative arts activates the medial prefrontal cortex and amygdala—regions central to adaptive emotional regulation. These findings suggest that creative expression and emotional processing share common neural pathways, reinforcing the therapeutic value of the arts. Furthermore, creative and reflective learning approaches, that is to say the pedagogical and developmental dimensions of creative practice, have been shown to support personal development, empathy, and a sense of belonging—key components of well-being (MacAskill et al., 2023). Practices such as embodied metaphor and expressive movement (Anderson, 2018; Gomes et al., 2020) not only enhance emotional awareness but also cultivate cultural humility and relational intelligence (Soulé et al., 2022). These insights are further substantiated by the World Health Organization's (WHO) comprehensive scoping review, which synthesizes evidence from over 3000 studies across the WHO European Region (Fancourt & Finn, 2019). The report identifies the arts as effective in both preventive and clinical contexts. The arts' capacity to engage aesthetic, emotional and relational dimensions simultaneously positions them as uniquely suited to address the complex, multifactorial nature of well-being. To put it simply, the report identifies two overarching domains in which the arts contribute to health: prevention and promotion, and management and treatment. Within these domains, arts engagement has been shown to enhance social cohesion, reduce loneliness, support human development, encourage health-promoting behaviours, and mitigate the effects of trauma and mental illness.

Complementing this, Fujiwara et al. (2014) offer a compelling economic valuation of the well-being impacts of cultural and physical engagement, using the Well-Being Valuation approach. Although this economic perspective is not the one favoured in the development of this chapter, it has nonetheless a very striking effect: Fujiwara et al. analysis of UK's landscape quantifies the subjective well-being benefits of activities such as arts participation, dance, music attendance, and sports, with values equivalent to thousands of pounds per individual, in annual income—underscoring simultaneously the substantial non-market value of cultural and physical practices. Adding further empirical nuance, in another UK setting's study, Wheatley and Bickerton (2017) analysed longitudinal data to explore how engagement in arts, culture, and sport correlates with subjective well-being across multiple domains. Their findings reveal that regular participation in art practices and sports is positively associated with life and leisure satisfaction, and general happiness. Interestingly, even infrequent engagement in cultural activities such as visiting museums or historical sites yields measurable well-being benefits. However, the study also highlights that these leisure experiences do not necessarily spill over into job satisfaction—suggesting that individuals compartmentalize work and leisure in their subjective evaluations of well-being. Wheatley and Bickerton also emphasize the importance of the frequency and type of engagement. Active participation—e.g., playing music or dancing—tends to require regular involvement to yield well-being benefits, while more 'passive' experience—e.g., attending concerts or visiting heritage sites—can be beneficial even when occasional. These findings reinforce the idea that the quality of leisure time, rather than its quantity alone, is central to deriving positive psychological outcomes.

Taken together, these findings invite a rethinking of mental health not as a purely clinical or cognitive domain, but as an integrative field in which body, mind, creativity, and emotion are inextricably linked. As digital technologies increasingly mediate our experiences—which can however be beneficial to initiate creative or mindful practices for beginners—the need to re-anchor well-being in embodied relational practices becomes urgent. Art and movement offer a distinctive modality that engages aesthetic, emotional, cognitive, and social dimensions simultaneously—providing both individual and collective pathways to healing. This chapter thus argues for a holistic paradigm of mental well-being—one that embraces the transformative potential of art and movement as embodied practices of care, connection, and meaning-making. In doing so, it goes along with the broader aims of this volume to explore how body-mind interactions can be harnessed to support flourishing, peace of mind and integrative mental health in the digital era.

THE WELL-BEING WITH ARTS FRAMEWORK FOR BODY-MIND ENGAGEMENT: OUTLINE OF THE PROJECT IN JAPAN

Based on the theoretical and empirical foundations outlined in the introduction, the *Well-Being with Arts* (WBA) project, that I finished building up in January 2024, is a concrete and interdisciplinary initiative designed to operationalize the principles of body-mind integration for more well-being, through holistic artistic practices. Coinciding with the WHO report's recommendation to foster studies in Asia about the effects of arts on mental health (Fancourt & Finn, 2019), I developed the project within the framework of Kyushu University's Institute for Asia and Oceanian Studies (Q-AOS, Japan) who granted competitive funds in March 2024 to the research module. Under my lead, the project gathers professors[1] from Kyushu University (Japan), Georgetown University (USA), Paris Cité University (France), Pau and Pays de l'Adour University (France), Trinity College Cambridge (UK), and the University of Udine (Italy). The researchers come from several backgrounds, such as arts and literatures, philosophy, psychiatry, psychosomatic medicine, psychology, psychopathology, and sports and health. The WBA project responds to the vital need for sustainable well-being strategies in the aftermath of the Covid-19 pandemic, but also to particularities related to therapy in the Japanese context. Indeed, Japan's evolving mental health landscape offers a compelling background for examining the role of the arts in promoting well-being. In recent years, Japan has experienced a notable increase in mental health concerns, particularly those linked to social anxiety and culturally specific conditions, such as *taijin kyôfushô* (Tei & Wu, 2021), literally translated as "anthropophobia" and related to group pressure in East Asian cultural contexts. These developments have prompted critical reflection on the country's conventional mental health infrastructure, which has historically emphasized institutional care and pharmacological treatment. As a result, many individuals receive only symptomatic relief through medication, without access to more holistic or sustained forms of psychological support. Despite growing public awareness of mental health issues, the uptake of psychotherapy in Japan remains thus limited. Among the existing therapies taught at the university level, art therapy is usually not included into conventional psychotherapy, nor proposed to state owned institutions' patients as a sustainable therapy. Moreover, cultural norms that prioritize emotional restraint and social conformity continue to discourage individuals from seeking help. This cultural backdrop contributes to a significant gap between the need for psychological care and the actual use of available services.

In response to these systemic and cultural challenges, Japanese health authorities have begun to explore alternative approaches to mental health care. A key development was the Ministry of Health, Labour and Welfare's 2003 policy initiative, which promotes a shift away from hospital-based treatment toward more community-oriented models, especially in the case of home-based psychiatric support, addressing severe forms of social withdrawal, such as the well-known phenomenon of *hikikomori* [shut-in, withdrawn person]. In Japan, where verbal disclosure is often inhibited by strict social norms, artistic expression offers an alternative channel for emotional articulation and identity formation. This is particularly relevant for individuals experiencing social anxiety, stress, and difficulties to share emotions in a constructive way. They may find in the arts a non-verbal, non-judgmental space for self-exploration and connection. By situating art and movement practices within a broader discourse on mental health reform and cultural sensitivity, the WBA project contributes to a growing body of work that positions art not merely as a supplement to clinical care, but as a vital component of holistic well-being, especially in the workplace.

The project's outline focuses on a two-folds definition of the term "well-being". Firstly, well-being shall be perceived as a state experienced by individuals and communities, and determined by intersectional factors such as environment, social relationships, and inner phenomena; the sense of purpose and meaning, the ability to contribute to the world, and the perceived quality of life are also key elements in the definition of well-being (WHO, 2021). Issues related to well-being can be addressed through art practices (Fancourt & Finn, 2019). Secondly, the definition given by the OECD, which receives the general agreement of the experts (Dolan & White, 2007; Stiglitz, Sen & Fitoussi, 2009; ONS, 2011; Takahashi et al., 2022), serves as a baseline for our research, stipulating that well-being can be defined as "good mental states, including all of the various evaluations, positive and negative, that people make of their lives, and the affective reactions of people to their experiences" (OECD, 2013, p. 10). That is why the project supports the Sustainable Development Goals, especially SDG 3 (Good Health and Well-Being), and contributes to the broader academic discourse on the transformative potential of art-based interventions. The WBA module is grounded in a dual mission: to promote the emotional, psychological, and physical benefits of holistic arts—including performance, sound, text, visual arts, and "arts of balance", e.g., yoga—and to generate empirical insights into how these practices foster resilience, reduce stress, and enhance community well-being. The project's vision is both inclusive and transdisciplinary, drawing on cross-cultural knowledge systems from East Asia, Europe, and the Indo-Pacific, to explore how embodied artistic practices can support individual and collective flourishing.

Two interrelated research axes structure the WBA project. The first focuses on the cultural and philosophical dimensions of the arts, examining how body-mind practices are shaped by and contribute to transnational circulations of knowledge and aesthetics. This axis investigates how practitioners and audiences co-create meaning and well-being through artistic engagement, particularly in contexts where traditional and contemporary forms intersect. The second axis is empirical, centred on the collection and analysis of data from on-site practices of Art-Yoga. These yoga sessions, a Vinyasa style practice, are designed by me with music, dance, visual arts, and literary images, to evoke emotional responses and foster a sense of peacefulness and awareness. I firstly coined the term "Art-Yoga" after studying Vinyasa yoga, Hatha Yoga, and Aerial yoga, and passing an internationally recognised yoga teacher's exam (Yoga Alliance RYT-200, Japan). By using this term, I was trying to acknowledge the importance of music, dance, literary images to foster a better sense of peacefulness and contentment for the participants in my yoga lessons. It draws from my long-term research in poetry and arts, intermedia studies, and embodied practices, further developed by my personal experience of art practices: twelve years of music theory, piano study and choir performance at the Conservatoire in France, three years of theatre practice, and four years of classical and contemporary dance, both in the US and in France, also participating in several multiday workshops held by famous choreographers based in France—David Rolland, Hervé Robbe, Aurélie Berland and Joanne Leighton. Since 2007, I also led numerous intermedia projects for the French National Education, in collaboration with writers and artists—e.g., dance-contact self-expression, stage performance, dance and literature, cinema and literature, visual arts and literature.

In the WBA's yoga pilot-study, surveys, interviews, using psychological and health literacy's scales, are employed to assess participants' experience, with a focus on relaxation, emotional release, cultural and body-mind engagements. The implementation strategy is participatory and inclusive, emphasizing accessibility across nationalities, genders, and levels of proficiency. Weekly sessions are offered in English and are free of charge for Kyushu University's faculty members, staff, students, and planned to be open to the local community. This practice is complemented by international symposiums for academics, additionally inviting non-academics to share their valuable knowledge. A series of interdisciplinary seminars is given by scholars and eminent professors, both for the specialized audience and the students—in the latter case, with educational purposes—but also for the general audience, in order to disseminate the scientific information. The project includes partnerships with academic institutions across East Asia, Europe, and North America, fostering a multilateral exchange on holistic well-being, and opened to developments in other parts of the world, as shown by the implementation of a related project in Istanbul, Türkiye.

Methodologically, the WBA project integrates qualitative and quantitative approaches. Theoretical and praxis analysis of artistic and literary practices is combined with psychological assessments, and behavioural evaluations. This triangulation enables a nuanced understanding of how holistic arts practices influence well-being, both subjectively and socially, but also epistemologically. The project simultaneously aims to develop new measurement protocols and contribute to the creation of open-access resources, including peer-reviewed publications, and digital archives. Finally, the project illustrates how academic research can be mobilized to address real-world challenges through culturally sensitive, interdisciplinary, and community-engaged practices. It offers a replicable model for integrating arts and health in higher education and public life, and aims at demonstrating how body-mind connections, when nurtured through the arts, can lead to more resilient, connected, and healthy societies.

ART-YOGA IN ISTANBUL: A WELL-BEING WITH ARTS CASE STUDY

In February-March 2025, in collaboration with Prof. Dr. Barış Çoban, Dean of the Faculty of Arts and Sciences at Doğuş University, Istanbul, and Head of the Department of Communication Sciences, I was invited to lead an educational program with theoretical and practical training in "Well-Being with Arts", associated with data collection during a two-months Art-Yoga session. The project was named *Well-Being with Art-Yoga in the Istanbul Context* and constitutes a case study that gives concrete insights, to better understand the potential of combined art and movement in terms of well-being. This study was conducted within the complex and often adverse socio-political climate of Türkiye, as detailed in the European Commission's *Türkiye Report* (2024). The country continues to experience significant democratic backsliding, with weakened institutional checks and balances under a highly centralized presidential system. Civil society operates under increasing constraints, with human rights defenders, academics, and artists frequently subjected to judicial harassment and censorship. Freedom of expression, gender equality, and minority rights—particularly for women, LGBTIQ individuals, and Kurdish communities—remain areas of critical concern, according to the European Union's report. The judiciary lacks independence, and the rule of law is inconsistently applied, contributing to a pervasive sense of insecurity and mistrust. These systemic pressures compounded by economic instability and prominent levels of social polarization, directly affect the psychological well-being and expressive freedom of individuals, particularly within academic and creative communities. In this context, the implementation of an Art-Yoga intervention aiming at enhancing well-being must be understood not only as a therapeutic practice but also as a subtle form of resilience and self-affirmation against a backdrop of structural repression and social precarity.

Despite their distinct cultural and geographic contexts, Japan and Türkiye exhibit notable similarities in terms of subjective well-being. Both countries consistently report life satisfaction scores below the OECD average, reflecting moderate to low levels of perceived well-being among their populations. Cultural norms play a significant role in shaping these perceptions. In Japan, values such as social harmony and modesty may lead individuals to understate their happiness, while in Türkiye, strong familial and communal ties often mitigate economic stressors, though political and financial instability can negatively impact overall well-being. Both societies have also strong patriarchal ties and social hierarchies that impact the relationships between people and across genders. Economic factors, including job insecurity in Japan—especially for women—and inflation in Türkiye, are prominent contributors to public sentiment. Additionally, both societies emphasize the importance of reduced outspoken social relationships, which serve as protective factors. Simultaneously, rapid urbanization with small apartments in concrete buildings, and evolving lifestyles, are challenging the need for a breathable environment and the traditional support systems. Mental health awareness is gradually increasing in both countries, yet stigma remains a barrier to widespread acceptance and access to care. These shared dynamics underscore the complex interplay between cultural, economic, and social factors in shaping subjective well-being across diverse societies, and allowed us to implement the project in Istanbul.

In terms of method, the Art-Yoga program conducted in Istanbul invited participants into a multisensory and emotionally immersive experience, combining dance-like movement, music, and poetic imagery. The interventional pilot study aimed to assess accurate mood changes before and after Art-Yoga lessons. This summative assessment additionally focused on evaluating the effectiveness of the yoga program after implementation, as recommended by the scholars (Emery, 2009; Fynn et al., 2020).

Participants

Volunteering participants were PhD students, lecturers, and faculty members at Doğuş University, Istanbul. Attendance was encouraged for at least nine lessons to enable a comprehensive evaluation of the Art-Yoga program's effects over time. The sample was predominantly women aged 20-40 (approximately 3:1 female-to-male ratio), a distribution the study interprets in light of local gendered perceptions of yoga and comfort levels in mixed settings. One male participant (49 years old) with more than 20 years of university service took part, while most female participants had fewer than five years of service (~78%). Prior to the Art-Yoga session, 22 pre-lesson questionnaires were collected: 68% of questionnaires show that respondents did not practice yoga regularly or at all, while 55% reported more regular experience with meditation or mindfulness; several participants were beginners or carried negative prior experiences with yoga, which positioned the session as an opportunity for a reframed introduction to the practice.

Measures

Quantitative Measures: Mood changes were assessed using the Profile of Mood States (POMS), Revised Version 15.2, a validated 40-item instrument commonly used to measure transient emotional states in contemplative and mind-body interventions. This abbreviated format was intentionally selected to minimize interference with the relaxing effects of the sessions and to avoid cognitive overload after practice. The scale has been previously validated for assessing short-term mood fluctuations and has been used in research on meditation and related practices (e.g., Rangasamy et al., 2019). The study did not develop any new items or altered instruments; rather, it employed the standardized tool to ensure reliability and comparability with existing psychological research on body-mind practices.

Qualitative Measures: To complement the quantitative assessment, a semi-structured interview guide was developed following a state-of-the-art review in art therapy and informed by elements of the Warwick-Edinburgh Mental Well-Being Scales (WEMWBS). The guide explored domains such as self-expression, emotion regulation, and overall well-being, enabling deeper insight into participants' experiential and emotional processes. This tool provided the qualitative framework later used to contextualize and interpret the POMS-based mood changes observed during the intervention.

Procedures

The Istanbul implementation offered a two-month educational program combining theoretical framing (Well-Being with Arts) and weekly Art-Yoga lessons. Each lesson invited a multisensory experience—dance-like movement, music, and poetic imagery/voice guidance—with pose modifications for all levels and a supportive, non-judgmental atmosphere. Immediately before each lesson, participants completed the POMS (pre); immediately after, they completed the POMS (post). A total of 27 post-lesson questionnaires were retrieved (exceeding the 22 pre-session forms because some attendees arrived late, after the pre-assessment), reflecting real-world lesson timing while preserving measurement of post-practice states.

Pre-interviews were conducted before the program to map baseline practices (e.g., journaling, walking, meditation, music, movement) and expressive constraints; post-interviews followed the program to elicit perceived changes (e.g., reductions in tension/overload; increases in clarity, creativity, and connection).

Analysis

For the quantitative data, pre- and post-lesson POMS responses were summarized descriptively and compared to examine direction and magnitude of immediate mood shifts commonly targeted in pilot, practice-proximal evaluations. Given the exploratory scope of a field-based chapter study, emphasis was on interpretable pre-post differences across negative (e.g., tension, anxiety, fatigue, anger, sadness, confusion, unease) and positive (e.g., liveliness, pride, competence) mood states.

As for the qualitative data, interview transcripts were read iteratively and coded for recurrent patterns, generating thematic summaries around four integrative dimensions: music as emotional catalyst; dance/creativity and expressive release; the role of poetic voice/imagery; and translational effects into daily academic and personal life. These themes were used to contextualize and triangulate the quantitative mood shifts observed in lesson-level data.

Mood evaluation before the Art-Yoga lessons

Before the Art-Yoga session, many participants reported feeling tense and anxious. Specifically, 86% of participants felt tense, while 73% felt anxious. The prevalence of these feelings suggests a need for interventions that can help reduce stress and promote relaxation. A significant number of participants felt worn out and fatigued, due to the demand of their familial and professional roles, and of their research, and the lack of sufficient rest or recreational activities. Fatigue and exhaustion were reported by 68% of participants, among which 22% being extremely or a lot exhausted, and 27% extremely or a lot of fatigued. Feelings of anger, unhappiness, and sadness were also common among the participants. Anger was expressed by 55% of participants, unhappiness by 68%, and sadness by 45,5%. These emotions can be linked to numerous factors such as personal issues, work-related challenges, socio-political context, or general dissatisfaction. Moreover, the study was held in Istanbul during a major political turmoil, after the arrest of Istanbul's democrat mayor Ekrem İmamoğlu, who was the main challenging leader for the next presidential elections, leading to huge protests of millions of people in the streets of Istanbul and in many cities across the country, also with thousands of people being arrested during several months, both protesters and democrat politicians, all supporters of İmamoğlu's release. Some participants of the yoga study thus expressed being sometimes confused and uneasy, which might reflect uncertainty or lack of clarity in their current situation. Confusion was reported by 68% of participants, and unease by 73%. This state of mind can affect decision-making, student-aimed transmission, research achievements, and overall mental stability, underscoring the need for practices that enhance focus and clarity. On the long term, addressing these emotions is crucial for improving mental health and fostering a positive outlook. Despite the prevalence of negative moods, there were also reports of positive feelings such as liveliness, pride, and competence. Liveliness and pride were still expressed by 68% of participants, among which the majority however valued their level as little or moderate. Competence was expressed by 59%, among which the majority appreciated it likewise as little or moderate. These positive states are nevertheless important as they can counterbalance part of the negative emotions and contribute to a more nuanced mood profile.

Self-expression, Emotion Regulation, and Global Well-Being Interviews

Self-expression varied widely across participants, with clear distinctions between verbal and written modes, and between public and private spheres. While a male participant, particularly in leadership roles, described himself as generally transparent and comfortable expressing emotions verbally—especially in trusted relationships—female participants, particularly younger ones, often relied on journaling as a primary outlet. Writing served as a space for emotional honesty, reflection, and sometimes gentle self-deception, as one participant noted she would "make things a little bit more pinky… it is about hope". The gendered divergence in expressive style was also shaped by professional context. Participants across the board expressed caution in emotional expression within the workplace, often drawing a line between personal authenticity and personal restraint. The tension between inner emotional life and external presentation was a recurring theme, particularly among women navigating academic hierarchy.

Emotional regulation strategies ranged from structured practices like journaling, walking, and meditation, to sensory and spontaneous activities such as dancing, listening to music or engaging in self-massage, e.g., face yoga. These practices often served as transitional rituals, helping participants move from stress to calm, or from emotional overload to clarity. Younger women tended to describe bodily and emotional release through music and movement, while more mature women leaned toward quiet, restorative routines like walking in nature or engaging in self-care practices. A senior male participant emphasized cognitive and social strategies, such as reading, philosophical reflection, and dialogue with trusted friends. However, several participants—particularly those in early-career academic roles—expressed difficulties in maintaining these practices. Overwork, emotional fatigue, and urban disconnection were cited as barriers to consistent self-care. One participant admitted, “I always postpone finding solutions for these problems”, highlighting the gap between emotional need and lived reality.

When asked about their overall well-being, participants often describe a delicate and dynamic balance, influenced by physical health, emotional resilience, and relational support. Few considered their lives fully balanced. Younger female participants described their lives as work-dominated, with physical and emotional well-being often side-lined. More mature participants, male and female, while more reflective, also acknowledged the toll of institutional dysfunction and social unrest. Happiness and peacefulness were frequently described as interconnected and culturally entangled: in the Turkish context, several participants noted that these mental states are not easily separated—“If you are happy, also you are peaceful.” This is a specific cultural trait in the Turkish language and perception of both states.

Mood Evaluation after the Art-Yoga lessons

After each Art-Yoga lesson, the volunteering participants reported significant improvements in their mood states. The prevalence of tension and anxiety decreased substantially, with only 22% of participants feeling a little tense, 22% a little anxious, 26% a little restless, and 18,5% moderately helpless. This suggests that the Art-Yoga lessons were effective in reducing stress and promoting relaxation. Fatigue and exhaustion also saw a notable reduction, with only 11% of participants reporting moderate fatigue and exhaustion. After discussion with the participants, it appears that the remaining percentage of fatigue and exhaustion is related to the fact that a substantial number of the participants did not practice any sport at all or did not practice sport regularly. The English-language nuances might also have been a barrier in understanding the scale’s items for many of the participants for whom it was not a mother tongue, nor a fluently mastered language, sometimes leading to a confusion between mental fatigue and exhaustion, and healthy sport’s tiredness. However, this improvement highlights the rejuvenating and energizing effects of the Art-Yoga classes.

Negative emotions such as anger, unhappiness, and sadness were less common after the lessons. A little anger was expressed by 15% of participants, unhappiness by 7%, and sadness by 11%, which might also be related to the social and political context in Istanbul at the time of the study, as shown by all the pre-interviews. These reductions indicate however that the Art-Yoga classes helped in addressing negative emotions and fostering a more positive outlook. Confusion and unease also decreased, with only 7,5% of participants feeling moderately confused and 22% feeling a little uneasy, suggesting an enhancement in mental clarity and stability. Positive feelings such a liveliness, pride, and competence increased after the practice. Liveliness and pride were expressed by 100% of participants, among which 70% were expressing feeling a lot or extremely lively, and 56% a lot or extremely proud. Competence was also expressed by 89% of participants.

Interviews about the Art-Yoga's Effects

The qualitative responses revealed a progression from emotional tension to clarity, from routine to creativity, and from isolation to connection. This synthesis is organized into four thematic sections, each reflecting a core dimension of the participants' lived experiences.

Music as Emotional Catalyst

Music was described as a central emotional driver of the Art-Yoga session. It did not merely accompany the practice: it shaped its emotional trajectory. The oldest participant, a male senior professor in his late 40s, described music as "the most effective thing for [him] to feel something". He associated the initial meditative music with a sense of emotional safety, the soft piano with gentle introspection, and the rhythmic and dynamic music with excitement, freedom, and confidence. These transitions helped him move from a state of mental fatigue to one of creative alertness.

Middle-aged female participants emphasized the emotional resonance of familiar music. One noted, "If I knew the song before… I really felt it", suggesting that recognition triggered emotional warmth, trust, and cultural intimacy. Turkish songs evoked nostalgia, comfort, and emotional grounding, while unfamiliar music was less effective, unless paired with evocative imagery mediated by the vocal guidance. A literature professor in her early 40s offered a more precise interpretation. She cited Mitski's "My Love Mine All Mine" song and Yiruma's piano compositions as evoking compassion, peace, and emotional clarity. Instrumental music helped her "escape the world", allowing her to enter a state of focused serenity.

The youngest participant, a woman in her late 20s, described music as a source of emotional activation. She responded strongly to nature sounds—especially fire and water—which helped her shift from urban stress to inner calm. "We feel ourselves in the flow of the music", she said, describing how music also helped her reconnect with her body and regulate her mood.

Dance, Creativity, and Emotional Expression

Art-Yoga was widely experienced as a space for expressive movement and emotional release. Participants described the lessons as liberating, non-judgmental, and creatively stimulating. The senior male participant, who had never practiced yoga before, reflected: "I'm not a good dancer, but it was perfect for me to feel the dancing motion… it's dreamy". He described flame and water-inspired movements and imagery as evoking lightness, imagination, and self-esteem, and noted that the non-compulsory nature of the movements allowed him to feel free from performance pressure.

Middle-aged women described the lessons as emotionally freeing, especially in contrast to the rigidity of academic life and the difficulties of women in a highly patriarchal society. One participant, despite a knee injury that prevented her from entering each movement the way she would have liked to, found the watery warm-up movements and images deeply expressive. She described feeling relief, gentle joy, and a sense of inner spaciousness. The lessons helped her feel more relaxed, creative, and emotionally attuned, even enhancing her academic writing. The youngest participant expressed the most vibrant response, describing the dance-like movements as "alive and flowing". She associated hip movements and wing-like dance gestures with release, confidence, and emotional clarity. Coming from a smaller town, these gestures helped her process the stress of urban adaptation in a huge city, and reconnect with her inner rhythm. She felt more open and emotionally connected, both in her lectures at a vocational school and in her personal life. Finally, a mid-career professor offered a poetic reflection, comparing the savasana pose to "going on the sea" or "floating in an airport display". These metaphors apprehended the effortless flow, emotional detachment, and deep relaxation she experienced. The lessons helped her silence her inner critic and reconnect with her creative self, describing a shift from self-doubt to contentment.

The Power of Poetry and Voice

My voice, rhythm, and use of imagery were described as essential to the emotional and imaginative depth of the lessons. Participants emphasized how verbal guidance helped them access inner landscapes and emotional clarity. The senior male participant described the voice "like the call of a nymph", guiding him through elemental metaphors—water, wind, flame—that triggered personal memories, emotional insight, and a sense of connection to the world. The imagery of the roots of the chestnut tree from ancient Turkish poetry, and the metaphor of the Marmara Sea helped him see his environment "from a more emotional point of view", transforming familiar places into symbols of grounding and flow.

Middle-aged participants found the voice grounding and supportive. One admitted, "I'm not good at imagination", but noted that the use of local imagery, like the Marmara Sea's quiet flow, helped her focus and feel emotionally anchored in her city. The voice became a catalyst for emotional presence, helping her shift from mental overactivity to embodied awareness. The youngest participant connected deeply with symbolic language. For example, when she heard: "Feel your roots in the ground", a guidance that was related to a famous Turkish poem evoking Istanbul, it helped her relate to the city and feel more rooted, secure, and emotionally stable, despite feeling herself a bit lonely in this town where she just moved in. The fire imagery reminded her of "the energy of life and the fire of life in [her]", enhancing her sense of vitality, motivation, and inner strength. Finally, a mid-career professor praised the voice as "naturally beautiful", noting its ability to "slow down the flow around" and facilitate concentration, emotional containment, and aesthetic pleasure. The sound of the singing bowl, used at the beginning and end of each lesson, marked a symbolic threshold toward a meditative state, helping her disconnect from external stress and enter a space of inner stillness.

Transformative Effects on Daily Life

Participants described a profound shift in their perceptions of the world, their emotional states, and their interactions with others. The youngest participant said: "I was more like a grave, but now I'm more like a sun, a rainbow". This transformation extended into her daily routines, where she felt more energetic, present, and emotionally open. She described improved sleep, emotional regulation, and a greater sense of joy in teaching. Middle-aged participants described the lessons as emotional refuges. One reflected: "These lessons are a kind of exit, releasing, an exit from the reality." She noticed that her colleagues perceived her as more relaxed, positive, and approachable, reinforcing the internal changes she experienced. She described a shift from irritability to calm, and from emotional fatigue to resilience. A senior professor described a shift from exhaustion to balance. "Just an hour can do something different in a workday", she noted. She became more patient, empathetic, and self-compassionate, especially in professional settings, because she also bears heavy administrative responsibilities. She reported feeling more creative, focused, and emotionally available in her research, and in reaction to administrative issues. Also bearing heavy administrative duties, the senior male participant described a dramatic change in mindset: "I got the power to change my mental state by using something that I have been voluntarily part of." He began to see the world more positively, felt more hopeful, and described a new sense of agency in shaping his emotional life. He also began to share the benefits of Art-Yoga with others, becoming a source of inspiration and emotional leadership in his academic environment.

Across all profiles, participants reported increased happiness and peacefulness, with self-reported scores rising from 3-4 before the program to 8-10 after. They described themselves as being at "a good start", "a beginner", or "living more slowly" on their path to balance. The practice fostered emotional clarity, self-compassion, and a renewed sense of agency. They also reported feeling the practice beneficial in the workplace to lessen the tensions and increase their creativity and clarity of mind. Afterwards, one of them started practicing yoga on a regular basis in a studio, while the others insisted on the fact they wished to perpetuate the regularity they implemented with the Art-Yoga session.

The Istanbul Case: Synthesis

The prospective interventional pilot study conducted in Istanbul demonstrated the effectiveness of Art-Yoga in improving mood states among participants in academic settings. The repeated measurement approach provided robust evidence for the study's conclusions, showing significant reductions in negative mood states such as tension, anxiety, fatigue, anger, unhappiness, sadness, confusion, and unease. Additionally, positive mood states such as liveliness, pride, and competence increased after the Art-Yoga lessons. The significant mood improvements observed in this study can compare with the results of other studies that have used the reduced POMS scale, e.g., for meditation (Rangasamy et al., 2019), reinforcing its credibility as a tool for evaluating mood states during Art-Yoga practices.

The post-practice interviews reveal that Art-Yoga served as a transformative experience for participants, offering a space for emotional release, creative exploration, and personal growth. Music, movement, voice, and imagery worked together to create a practice that was emotionally resonant and personally meaningful, sometimes directly linked to Turkish cultural references. Participants navigated their emotional landscapes with greater ease, found new ways to express themselves, and experienced a shift in how they related to others and the world around them. The practice helped them reconnect with their bodies, regulate their emotions, and cultivate a sense of peace and vitality. Art-Yoga emerged not merely as a modern variation of traditional yoga, but as a redefinition—one that integrates artistic and cultural sensibilities with emotional depth, thus not focusing on the strict alignment of the body[2] like in Iyengar lineage, or on the physical performance like in fitness yoga or Ashtanga yoga, nor on the spiritual aspect like in some forms of Bhakti yoga. Nonetheless, like many forms of yoga, it offers participants a sanctuary in which to explore, heal, and transform.

These findings highlight the potential of Art-Yoga as an effective intervention for promoting mental health and well-being, particularly in reducing stress and enhancing positive emotions. The study's results offer valuable insights for designing new and more accurate interventions that leverage activities, like Art-Yoga, to improve overall well-being. The collaboration with a local institution provided a supportive environment for this educational program, emphasizing the importance of integrating theoretical and practical training for more well-being at university, while also helping me develop a framework tailored to the cultural context of Türkiye. Overall, the *Well-Being with Art-Yoga in the Istanbul Context* project successfully demonstrated that Art-Yoga can be a valuable tool in Turkish academic settings where stress and negative emotions are prevalent too, especially when looking at the increasing number of tasks and short-term achievements expected nowadays.

Toward Broader Implementation

The Istanbul findings also highlight the potential scalability of Art-Yoga in institutional contexts. Because the lessons require minimal equipment and can be adapted across languages, cultural references, and physical abilities, the model can be integrated into university well-being programs, staff development initiatives, or community outreach. Future phases of the WBA project include designing training modules and a reproducible session blueprint to support facilitators in different institutions. This approach positions Art-Yoga as an accessible, culturally sensitive, and sustainable resource for mental-health promotion.

UNDERSTANDING THE MECHANISMS AT STAKE IN MINDFUL ART-BASED PRACTICES

As demonstrated by the impact of modern activities on human well-being and the recent desire to foster a more peaceful lifestyle, the interplay between ancient yogic wisdom and modern art-based practices presents an interesting way to explore human experience. By examining body-mind practices as a bridge that connects these seemingly distant spaces, it can be of use to question the relationships between the philosophies and ethical imperatives of ancient traditions, and the functionalities of the contemporary world.

From Ancient Yogic Wisdom to Holistic Well-Being

Yogic philosophies offer a structured system linking metaphysics, ethics, and self-realization. Foundational texts such as the *Patañjali Yoga Sūtras* and the *Bhagavad Gītā* articulate a worldview in which physical practice, ethical guidance, and inner awareness support mental clarity and well-being (Vivekananda, 2018; Zaehner, 1979). Compiled between the 2nd century BCE and the 4th century CE, the *Yoga Sūtras* describe the eight-limbed path (*a ā ga yoga*), integrating ethical foundations, postures, breath regulation, concentration, and meditation as a progressive refinement of consciousness. Their aim is to stabilize the mind, distinguish transient mental activity (*citta*) from the deeper self (*puru a*), and guide practitioners toward liberation through disciplined practice and discernment.

The *Bhagavad Gītā*, composed between the 5th and 2nd centuries BCE as part of the *Mahābhārata*, likewise harmonizes embodied action and spiritual insight (Zaehner, 1979). Through its dialogue between K a and Arjuna, it introduces the complementary paths of action (*karma yoga*), knowledge (*jñāna yoga*), and devotion (*bhakti yoga*). The principle of *ni kāma karma*—acting without attachment to outcomes—reconciles worldly engagement with inner freedom. Together, these texts present a holistic framework in which ethical action, contemplative practice, and embodied awareness support personal transformation.

These sources are included here to emphasize that yoga has always been more than physical exercise: it is a philosophical and experiential inquiry into reality, consciousness, and human flourishing. Their emphasis on presence, awareness, and emotional clarity resonates strongly with contemporary mindfulness research, notably the work of Kabat-Zinn and Langer, who frame mindful attention as an intentional, non-judgmental engagement with thoughts, sensations, and environments (Kabat-Zinn, 2016; Langer, 2014). This positioning highlights how yogic traditions inform modern understandings of meta-awareness, resilience, and balanced living.

The multidimensional nature of yoga—linking posture, breath, meditation, and ethical reflection—mirrors contemporary psychological approaches to stress and emotional regulation. Modern therapeutic modalities increasingly incorporate yogic and mindful practices to support diverse populations, including those experiencing chronic stress or trauma (Groessl et al., 2008; Perera, 2024). The transformative narratives found in ancient texts also converge with modern theories of human development, suggesting that embodied, reflective practices can foster self-awareness and psychological growth (Ranisha & Kumari, 2024; Ranisha et al., 2024). As global interest in mindfulness expands, these traditions continue to offer a meaningful framework for cultivating resilience and holistic health. Their integration into contemporary body-mind interventions — such as the WBA Art-Yoga study (Clonts et al., 2026) — demonstrates how ancient wisdom and modern psychology can mutually enrich approaches to well-being (Gamage et al., 2024).

Body-Mind Engagement in Art-Yoga: An Autopoietic Machine

Based on the ancient Greek πο ησις [*poiesis*: creation, production, tailor] and α τ ς [*autos*: oneself, self-], the expression of "autopoietic machine" comes from the enactive theory. The enactive approach is particularly interesting for studying the body-mind engagement in the Art-Yoga practice, as this approach highlights the cognitive relevance of an embodied and multidisciplinary experience of life. Indeed, a mindful practice can be understood as a way to grasp firstly the idea of the fragmentation of the self, idea that can also be found in the cognitivism and connectivism theories. The difficulty to seize a unified self puts into question the Cartesian conception of a *res cogitans* [mental substance, 'thinking thing'] that leaves aside the experiential nature of the self, the processes of the thought in action, and its lived relations with the body. If there is a self, body-mind practices first highlight its incessant bifurcations, instability, and multiple forms, particularly by emphasizing cognitive processes through the experience of thought progression and its relationship to practice in motion, in relation to a specific environment. The latter tends to lead to an absence of discrimination between the self and the non-self, that is neither the disembodied *cogito* [I think] as in the Cartesian tradition, and neither the transcendent self as in the Kantian thought. It might be closer to David Hume's *Treatise of Human Nature*, when having the sensation that perceived exteriority is neither continuous nor separate. The worldly and universal components are constantly acting on each other, in a perpetual circulation and by interpretative phenomena in movement. In the digital age, where the AI has now a predominant place, the human body-mind and the environment altogether create nonetheless an infinite body that is a system and that questions the metaphysic knowledge through the body-mind experience, without excluding the relationship to the digital components of the recent changing human experience.

These processes involve recognizing a cognitively valid practice for experiencing other forms of life than those approved by the norm—challenged e.g., in many artistic and literary approaches. This praxis positioning does not oppose the cognitive sciences of the mid-20th century but rather proposes an advancement. Indeed, succeeding philosophy and psychology in describing psychic phenomena, cognitive sciences emerged between 1943 and 1953 under the name of cybernetics. Francisco Varela, Evan Thompson, and Eleanor Rosch wrote in *The Embodied Mind—Cognitive Science and Human Experience* (p. 38): "these cyberneticians felt a calling to express the processes underlying mental phenomena in explicit mechanisms and mathematical formalisms." Then, from 1956, they took the name of cognitive sciences, under the incentive of Herbert Simon, Noam Chomsky, Marvin Minsky, and John McCarthy. The idea that cognition is the processing of information through physical and symbolic computations, in other words, through the manipulation of symbols, gradually took shape. Nonetheless, within this background, the cognitive experience proposed by body-mind practices, such as the Art-Yoga, is achieved through different means than the study of the brain perceived as a deductive machine by Western cybernetics and post-war cognitivism.

In other modern cultures with different philosophical background, it seems evident that psychoanalysis and cognitivism are not the only means of accessing the depths of the human being in relation to perceived exteriority. For instance, in a predominantly Mahayana-Buddhist Japan, the "liberation of the individual from their ego" [: *satori*] and the "awakening to a self with which one is in harmony" [: *ikigai*] are also valid ways of experiencing the uncertainties, impermanence, and instability of the "human heart, mind, and intention" [: *kokoro*], and even for alleviating the mental agitations and the physical tensions that arise from them. Rooted notably in Mahayana Buddhism and phenomenology, the enactive approach proposed essentially by the biologists and neuroscientists Maturana and Varela is more specifically relevant for studying the relationships between the body and the mind, including the experience of the physical and mental "vibrations"—e.g., brain waves related to moods, effects of sound on body and mind, etc.—and of the multiplicity of the self, potentially contradictory but non-exclusive. In fact, the processes and dynamic relationships generated in mindful practices are similar to those of the autopoietic machine defined by Maturana and Varela. Referring to the organization of living beings, they firstly used the term "autopoiesis" in a publication from 1972:

> *An autopoietic machine is a machine organized (defined as a unity) as a network of processes of production (transformation and destruction) of components that produces the components which: (i) through their interactions and transformations continuously regenerate and realize the network of processes (relations) that produced them ; and (ii) constitute it (the machine) as a concrete unity in the space in which they (the components) exist by specifying the topological domain of its realization as such a network. (Maturana & Varela, p. 79)*

The perception of an autopoietic machine revolves around the idea of self-creation and self-maintenance. An autopoietic machine encompass in its processes an organization as a unity, a continuous regeneration, and a concrete unity. It is organized as a single entity, defined by a network of processes that produce, transform, and destroy its components. Then, the components of the machine interact and transform in such a way that they continuously regenerate and realize the network of processes that produced them. This means the machine is self-sustaining and self-regenerating. Finally, the components of the machine constitute it as a concrete entity in the space where they exist. They define the topological domain—that is to say, the spatial structure—of the machine's realization as a network. This network of processes produces the components that, in turn, regenerate the network, ensuring the system's continuity and integrity. Like in the cellular process of autopoiesis, a holistic perception of life constantly delineates its own shifting boundaries by refusing to be confined to a single categorization. It involves shedding a total dissociation such as that between body and mind, or between abstraction and experience, or even between human life and machine, which is a recurrent question in the digital age. Ideally, what is internal and external to body-mind practices is determined only by its own dynamics, in the sense of form, and not imposed by normative and nomenclatural processes. Thus, these autogenerations foster a cognitive value. According to researcher Letícia Renault, one indeed finds in the enactivism of

Maturana and Varela the idea that cognitive functioning "establishes a circularity between perception and action. Such circularity rejects the idea that cognition has a purely representational role and highlights the co-dependence between the object that is known and the subject who knows." (Renault, 2020, p. 145) Furthermore, in Varela's view, "perception does not correspond to the representation of intrinsic qualities of the world, but is a function of the organism's activity itself." (Renault, p. 145) Thus, being human—and not a robot—is not the symbolic processing of a knowledge external to oneself, as shown by the back-and-forth movements, penetrations, and mutual transformations at all levels. This global system in which the human being lives is produced by embracing experience, in interaction with the environment in which it is realized. This knot is called by Varela, Thompson, and Rosch "the human life-world" (p. 13).

CONCLUSION

This chapter has explored the transformative potential of creativity and movement—particularly through embodied, art-based practices—as integrative modalities for cultivating peace of mind and promoting mental health. Artistic engagement, when interwoven with mindful body-mind practices, offers a powerful tool for fostering emotional resilience, cognitive flexibility, and holistic well-being. Drawing from interdisciplinary research and ancient wisdom traditions, the investigation in the chapter shows that the body is not a passive vessel but an active participant in shaping emotional and cognitive experience. The arts—defined here expansively to include literature, music, dance, performance, and visual expression—engage symbolic, sensory, and relational dimensions simultaneously, making them particularly suited to address the multifactorial nature of mental health. This convergence of disciplines affirms the need for a reimagined therapeutic landscape—one that embraces the expressive, the embodied, and the relational.

It is within this context that the *Well-Being with Arts* (WBA) project finds its resonance. First implemented in Japan, the project responded to culturally specific challenges such as emotional restraint, social anxiety, and limited access to holistic therapies. By introducing Art-Yoga as a non-verbal and open-ended practice, it created a space where movement, music, visual art, and literary images, could support emotional articulation and psychological care. This approach was not only therapeutic but also culturally sensitive, offering a gentle reconfiguration of mental health support within academic settings. The Istanbul case study, conducted in early 2025, extended this vision into a politically and socially constrained environment. Participants—faculty and students—engaged in a multisensory experience that combined dance-like movement, evocative music, and poetic imagery. The results were striking: tension and anxiety dropped from over 70% to just 22%, fatigue and exhaustion were reduced to 11%, and negative emotions such as anger, sadness, and confusion saw significant declines. Simultaneously, positive states such as liveliness, pride, and competence surged, with 100% of participants reporting increased vitality and 89% feeling more capable and confident.

These outcomes were not incidental but deeply intertwined with the structure of the practice. Music shaped the emotional rhythm of each lesson—according to the participants, meditative tones fostered safety, soft piano invited introspection, and dynamic compositions activated energy and confidence. Dance-like movement, inspired by elemental metaphors such as water and flame, enabled expressive embodiment and emotional release. Poetic imagery and voice guidance anchored attention and evoked symbolic depth, transforming familiar spaces into landscapes of emotional resonance thanks to poetic evocations related to Istanbul's culture. Together, these artistic modalities did not merely accompany the yoga: they constituted its expressive and therapeutic core, transforming the lessons into a multimodal experience of being.

This combination of mindful movement and arts reflects the autopoietic nature of body-mind practices, as conceptualized by Maturana and Varela. The Art-Yoga lessons functioned as self-organizing systems—networks of sensation, movement, and meaning that continuously regenerated themselves through interaction. Participants did not passively receive therapeutic input: they actively co-created their experience through embodied engagement and cultural relation. The practice thus exemplifies an enactive model of cognition, where perception and action are circularly linked, and where the boundaries between self and environment dissolve into a dynamic ecology of transformation. Moreover, this approach resonates with ancient yogic philosophies, which harmonize physical discipline, ethical conduct, and spiritual insight. Foundational texts such as the *Patanjali Yoga Sutras* and the *Bhagavad Gita* articulate a path toward liberation that is grounded in embodied awareness and conscious action. The Art-Yoga practice, while contemporary in form, echoes these principles: it fosters one-pointed attention, emotional clarity, and a sense of inner spaciousness. It is not merely a therapeutic intervention, but a modern art of living—a pedagogical and philosophical practice that invites individuals to inhabit their lives more fully, with compassion, creativity, and presence.

To deepen this reflection, inspired by the Francophone poet Ghérasim Luca's expression of "phylogenic weddings/unions" [*noces phylogéniques*], a conceptual shift could be proposed. This poetic image gestures toward a vision of interconnectedness that transcends species, systems, and temporalities. It reminds us that experience is not isolated within the individual but accumulated within the collective—marked by historical traces and shaped by evolutionary continuities. Within this framework, mindful movement and embodied creativity become practices of release: they help loosen the ontogenetic residues of personal conditioning and invite us into a wider ecology of being. Such a vision sustains the idea of a plasticity of the body-mind system, relying on its capacity for metamorphosis through relational, enactive processes. These practices do not seek to represent the world from a distance, but to inhabit it intimately, through movement, breath, rhythm, beauty, and imagination. They offer a way of living that is attuned to multiplicity, interdependence, and transformation. To conclude, this chapter suggests that well-being is not a static state to be achieved, but a continuous unfolding, and a poetic and embodied process of becoming. Through the lens of "phylogenic unions", we are invited to reimagine mental health not as a clinical endpoint, but as a shared, evolving condition, one that honours the complexity of human experience and the generative potential of body-mind interactions. In this light, well-being with arts becomes not only a therapeutic strategy, but a creative and relational path toward peace of mind in an increasingly complex world.

Scalability and Institutional Adaptation

Beyond individual interventions, the Art-Yoga framework lends itself to broader institutional integration. Its low material demands, cultural adaptability, and multimodal structure make it suitable for implementation in universities, community centers, and workplace wellness programs. The WBA project is currently exploring the creation of facilitator guidelines and open-access resources that would allow non-specialist educators and practitioners to adopt the method in diverse settings. Such developments underscore the potential of Art-Yoga to contribute to long-term, systemic well-being strategies within academic and cultural institutions.

REFERENCES

Anderson, R. C. (2018). Creative engagement: Embodied metaphor, the affective brain, and meaningful learning. *Mind, Brain and Education : the Official Journal of the International Mind, Brain, and Education Society, 12*(2), 72–81. DOI: 10.1111/mbe.12176

Barnett, K. S., & Vasiu, F. (2024). How the arts heal: A review of the neural mechanisms behind the therapeutic effects of creative arts on mental and physical health. *Frontiers in Behavioral Neuroscience, 18*, 1–15. DOI: 10.3389/fnbeh.2024.1422361 PMID: 39416439

Clonts, C., Kishimoto, H., NIU, T., Kawata, N., & Yokota, F. (2026). Art-Yoga for well-being, awareness and self-care in higher education: First data analysis of a pilot study in a Japanese university. [Bulletin of KIKAN Education], 12, 131-147. DOI: 10.15017/7405176

Dolan, P., & White, M. P. (2007). How can measures of subjective well-being be used to inform public policy? *Perspectives on Psychological Science, 2*(1), 71–85. DOI: 10.1111/j.1745-6916.2007.00030.x PMID: 26151920

Emery, C. (2009). Research Design for Evaluation Studies. In Verhagen, E., van Mechelen, W. (eds.), Oxford Academic, Sports Injury Research. DOI: 10.1093/acprof:oso/9780199561629.003.013

European Commission. (2024). *Türkiye Report. 2024 Communication on EU enlargement policy*. EU Publishing.

Fancourt, D., & Finn, S. (2019). What is the evidence on the role of the arts in improving health and well-being? A scoping review. WHO Regional Office for Europe. *Health Evidence Network Synthesis, 67*, 1–133.

Fujiwara, D., Kudrna, L., & Dolan, P. (2014). Quantifying and Valuing the Well-Being Impacts of Culture and Sport. UK Government Department of Culture and Sport Report. 1-45.

Fynn, J., Hardeman, W., Milton, K., Murphy, J., & Jones, A. (2020). A systematic review of the use and reporting of evaluation frameworks within evaluations of physical activity interventions. *The International Journal of Behavioral Nutrition and Physical Activity, 17*(107), 1–17. DOI: 10.1186/s12966-020-01013-7 PMID: 32831111

Gamage, B., Gamage, M. N., Perera, N. M., Kodikara, C. S., Wijeratne, J. U. M., Seneviratne Alles, S. M. D. P., Kumaran, T., Jeewandara, J. M. C., & Mahawithanage, S. T. C. (2024). Impact of mindfulness-based tri-modal prehabilitation on functional recovery and selected surgical outcomes of patients with colorectal cancer admitted to surgical hospital wards. *BMJ Open*, *14*. Advance online publication. DOI: 10.1136/bmjopen-2023-080192 PMID: 39806718

Gomes, N., Cochet, S., & Guyon, A. (2020). Dance and embodiment: Therapeutic benefits on body-mind health. *Journal of Interdisciplinary Methodologies and Issues in Science*, *9*, 1–23. DOI: 10.18713/JIMIS-02072021-9-4

Groessl, E. J., Weingartn, K. R., Aschbacher, K., Pada, L., & Baxi, S. (2008). Yoga for veterans with chronic low-back pain. *Journal of Alternative and Complementary Medicine (New York, N.Y.)*, *14*(9), 1123–1129. DOI: 10.1089/acm.2008.0020 PMID: 18991515

Kabat-Zinn, J. (2016). *Mindfulness for Beginners*. Sounds True Editions.

Langer, E. J. (2014). *Mindfulness*. Da Capo Press.

MacAskill, W., Chua, W. J., Woodall, H., & Pinidiyapathirage, J. (2023). Beyond the Written Reflection: A Systematic Review and Qualitative Synthesis of Creative Approaches to Reflective Learning Amongst Medical Students. *Perspectives on Medical Education*, *12*(1), 361–371. DOI: 10.5334/pme.914 PMID: 37720690

Maturana, H., & Varela, F. (1980). *Autopoiesis and Cognition*. D. Reidel Publishing Company.

OECD. (2013). *OECD Guidelines on Measuring Subjective Well-Being*. OECD Publishing., DOI: 10.1787/9789264191655-

ONS. (2011). *ONS Opinions and Lifestyle Survey—Well-Being Module*. ESDS UK Government Publishing.

Perera, R. (2024). Mat to Clinic: A Systematic Review on Role of Therapeutic Yoga in Clinical Management of Mental Disorders and Wellbeing Promotion in Integrative Health Care. SICASH 2024, SLIIT International Conference on Advancements in Sciences and Humanities Proceedings, 420-225.

Rangasamy, V., Susheela, A.T., Mueller, A., Chang, T.F.H., & Sadhasivam, S., & Subramaniam*, B. (2019). The effect of a one-time 15-minute guided meditation (Isha Kriya) on stress and mood disturbances among operating room professionals: A prospective interventional pilot study. *F1000 Research*, *8*, 335. DOI: 10.12688/f1000research.18446.1 PMID: 32665843

Ranisha, K., & Kumari, S. (2024). Effect of a yogic stress management technique (cyclic meditation) on stress, mindfulness, and well-being: A systematic review. *Yoga Mimamsa*, *56*(2), 129–140. DOI: 10.4103/ym.ym_51_24

Ranisha, K., Kumari, S., & Dwivedi, U. (2024). Human Development Model Based on Yogic Wisdom for Well-being and Self-actualization: A Conceptual Framework. *Journal of Human Values*, *30*(2), 202–213. DOI: 10.1177/09716858231210598

Renault, L. (2020). L'approche énactive et la place de l'altérité – Dialogue entre Varela et Buber. *Journal of French and Francophone Philosophy—Revue de la philosophie française et de langue française*, vol. XXVIII, n° 1/2020, 143-166.

Rodríguez-Jiménez, R.-M., Carmona, M., García-Merino, S., Díaz-Rivas, B., & Thuissard-Vasallo, I. J. (2022). Stress, subjective well-being and selfknowledge in higher education teachers: A pilot study through bodyfulness approaches. *PLoS One*, *17*(12), 1–34. DOI: 10.1371/journal.pone.0278372 PMID: 36520842

Soulé, I., Littzen-Brown, C., Vermeesch, A.L.*, & Garrigues, L. (2022). Expanding the Mind–Body–Environment Connection to Enhance the Development of Cultural Humility. International Journal of Environmental Research and Public Health, 19 (20): 13641, 1-8. DOI: 10.3390/ijerph192013641

Stiglitz, J., Sen, A., & Fitoussi, J.-P. (2009). The Measurement of Economic Performance and Social Progress Revisited. French State commissioned report from the CMEPSP, 1-63.

Swami Vivekananda. (2018). *Raja Yoga: Being Lectures by the Swami Vivekananda, with Patanjali's Aphorisms, Commentaries and a Glossary of Terms*. Routledge.

Takahashi, T., Asano, S., Uchida, Y., Takemura, K., Fukushima, S., Matsushita, K., & Okuda, N. (2022). Effects of forests and forest-related activities on the subjective well-being of residents in a Japanese watershed: An economic analysis through the capability approach. *Forest Policy and Economics*, *139*, 1–12. DOI: 10.1016/j.forpol.2022.102723

Tei, S., & Wu, H. Y.-J. (2021). Historical Reflection on Taijin-kyôfushô during Covid-19: A Global Phenomenon of Social Anxiety? *History and Philosophy of the Life Sciences*, *43*(2), 60. DOI: 10.1007/s40656-021-00392-9 PMID: 33864152

Van Bael, K., Ball, M., Scarfo, J., & Suleyman, E. (2023). Assessment of the mind-body connection: Preliminary psychometric evidence for a new self-report questionnaire. *BMC Psychology*, *11*(309), 1–21. DOI: 10.1186/s40359-023-01302-3 PMID: 37803484

Varela, F., Thompson, E., & Rosch, E. (2016). *The Embodied Mind—Cognitive Science and Human Experience*. MIT Press. Revised Edition [1991].

Wheatley, D., & Bickerton, C. (2017). Subjective well-being and engagement in arts, culture, and sport. *Journal of Cultural Economics*, *41*, 23–45. DOI: 10.1007/s10824-016-9270-0

WHO. (2021). *Health Promotion Glossary of Terms 2021*. WHO Publishing.

Zaehner, R. C. (1979). *The Bhagavad Gita, with a commentary based on the original source*. Oxford University Press.

ENDNOTES

1 I would like to thank Cardilli, L., Chol, I., Hasuzawa, S., Huang, Z., Khalfa, J., Kishimoto, H., Spielmann, G., Takayanagi, S., Thibierge, S., Yang, Y., Yoshihara, K., for their involvement in the WBA project's team and for swiftly agreeing to join me into this new research path.

2 Even though the practice was carried out safely—with plenty of pose modifications for all levels—and was gently supervised in a supportive, non-judgmental way.

Compilation of References

Acosta, A. (2020, June 3). *The science and philosophy of OM*. Iyengar Yoga London. https://iyengaryogalondon.co.uk/the-science-and-philosophy-of-om-aum/

Adams, T. E., Ellis, C., & Jones, S. H. (2015). *Autoethnography. Understanding qualitative research*. Oxford University Press.

Adler, M. G., & Fagley, N. S. (2005). Appreciation: Individual differences in finding value and meaning as a unique predictor of subjective well-being. *Journal of Personality, 73*(1). Advance online publication. DOI: 10.1111/j.1467-6494.2004.00305.x PMID: 15660674

Affleck, G., & Tennen, H. (1996). Construing Benefits from Adversity: Adaptational Significance and Dispositional Underpinnings. *Journal of Personality, 64*(4). Advance online publication. DOI: 10.1111/j.1467-6494.1996.tb00948.x PMID: 8956517

Ago, Y. (2009). Treatment of psychosomatic disorders—overview. [in Japanese] In Kubo, C. (Ed.), *Standard textbook of psychosomatic medicine* (3rd ed., pp. 238–245). Igaku-Shoin.

Ahern, S. (2024). Affect Theory and Literary Criticism. *Emotion Review, 16*(2), 96–106.

Ahmed, S. (2020). Happy Objects. In Gregg, M., & Seigworth, G. J. (Eds.), *The Affect Theory Reader* (pp. 29–51). Duke University Press.

Albertini, C. (2012). *Arteterapia nel trattamento delle psiconevrosi. Fobie e situazioni traumatiche trattate in un contesto arteterapeutico e psicoterapeutico* [Art therapy in the treatment of psychoneurosis. Phobias and traumatic situations treated in an art-therapeutic and psychotherapeutic context]. Cleup.

Alfrey, A., Field, V., Xenophontes, I., & Holttum, S. (2021). Identifying the mechanisms of poetry therapy and associated effects on participants: A synthesised review of empirical literature. *The Arts in Psychotherapy, 75*. Advance online publication. DOI: 10.1016/j.aip.2021.101832

Allen, M., & Sakamoto, R. (2013). War and peace: War memories and museums in Japan. *History Compass, 11*(12), 1047–1058.

Alschuler, M. (2006). Poetry, the Healing Pen. In Brooke, S. (Ed.), *Creative Therapies Manual* (pp. 253–262). Charles C Thomas Publisher Ltd.

Álvarez-Pérez, Y., Rivero-Santana, A., Perestelo-Pérez, L., Duarte-Díaz, A., Ramos-García, V., Toledo-Chávarri, A., Torres-Castaño, A., León-Salas, B., Infante-Ventura, D., González-Hernández, N., Rodríguez-Rodríguez, L., & Serrano-Aguilar, P. (2022). Effectiveness of mantra-based meditation on mental health: A systematic review and meta-analysis. *International Journal of Environmental Research and Public Health, 19*(6), 3380. DOI: 10.3390/ijerph19063380 PMID: 35329068

American Psychiatric Association. (2022). *Diagnostic and statistical manual of mental disorders, text revision DSM-5-TR. English edition*. American Psychiatric Association Publishing.

Amore, M., Antonella, C., Bettini, E., Boracchia, L., Innamorati, M., Montali, A., Parisoli, C., Pisi, R., Ramponi, S., & Chetta, A. (2013). Disease control in patients with asthma is associated with alexithymia but not with depression or anxiety. *Behavioral Medicine (Washington, D.C.), 39*(4), 138–145. https://www.tandfonline.com/doi/10.1080/08964289.2013.818931 PMID: 24236811

Anders, G. (1935–1936). [Günther Stern] (1935). Une interprétation de l'a posteriori. *Recherches Philosophiques, IV*, 65–80.

Anders, G. (1936–1937). [Günther Stern] (1937). Pathologie de la liberté. *Recherches Philosophiques, VI*, 22–54.

Anderson, R. C. (2018). Creative engagement: Embodied metaphor, the affective brain, and meaningful learning. *Mind, Brain and Education : the Official Journal of the International Mind, Brain, and Education Society, 12*(2), 72–81. DOI: 10.1111/mbe.12176

Ando, S., Yamaguchi, S., Aoki, Y., & Thornicroft, G. (2013). Review of mental-health-related stigma in Japan. *Psychiatry and Clinical Neurosciences, 67*(6), 471–482. DOI: 10.1111/pcn.12086 PMID: 24118217

Angeli-Gordon, J. M. (2025). Ancestral parenting: Reclaiming Māori child-rearing practices in the wake of colonial disruption. *Genealogy*, *9*(2), 36. DOI: 10.3390/genealogy9020036

Antoine, P. (2011). *Quand le voyage devient promenade*. PUPS.

An, X., Bandler, R., Öngür, D., & Price, J. L. (1998). Prefrontal cortical projections to longitudinal columns in the midbrain periaqueductal gray in macaque monkeys. *The Journal of Comparative Neurology*, *401*(4), 455–479. https://onlinelibrary.wiley.com/doi/10.1002/(SICI)1096-9861(19981130)401:4%3C455:AID-CNE3%3E3.0.CO;2-6 PMID: 9826273

Arbo, A. (2004). Breve storia del rumore, da Rousseau a Grisey. *Musicalia. Annuario internazionale di studi musicologici*, *1*, 29–51. http://www.libraweb.net/riviste.php?chiave=52&h=432&w=300

Arendt, H. (1998). *The Human Condition*. The University of Chicago Press.

Aristotle. (1932). *Poetics*. In *Aristotle in 23 volumes* (Vol. 23). Harvard University Press. http://data.perseus.org/texts/urn:cts:greekLit:tlg0086.tlg034.perseus-eng1

Arndt, S., Naguschewski, D., & Stockhammer, R. (Eds.). (2007). *Exophonie: Anderssprachigkeit (in) der Literatur*. Kulturverlag Kadmos.

Artières, P. (2013a). *Reconstitution, jeux d'histoire*. Manuella éditions.

Artières, P. (2013b). *Vie et Mort de Paul Gény*. Seuil.

Atkinson, , RFlint, , J. (2001). Accessing hidden and hard-to-reach populations: Snowball research strategies. *Social Research Update, 33*(1). Retrieved from http://sru.soc.surrey.ac.uk/SRU33.html

Atkinson, M. (2017). *The Poetics of Transgenerational Trauma*. Bloomsbury Academic & Professional.

Azuma, N. (2020). Seishinka ni okeru shintai kousoku: jinken no shiten kara (Physical restraint in psychiatry: human rights considerations). *Seishin Shinkeigaku Zasshi. Psychiatria et Neurologia Japonica*, *122*(12), 946–954.

Bacon, , A. MCharlesford, , JHyland, , MPuskas, , THughes, , P. (2025). Finding silver linings in the covid-19 pandemic: A 2-wave study in the UK. *Psychological Reports,* 128(6), 4120-4138.

Bahloul, J. (1992). *La maison de mémoire, ethnologie d'une demeure judéo-arabe en Algérie (1937-1961)*. Editions Métailié.

Banasik, J., Williams, H., Haberman, M., Blank, S. E., & Bendel, R. (2011). Effect of Iyengar yoga practice on fatigue and diurnal salivary cortisol concentration in breast cancer survivors. *Journal of the American Academy of Nurse Practitioners, 23*(3), 135–142. DOI: 10.1111/j.1745-7599.2010.00573.x PMID: 21355946

Barba, E., & Savarese, N. (1996). *L'arte segreta dell'attore: Un dizionario di antropologia teatrale*. Argo.

Barbaresi, M., Nardo, D., & Fagioli, S. (2025). Physiological entrainment: A key mind–body mechanism for cognitive, motor and affective functioning, and well-being. *Brain Sciences, 15*(1), 3. DOI: 10.3390/brainsci15010003 PMID: 39851371

Barnes, V. A. (2018). Transcendental Meditation and treatment for post-traumatic stress disorder. *The Lancet. Psychiatry, 5*(12), 946–947. DOI: 10.1016/S2215-0366(18)30423-1 PMID: 30449710

Barnett, K. S., & Vasiu, F. (2024). How the arts heal: A review of the neural mechanisms behind the therapeutic effects of creative arts on mental and physical health. *Frontiers in Behavioral Neuroscience, 18*, 1–15. DOI: 10.3389/fnbeh.2024.1422361 PMID: 39416439

Barr, , E. ARaybin, , J. LBennett, , C. RSmith, , M. C. (2024). Silver Linings: A principle-based concept analysis examining the emergence of positive changes that accompany adversity. *International Journal of Nursing Studies Advances*, 7, 100243.

Barrett, L. F. (2017). The theory of constructed emotion: An active inference account of interoception and categorization. *Social Cognitive and Affective Neuroscience, 12*(1), 1–23. PMID: 27798257

Barthes, R. (1980). *La Chambre claire: Note sur la photographie*. Gallimard.

Baumeister, R. F., & Leary, M. R. (1995). The need to belong: Desire for interpersonal attachments as a fundamental human motivation. *Psychological Bulletin, 117*(3), 497–529. DOI: 10.1037/0033-2909.117.3.497 PMID: 7777651

Behrens, K. Y. (2004). A multifaceted view of the concept of *amae*: Reconsidering the indigenous Japanese concept of relatedness. *Human Development, 47*(1), 1–27. DOI: 10.1159/000075366

Behrmann, M., & Plaut, D. C. (2014). Bilateral Hemispheric Processing of Words and Faces: Evidence from Word Impairments in Prosopagnosia and Face Impairments in Pure Alexia. *Cerebral Cortex (New York, N.Y.), 24*(4), 1102–1118. DOI: 10.1093/cercor/bhs390 PMID: 23250954

Bellizzi, K. M., & Blank, T. O. (2006). Predicting posttraumatic growth in breast cancer survivors. *Health Psychology, 25*(1). Advance online publication. DOI: 10.1037/0278-6133.25.1.47 PMID: 16448297

Beshai, S., Tesar, E., & Brown, L. (2024). Mindfulness and CBT: A conceptual integration bridging clinical science and contemplative meditation. *Frontiers in Psychology, 15*, 1489798. DOI: 10.3389/fpsyg.2024.1489798 PMID: 39723397

Bianconi, L. (2008). La forma musicale come scuola dei sentimenti. In La Face Bianconi, G., & Frabboni, F. (Eds.), *Educazione musicale e formazione* (pp. 85–120). FrancoAngeli.

Bisceglia, A. (2023, March 15). *Pittura e Poesia | Opere | Le Gallerie degli Uffizi*. Le Gallerie degli Uffizi. https://www.uffizi.it/opere/pittura-e-poesia

Blackie, , L. E. RWeststrate, , N. MTurner, , KAdler, , J. MMcLean, , K. C. (2023). Broadening our understanding of adversarial growth: The contribution of narrative methods. *Journal of Research in Personality, 103*. Advance online publication. DOI: 10.1016/j.jrp.2023.104359

Boals, , ABedford, , L. ACallahan, , J. L. (2019). Perceptions of change after a trauma and perceived posttraumatic growth: A prospective examination. *Behavioral Sciences, 9*(1). https://doi.org/10.3390/bs9010010

Bohlmeijer, , EWesterhof, , G. (2021). The model for sustainable mental health: future directions for integrating positive psychology into mental health care. *Frontiers in psychology, 12*, 747999.

Bonardel, F. (2023). *Entre mystiques et magiciens*. Fage.

Bonnechère, B. (2017). Revalidation physique, entraînez le cerveau. *Medecine Sciences, 33*, 887–890. PMID: 28994385

Borgdorff, H. (2012). *The Conflict of the Faculties: Perspectives on Artistic Research and Academia*. Leiden University Press.

Bormann, J. E. (2010). Mantram repetition: A "portable contemplative practice" for modern times. In Plante, T. G. (Ed.), *Contemplative practices in action: Spirituality, meditation, and health* (pp. 78–99). ABC-CLIO.

Bormann, J., Liu, L., Thorp, S., & Lang, A. J. (2012). Spiritual Wellbeing Mediates PTSD Change in Veterans with Military-Related PTSD. *International Journal of Behavioral Medicine, 19*, 496–502. DOI: 10.1007/s12529-011-9186-1 PMID: 21874605

Bourges-Celaries, A. (2024a). *L'exophonie chez les autrices Shimazaki Aki, Tawada Yōko et Sekiguchi Ryōko* [Exophony in the works of authors Shimazaki Aki, Tawada Yōko, and Sekiguchi Ryōko] [Doctoral dissertation, University of Montréal]. Papyrus. DOI: 10.71781/14100

Bourges-Celaries, A. (2024b). Des espaces japonais du français. In M. O. M., Hertrampf & D., Mistreanu (Eds), *Langue(s) et espaces dans les xénographies féminines en français*. 55–68. AVM Verlag.

Boyd, J. E., Lanius, R. A., & McKinnon, M. C. (2017). Mindfulness-based treatments for post-traumatic stress disorder: A review of the treatment literature and neurobiological evidence. *Journal of Psychiatry & Neuroscience : JPN*, *43*(1), 7–25. DOI: 10.1503/jpn.170021 PMID: 29252162

Braun, V., & Clarke, V. (2006). Using thematic analysis in psychology. *Qualitative Research in Psychology*, *3*(2), 77–101. DOI: 10.1191/1478088706qp063oa

Bride, O. M., Dunwoody, L., Lowe-Strong, A., & Kennedy, S. M. (2008). Examining adversarial growth in illness: The factor structure of the silver lining questionnaire (SLQ-38). *Psychology & Health*, *23*(6). Advance online publication. DOI: 10.1080/14768320701356540 PMID: 25160809

Brooke, R. (2017). An Archetypal Approach to Treating Combat Post-Traumatic Stress Disorder. In Downing, D., & Mills, J. (Eds.), *Outpatient Treatment of Psychosis. Psychodynamic Approaches to Evidence-Based Practice* (pp. 171–195). Karnak.

Buccino, D. (2005). *Ma vero* [Unpublished dossier]. Retrieved from http://www.dariobuccino.com

Buccino, D. (2006). *Sistema HN* [Online article]. Retrieved from http://www.dariobuccino.com

Buric, I., Farias, M., Jong, J., Mee, C., & Brazil, I. A. (2017). What is the molecular signature of mind–body interventions? A systematic review of gene expression changes induced by meditation and related practices. *Frontiers in Immunology*, *8*, 670. Advance online publication. DOI: 10.3389/fimmu.2017.00670 PMID: 28670311

Burke, A., Lam, C. N., Stussman, B., & Yang, H. (2017). Prevalence and patterns of use of mantra, mindfulness and spiritual meditation among adults in the United States. *BMC Complementary and Alternative Medicine*, *17*(1), 316. DOI: 10.1186/s12906-017-1827-8 PMID: 28619092

Büssing, A., Ostermann, T., Lüdtke, R., & Michalsen, A. (2012). Effects of yoga interventions on pain and pain-associated disability: A meta-analysis. *The Journal of Pain*, *13*(1), 1–9. DOI: 10.1016/j.jpain.2011.10.001 PMID: 22178433

Butler, J., & Jaffe, S. (2021). Challenges and Gratitude: A diary study of software engineers working from home during Covid-19 Pandemic. *Proceedings - International Conference on Software Engineering*. DOI: 10.1109/ICSE-SEIP52600.2021.00047

Calhoun, L. G., & Tedeschi, R. G. (1999). Facilitating Posttraumatic Growth: A Clinician's Guide. In *Personality and Clinical Psychology Series*.

Campbell, J. (1993). *Creative art in groupwork*. Speechmark Publishing.

Capuron, L., Pagnoni, G., Demetrashvili, M., Woolwine, B. J., Nemeroff, C. B., Berns, G. S., & Miller, A. H. (2005). Anterior cingulate activation and error processing during interferon-alpha treatment. *Biological Psychiatry*, *58*(3), 190–196. DOI: 10.1016/j.biopsych.2005.03.033 PMID: 16084839

Carlat, D. (1998). *Gherasim Luca l'intempestif*. José Corti.

Carson, J. W., Carson, K. M., Jones, K. D., Bennett, R. M., Wright, C. L., & Mist, S. D. (2010). A pilot randomized controlled trial of the Yoga of Awareness program in the management of fibromyalgia. *Pain*, *151*(2), 530–539. DOI: 10.1016/j.pain.2010.08.020 PMID: 20946990

Carson, J. W., Carson, K. M., Jones, K. D., Mist, S. D., & Bennett, R. M. (2012). Follow-up of yoga of awareness for fibromyalgia: Results at 3 months and replication in the wait-list group. *The Clinical Journal of Pain*, *28*(9), 804–813. DOI: 10.1097/AJP.0b013e31824549b5 PMID: 22751025

Case, C., Dalley, T., & Reddick, D. (2022). *The handbook of art therapy*. Routledge. (Original work published 1992)

Casey, P., & Bailey, S. (2011). Adjustment disorders: The state of the art. *World Psychiatry; Official Journal of the World Psychiatric Association (WPA)*, *10*(1), 11–18. DOI: 10.1002/j.2051-5545.2011.tb00003.x PMID: 21379346

Cassin, B. (2015). *La nostalgie* [Nostalgia]. Pluriel.

Cavicchi, D. (2002). From the bottom up: Thinking about Tia DeNora's Music in Everyday Life. *Action, Criticism, and Theory for Music Education*, *1*(2). https://act.maydaygroup.org/volume-1-issue-2

Center for Substance Abuse Treatment. (2014a). *Trauma-informed care: A sociocultural perspective (Chapter 1)*. In *TIP 57: Trauma-informed care in behavioral health services* (Treatment Improvement Protocol [TIP] Series, No. 57). Substance Abuse and Mental Health Services Administration. https://www.ncbi.nlm.nih.gov/books/NBK207195/

Center for Substance Abuse Treatment. (2014b). *Understanding the impact of trauma (Chapter 3).* In *TIP 57: Trauma-informed care in behavioral health services* (Treatment Improvement Protocol [TIP] Series, No. 57). Substance Abuse and Mental Health Services Administration. https://www.ncbi.nlm.nih.gov/books/NBK207191/

Chacon, Q. (2020). *La Préparation mentale au service du sportif blessé.* Master thesis, STAPS, Université de Bretagne.

Chadefaud, C. (1993). *L'écrit dans l'Égypte ancienne* [*Writing in ancient Egypt*]. Hachette.

Champagne-Langabeer, T., Ratcliff, C. G., Bakos-Block, C., Vega, F., Cardenas-Turanzas, M., Malik, A., & Korupolu, R. (2025). Evaluating the meditation practices and barriers to adopting mindful medicine among physicians. *American Journal of Lifestyle Medicine*. Advance online publication. DOI: 10.1177/15598276251323850 PMID: 40092531

Chang, H. (2008). *Autoethnography as Method.* Routledge., DOI: 10.4324/9781315433370

Chen, E., Fisher, E. B., Bacharier, L. B., & Strunk, R. C. (2003). Socioeconomic status, stress, and immune markers in adolescents with asthma. *Psychosomatic Medicine*, *65*(6), 984–992. https://journals.lww.com/bsam/abstract/2003/11000/socioeconomic_status,_stress,_and_immune_markers.9.aspx PMID: 14645776

Chevalier, O. (2024). Jeanne Barret, Hester Stanhope et Alexandra David-Néel: Les exploratrices au prisme du passing. *TRANS*, *29*. Advance online publication. DOI: 10.4000/trans.9058

Chida, Y., Sudo, N., Sonoda, J., Hiramoto, T., & Kubo, C. (2007). Early-life psychological stress exacerbates adult mouse asthma via the hypothalamus-pituitary-adrenal axis. *American Journal of Respiratory and Critical Care Medicine*, *175*(4), 316–322. DOI: 10.1164/rccm.200607-898OC PMID: 17110645

Chijiwa, T., Oka, T., Tominaga, M., Matsumura, S., Tsuzuki, S., Iida, H., & Fuchigami, T. (2015). Prior chronic stress induces persistent polyI:C-induced allodynia and depressive-like behavior in rats: Possible involvement of glucocorticoids and microglia. *Physiology & Behavior*, *147*, 264–273. https://www.sciencedirect.com/science/article/abs/pii/S0031938415002577?via%3Dihub PMID: 25936823

Chklovski, V. (2008). *L'art comme procédé*. Editions Allia.

Cinelli, G. (2022). *Le guerre di Mario Rigoni Stern. Trauma, racconto, guarigione* [The Wars of Mario Rigoni Stern. Trauma, Narrative, and Healing]. Morlacchi.

Ciompi, L., & Hoffmann, H. (2004). Soteria Berne: An innovative milieu therapeutic approach to acute schizophrenia based on the concept of affect-logic. *World Psychiatry; Official Journal of the World Psychiatric Association (WPA), 3*(3), 140–146. PMID: 16633478

Cirillo, F., Spina, G., Irrera, M., Bozzola, E., Mascolo, C., Gargiullo, L., Burla, V., Roversi, M., Carlevaris, C. M., Dusi, S., Pretelli, I., & Marchili, M. R. (2025). The Impact of Expressive Arts Therapy on Alexithymia Levels in Adolescent Inpatients with Severe Anorexia Nervosa. *Children (Basel, Switzerland), 12*(10). PMID: 41153576

Clauw, D. J. (2014). Fibromyalgia: A clinical review. *Journal of the American Medical Association, 311*(15), 1547–1555. DOI: 10.1001/jama.2014.3266 PMID: 24737367

Clonts, C. (2021). La Poésie Pratique de Ghérasim Luca. *Études des Lettres Françaises*, 56, 15–32. DOI: 10.20767/ELFK.56.0_15

Clonts, C., Kishimoto, H., NIU, T., Kawata, N., & Yokota, F. (2026). Art-Yoga for well-being, awareness and self-care in higher education: First data analysis of a pilot study in a Japanese university. [Bulletin of KIKAN Education], 12, 131-147. DOI: 10.15017/7405176

Clonts, C. (2016). L'Avant–garde bucarestoise: Alge, de la revue à l'affiche. In *LiVres de pOésie Jeux d'eSpace* (pp. 279–305). Honoré Champion.

Clonts, C. (2020). *Gherasim Luca: Texte, Image, Son*. Peter Lang. DOI: 10.3726/b17339

Clough, P. T. (Ed.). (2007). *The Affective Turn*. Duke University Press.

Clüver, C. (2018). On Gazers' Encounters with Visual Art: Ekphrasis, Readers, 'Iconotexts'. In Kennedy, D., & Meek, R. (Eds.), *Ekphrastic Encounters: New Interdisciplinary Essays on Literature and the Visual Arts* (pp. 237–256).

Cole, E. (1967). *House of Bondage*. Ridge Press/Random House.

Collins, R. L., Taylor, S. E., & Skokan, L. A. (1990). A Better World or a Shattered Vision? Changes in Life Perspectives Following Victimization. *Social Cognition, 8*(3). Advance online publication. DOI: 10.1521/soco.1990.8.3.263

Cometa, M. (2024). *The Literary Life of Pictures: A Theory of Description* (1st ed. 2024). Springer Nature Switzerland. DOI: 10.1007/978-3-031-52897-2

Confino, D., Einav, M., & Margalit, M. (2023). Post-traumatic growth: the roles of the sense of entitlement, gratitude and hope. *International Journal of Applied Positive Psychology*, *8*(2). Advance online publication. DOI: 10.1007/s41042-023-00102-9 PMID: 37361623

Cormio, , CMuzzatti, , BRomito, , FMattioli, , VAnnunziata, , M. A. (2017). Post-traumatic growth and cancer: a study 5 years after treatment end. *Supportive Care in Cancer*, *25*(4). https://doi.org/10.1007/s00520-016-3496-4

Corrao, S. (2005). L'intervista nella ricerca sociale [The interview in social research]. *Quaderni di Sociologia*, *38*, 147–171.

Correll, A. B., Correll, T. L., & Correll, M. C. (2024). Literary Prescriptions: Applying Bibliotherapy in a Psychotherapeutic Context. *Innovations in Clinical Neuroscience*, *21*(7-9), 15–21. PMID: 39329026

Craig, A. D. (2002). How do you feel? Interoception: The sense of the physiological condition of the body. *Nature Reviews. Neuroscience*, *3*(8), 655–666. DOI: 10.1038/nrn894 PMID: 12154366

Critchley, H. D., Corfield, D. R., Chandler, M. P., Mathias, C. J., & Dolan, R. J. (2000). Cerebral correlates of autonomic cardiovascular arousal: A functional neuroimaging investigation in humans. *The Journal of Physiology*, *523*(Pt 1), 259–270. DOI: 10.1111/j.1469-7793.2000.t01-1-00259.x PMID: 10673560

Critchley, H. D., Mathias, C. J., Josephs, O., O'Doherty, J., Zanini, S., Dewar, B. K., Cipolotti, L., Shallice, T., & Dolan, R. J. (2003). Human cingulate cortex and autonomic control: Converging neuroimaging and clinical evidence. *Brain*, *126*(Pt. 10), 2139–2152. DOI: 10.1093/brain/awg216 PMID: 12821513

Critchley, H. D., Tang, J., Smyth, S., Mathias, C. J., & Dolan, R. J. (2005). Anterior cingulate activity during error and autonomic response. *NeuroImage*, *27*(4), 885–895. DOI: 10.1016/j.neuroimage.2005.05.047 PMID: 15996878

Critchley, H. D., Wiens, S., Rotshtein, P., Öhman, A., & Dolan, R. J. (2004). Neural systems supporting interoceptive awareness. *Nature Neuroscience*, *7*(2), 189–195. DOI: 10.1038/nn1176 PMID: 14730305

Crothers, S. M. (1916, September). Literary Clinic. *Atlantic Monthly*.

Cruz, D., Lichten, M., Berg, K., & George, P. (2022). Developmental trauma: Conceptual framework, associated risks and comorbidities, and evaluation and treatment. *Frontiers in Psychiatry*, *13*, 800687. DOI: 10.3389/fpsyt.2022.800687 PMID: 35935425

Csikszentmihalyi, M. (1990). *Flow: The psychology of optimal experience.* HarperCollins.

Cuijpers, P., Karyotaki, E., Weitz, E., Andersson, G., Hollon, S. D., & van Straten, A. (2014). The effects of psychotherapies for major depression in adults on remission, recovery and improvement: A meta-analysis. *Journal of Affective Disorders, 159*, 118–126. DOI: 10.1016/j.jad.2014.02.026 PMID: 24679399

Cushing, R., Braun, K., Alden, S., & Katz, A. (2018). Military-Tailored Yoga for Veterans with Post-traumatic Stress Disorder. *Military Medicine, 183*(5/6), e223–e231. PMID: 29415222

Daizen Victoria, B. (2006). *Zen at War.* Rowman and Littlefield.

Damasio, A. (2006). *Descartes' Error. Emotion, Reason and the Human Brain.* Vintage. (Original work published 1994)

Damasio, A. (2010). *Self Comes to Mind. Constructing the Conscious Brain.* Pantheon.

David-Néel, A. (1975). *Lettres à son mari. Journal de voyage 11 août 1904-31 décembre 1940.* Plon.

David-Néel, A. (1983). *Voyage d'une Parisienne à Lhassa: A pied et en mendiant, de la Chine à l'Inde à travers le Tibet.* Plon.

David-Néel, A. (2024). *Souvenirs d'une Parisienne au Thibet.* Plon.

David-Néel, A., & Aphur, Y. (2004). *Dieux et démons des solitudes tibétaines.* Plon.

de Almeida, I., & Nakao, G. (2021). Amae, an emotion to understand the Japanese psyche. [Otemon Gakuin University Business Society.]. *Otemon Business Management Review*, *27*(1), 145–154.

De Marinis, M. (2000). *In cerca dell'attore. Un bilancio del Novecento teatrale.* Bulzoni.

De Rogatis, T. (2018). *Elena Ferrante: Parole chiave.* Edizioni e/o.

Delaunay, J. (2015). Alexandra David-Néel: Bouddhisme et drapeau noir. *BALLAST: stand up, federate, initiate, 4*(1), 126-142.

Deleuze, G. (1981). *Francis Bacon—Logic of Sensation* (Vol. 1). La Différence.

Demanze, L. (2014). *Les vies romanesques d'Emmanuel Carrère.* Roman 20-50, 57(1), 5–14. https://doi.org/DOI: 10.3917/r2050.057.0005

Demanze, L. (2019). *Expériences de terrain, terrain d'expérimentation*. Revue critique de fixxion française contemporaine, 18, Article 18. https://doi.org/DOI: 10.4000/fixxion.1513

Demos, E. V. (2019). *The Affect Theory of Silvan Tomkins for Psychoanalysis and Psychotherapy: Recasting the Essentials*. Routledge.

Descartes, R. (1996). *Meditations on first philosophy: With selections from the objections and replies* (Cottingham, J., Ed. & Trans.). Cambridge University Press.

Despret, V. (2009). *Penser comme un rat*. Editions Quae.

Despret, V. (2015). *Au bonheur des morts. Récits de ceux qui restent*. La Découverte.

Despret, V. (2021). *Our Grateful Dead. Stories of Those Left Behind*. University of Minnesota Press.

Detrixhe, J. J. (2010). Souls in Jeopardy: Questions and Innovations for Bibliotherapy With Fiction. *The Journal of Humanistic Counseling, Education and Development*, *49*, 58–72. DOI: 10.1002/j.2161-1939.2010.tb00087.x

Devinsky, O., Morrell, M. J., & Vogt, B. A. (1995). Contributions of anterior cingulate cortex to behaviour. *Brain*, *118*(Pt 1), 279–306. DOI: 10.1093/brain/118.1.279 PMID: 7895011

Dewey, J. (1938). Logic: The theory of inquiry. In Boydston, J. A. (Ed.), *The later works of John Dewey, 1925–1953* (Vol. 12, pp. 1–528). Southern Illinois University Press.

Dewey, J. (1980). *Art as experience*. Perigee Books.

Dewey, J. (1997). *How we think*. Dover publications.

Dewey, J. (2005). *Art as Experience*. Penguin.

Diniz, , GKorkes, , LTristão, , L. SPelegrini, , RBellodi, , P. LBernardo, , W. M. (2023). The effects of gratitude interventions: a systematic review and meta-analysis. *Einstein (Sao Paulo)*, *21*.

Dixit, S. K., & Sinha, J. (n.d.) Efficacy of Gratitude Intervention in India: Distinctive Cross-Cultural Conceptions of Gratitude Matter. *Psychological Studies*.

Doi, T. (1973). *The Anatomy of dependence*. Kodansha International.

Dolan, P., & White, M. P. (2007). How can measures of subjective well-being be used to inform public policy? *Perspectives on Psychological Science*, *2*(1), 71–85. DOI: 10.1111/j.1745-6916.2007.00030.x PMID: 26151920

Dong, Y., Mak, M. H., Hepach, R., & Nation, K. (2025). Learning new words via reading: The influence of emotional narrative context on learning novel adjectives. *Quarterly Journal of Experimental Psychology, 78*(10), 2167–2180. DOI: 10.1177/17470218241308221 PMID: 39641281

Drewes, , JLanger, , P. CEbert, , JKleiber, , D., & Gusy, B. (2021). Associations between experienced and internalized HIV stigma, adversarial growth, and health outcomes in a nationwide sample of people aging with HIV in Germany. *AIDS and Behavior, 25*(4), 1037-1046.

Duan, C., & Hill, C. E. (1996). The current state of empathy research. *Journal of Counseling Psychology, 43*(3), 261–274. DOI: 10.1037/0022-0167.43.3.261

Duke, M. P., Lazarus, A., & Fivush, R. (2008). Knowledge of family history as a clinically useful index of psychological well-being and prognosis: A brief report. *Psychotherapy (Chicago, Ill.), 45*(2), 268–272. DOI: 10.1037/0033-3204.45.2.268 PMID: 22122420

Duro, J.-M. (2014). *I am a cloud*. Self-published.

Duro, J.-M. (2019). *Looking for my Japanese Family*. Self-published.

Eisenberger, N. I. (2012). The pain of social disconnection: Examining the shared neural underpinnings of physical and social pain. *Nature Reviews. Neuroscience, 13*(6), 421–434. DOI: 10.1038/nrn3231 PMID: 22551663

Eisenberger, N. I., Lieberman, M. D., & Williams, K. D. (2004). Why rejection hurts: A common neural alarm system for physical and social pain. *Trends in Cognitive Sciences, 8*(7), 294–300. DOI: 10.1016/j.tics.2004.05.010 PMID: 15242688

El Khoury-Malhame, M., Sfeir, M., Hallit, S., & Sawma, T. (2023). Factors associated with posttraumatic growth: Gratitude, PTSD and distress; one year into the COVID-19 pandemic in Lebanon. *Current Psychology (New Brunswick, N.J.)*. Advance online publication. DOI: 10.1007/s12144-022-04159-8 PMID: 36684466

Elias, A., & Brown, A. D. (2022). The role of intergenerational family stories in mental health and wellbeing. *Frontiers in Psychology, 13*. Advance online publication. DOI: 10.3389/fpsyg.2022.927795 PMID: 36237680

Emery, C. (2009). Research Design for Evaluation Studies. In Verhagen, E., van Mechelen, W. (eds.), Oxford Academic, Sports Injury Research. DOI: 10.1093/acprof:oso/9780199561629.003.013

Emmons, R. A., & McCullough, M. E. (2003). Counting blessings versus burdens: An experimental investigation of gratitude and subjective well-being in daily life. *Journal of Personality and Social Psychology, 84*(2), 377–389. PMID: 12585811

Espagne, M., & Werner, M. (Eds.). (1988). *Transferts. Les relations franco-allemandes dans l'espace francoallemand.* Éditions Recherche sur les civilisations.

European Commission. (2024). *Türkiye Report. 2024 Communication on EU enlargement policy.* EU Publishing.

Evans, J. (2012). *Philosophy for Life And Other Dangerous Situations.* Ebury Publishing.

Fagley, N. S. (2012). Appreciation uniquely predicts life satisfaction above demographics, the Big 5 personality factors, and gratitude. *Personality and Individual Differences, 53*(1). Advance online publication. DOI: 10.1016/j.paid.2012.02.019

Falk, E. B., O'Donnell, M. B., Cascio, C. N., Tinney, F., Kang, Y., Lieberman, M. D., Taylor, S. E., An, L., Resnicow, K., & Strecher, V. J. (2015). Self-affirmation alters the brain's response to health messages and subsequent behavior change. *Proceedings of the National Academy of Sciences of the United States of America, 112*(7), 1977–1982. DOI: 10.1073/pnas.1500247112 PMID: 25646442

Fancourt, D., & Finn, S. (2019). What is the evidence on the role of the arts in improving health and well-being? A scoping review. WHO Regional Office for Europe. *Health Evidence Network Synthesis, 67,* 1–133.

Fanon, F. (2004). *The Wretched of the Earth* (Philcox, R., Trans.). Grove Press. (Original work published 1961)

Fanon, F. (2020). *The Psychiatric Writings from Alienation and Freedom* (Khalfa, J., & Young, R. J. C., Eds.). Bloomsbury Academic.

Favret-Saada, J. (1977). *Les mots, la mort, les sorts.* Gallimard.

Ferber, R. (2007). What did Socrates know and how did he know it? In L. Brisson & M. Erler (Eds.), *Gorgias, Meno: Selected papers from the Seventh Symposium Platonicum* (pp. 263–267). Academia Verlag.

Ferrante, E. (1992). *L'amore molesto.* Edizionie/o.

Ferrante, E. (2016a). *Frantumaglia: A Writer's Journey* (A. Goldstein, Trans.; Unabridged and updated edition). Europa Editions.

Ferrante, E. (2016b). *La frantumaglia: Carte (1991-2003), Tessere (2003-2007), Lettere (2011-2016).* Edizioni e/o.

Ferrante, E. (2021). *I margini e il dettato*. Edizioni e/o.

Ferrante, E. (2006). *Troubling Love* (1st ed.). (Goldstein, A., Trans.). Europa Editions.

Ferrari, F. (2007). Socrate e la filosofia. In Ferrari, F. (Ed.), *Socrate tra personaggio e mito* (pp. 11–86). Rizzoli.

Finley, A. J., & Crowell, A. L. (2018). Self-affirmation enhances processing of negative stimuli among threat-prone individuals. *Social Cognitive and Affective Neuroscience, 13*(6), 569–580. DOI: 10.1093/scan/nsy045 PMID: 29873770

Fischer-Lichte, E. (2008). *The Transformative Power of performance. A new aesthetics*. Routledge.

Fischer-Lichte, E. (2008). *The transformative power of performance: A new aesthetics*. Routledge.

Fivush, R. (2008). Remembering and reminiscing: How individual lives are constructed in family narratives. *Memory Studies, 1*(1), 49–58. DOI: 10.1177/1750698007083888

Folkman, S. (1997). Positive psychological states and coping with severe stress. *Social Science & Medicine, 45*(8). Advance online publication. DOI: 10.1016/S0277-9536(97)00040-3 PMID: 9381234

Fondazione Isabella Scelsi. (n.d.). *Biography of Giacinto Scelsi*. Fondazione Isabella Scelsi. Retrieved from https://www.scelsi.it/en/biography/

Fornell, C., & Larcker, D. F. (1981). Fornell, C. and Larcker, D.F. (1981), "Evaluating structural equation models with unobservable variables and.pdf. *JMR, Journal of Marketing Research, XVIII*(February).

Fossion, P., Rejas, M. C., Servais, L., Pelc, I., & Hirsch, S. (2014). Transgenerational transmission of trauma in families of Holocaust survivors. *Journal of Affective Disorders, 171*, 48–53. PMID: 25285898

Foucault, M. (1984). *Le souci de soi*. Gallimard.

Fox, K. C. R., Nijeboer, S., Dixon, M. L., Floman, J. L., Ellamil, M., Rumak, S. P., Sedlmeier, P., & Christoff, K. (2014). Is meditation associated with altered brain structure? A systematic review and meta-analysis of morphometric neuroimaging in meditation practitioners. *Neuroscience and Biobehavioral Reviews, 43*, 48–73. DOI: 10.1016/j.neubiorev.2014.03.016 PMID: 24705269

Frank, A. J., & Wilson, E. A. (2020). *A Silvan Tomkins Handbook: Foundations for Affect Theory*. University of Minnesota Press. DOI: 10.5749/j.ctv182jthz

Frayling, C. 1993. Research in Art and Design. *Royal College of Art Research Papers* 1(1). https://researchonline.rca.ac.uk/id/eprint/384

Fredrickson, B. L. (2004). The broaden-and-build theory of positive emotions. *Philosophical Transactions of the Royal Society of London. Series B, Biological Sciences, 359*(1449), 1367–1378. PMID: 15347528

Fredrickson, B. L., Tugade, M. M., Waugh, C. E., & Larkin, G. R. (2003). What Good Are Positive Emotions in Crises? A Prospective Study of Resilience and Emotions Following the Terrorist attacks on the United States on September 11th, 2001. *Journal of Personality and Social Psychology, 84*(2). Advance online publication. DOI: 10.1037/0022-3514.84.2.365 PMID: 12585810

Freud, S. (1924). *Further recommendations in the technique of psycho-analysis: recollection, repetition, and working-through. Collected papers: clinical papers, papers on technique* (Riviere, J., Trans.). Hogarth Press.

Fritscher, L. (2023, November 9). Taijin kyofusho, a culture-bound social phobia. This form of anxiety is mostly found in Japan. *Verywellmind.* https://www.verywellmind.com/taijin-kyofusho-2671839

Fujiwara, D., Kudrna, L., & Dolan, P. (2014). Quantifying and Valuing the Well-Being Impacts of Culture and Sport. UK Government Department of Culture and Sport Report. 1-45.

Furini, F. (1626). *Pittura e Poesia* (Palazzo Pitti, Galleria Palatina, Sala di Berenice) [Oil painting on canvas]. https://www.uffizi.it/opere/pittura-e-poesia

Fu, Y., Yang, J., Bermúdez-Margaretto, B., Wang, H., Cordón, D. E. J., & Domínguez, A. (2025). From eye to cortex: Tracing the neurocognitive dynamics of bilingual novel word acquisition. *Brain and Language, 270*. Advance online publication. DOI: 10.1016/j.bandl.2025.105632 PMID: 40865422

Fynn, J., Hardeman, W., Milton, K., Murphy, J., & Jones, A. (2020). A systematic review of the use and reporting of evaluation frameworks within evaluations of physical activity interventions. *The International Journal of Behavioral Nutrition and Physical Activity, 17*(107), 1–17. DOI: 10.1186/s12966-020-01013-7 PMID: 32831111

Gadamer, H.-G. (2006). *Truth and method.* Continuum.

Gallagher, S. (2000). Philosophical Conceptions of the Self: Implications for Cognitive Science. *Trends in Cognitive Sciences, 4*(1), 14–21. PMID: 10637618

Gamage, B., Gamage, M. N., Perera, N. M., Kodikara, C. S., Wijeratne, J. U. M., Seneviratne Alles, S. M. D. P., Kumaran, T., Jeewandara, J. M. C., & Mahawithanage, S. T. C. (2024). Impact of mindfulness-based tri-modal prehabilitation on functional recovery and selected surgical outcomes of patients with colorectal cancer admitted to surgical hospital wards. *BMJ Open*, *14*. Advance online publication. DOI: 10.1136/bmjopen-2023-080192 PMID: 39806718

García, H., & Miralles, F. (2017). *Ikigai. The Japanese Secret to a Long and Happy Life*. Penguin.

García, H., & Miralles, F. (2017). *Ikigai: The Japanese secret to a long and happy life*. Penguin.

Gariglio, L. (2024). On fieldwork in the hybrid field: A "methodological novel" on ethnography, photography, fiction, and creative writing. *Qualitative Research*, *24*(2), 444–456. DOI: 10.1177/14687941221149584

Garth, S. J., & O'Donnell, V. (2015). *Propaganda and persuasion*. SAGE Publications.

Garvey, P. (2023). *Melanie Klein: A Contemporary Introduction* (1st ed.). Routledge. DOI: 10.4324/9781003215714

Gauvin, L. (Ed.). (2009). *L'écrivain francophone à la croisée des langues: Entretiens*. Karthala., DOI: 10.3917/kart.undef.2009.02

Gebhardt, L., & Masami, Y. (2014). *Literature and art after Fukushima. four approaches*. EBVerlag.

Ghanem, Z. Y. (2024). The process of healing individual and communal traumatic experiences through natural and cultural reconnection in Silko's *Ceremony*. *International Journal of Undergraduate Research and Creative Activities*, *16*(1), 6. DOI: 10.61809/2168-0620.1339

Gladstein, G. A. (1977). Empathy and counseling outcome: An empirical and conceptual review. *The Counseling Psychologist*, *6*(4), 70–79. 10.1177/001100007700600427

Gnoli, R. (1994). *Iniziazione= Kālacakra*. Adelphi.

Gomes, N., Cochet, S., & Guyon, A. (2020). Dance and embodiment: Therapeutic benefits on body-mind health. *Journal of Interdisciplinary Methodologies and Issues in Science*, *9*, 1–23. DOI: 10.18713/JIMIS-02072021-9-4

Goodkind, M., Eickhoff, S. B., Oathes, D. J., Jiang, Y., Chang, A., Jones-Hagata, L. B., Ortega, B. N., Zaiko, Y. V., Roach, E. L., Korgaonkar, M. S., Grieve, S. M., Galatzer-Levy, I., Fox, P. T., & Etkin, A. (2015). Identification of a common neurobiological substrate for mental illness. *JAMA Psychiatry*, *72*(4), 305–315. DOI: 10.1001/jamapsychiatry.2014.2206 PMID: 25651064

Gorelick, K. (1987). Greek tragedy and ancient healing. *Journal of Poetry Therapy*, *1*(1), 38–43.

Gotink, R. A., Meijboom, R., Vernooij, M. W., Smits, M., & Hunink, M. G. M. (2016). 8-week mindfulness based stress reduction induces brain changes similar to traditional long-term meditation practice—A systematic review. *Brain and Cognition*, *108*, 32–41. DOI: 10.1016/j.bandc.2016.07.001 PMID: 27429096

Gottschall, J. (2012). *The storytelling animal: How stories make us human*. Houghton Mifflin Harcourt.

Gouirir, M. (1998). L'observatrice, indigène ou invitée? Enquêter dans un univers familier. *Genèses*, *32*(1), 110–126. DOI: 10.3406/genes.1998.1527

Gramsci, A. (1992). *Selections from the prison notebooks of Antonio Gramsci* (Hoare, Q., & Nowell Smith, G., Eds.). International Publishers.

Green, K. (2020). *Rethinking Therapeutic Reading: Lessons from Senecca, Montaigne, Wordsworth and George Eliot*. Anthem Press.

Grensman, A., Acharya, B. D., Wändell, P., Nilsson, G. H., Falkenberg, T., Sundin, Ö., & Werner, S. (2018). Effect of traditional yoga, mindfulness-based cognitive therapy, and cognitive behavioral therapy, on health related quality of life: A randomized controlled trial on patients on sick leave because of burnout. *BMC Complementary and Alternative Medicine*, *18*(1), 80. Advance online publication. DOI: 10.1186/s12906-018-2141-9 PMID: 29510704

Gribaudi, G. (2005). *Guerra totale. Tra bombe alleate e violenze naziste. Napoli e il fronte meridionale 1940-1944*. Bollati Boringhieri.

Groessl, E. J., Weingartn, K. R., Aschbacher, K., Pada, L., & Baxi, S. (2008). Yoga for veterans with chronic low-back pain. *Journal of Alternative and Complementary Medicine (New York, N.Y.)*, *14*(9), 1123–1129. DOI: 10.1089/acm.2008.0020 PMID: 18991515

Grotowski, J. (2007). Dalla compagnia teatrale a L'arte come veicolo (1993). In Attisani, A., & Biagini, M. (Eds.), *J. Grotowski, Testi 1968-1998* (pp. 89–113). Bulzoni.

Grutman, R. (2019). *Des langues qui résonnent: L'hétérolinguisme au XIX*[e] *siècle québécois* [*Languages that resonate: Heterolingualism in 19*[th] *Century Quebec*]. Classiques Garnier.

Guaccero, D. (2005a). *"Un iter segnato". Scritti e interviste* (Mastropietro, A., Ed.). Ricordi-LIM.

Guaccero, D. (2005b). Postilla sul teatro musicale (1966). In Mastropietro, A. (Ed.), *D. Guaccero, "Un iter segnato". Scritti e interviste* (pp. 161–171). Ricordi-LIM.

Gualano, M. R., Bert, F., Martorana, M., Voglino, G., Andriolo, V., Thomas, R., Gramaglia, C., Zeppegno, P., & Siliquini, R. (2017). The long-term effects of bibliotherapy in depression treatment: Systematic eview of randomized clinical trials. *Clinical Psychology Review*, *58*, 49–58. DOI: 10.1016/j.cpr.2017.09.006 PMID: 28993103

Guanti, G. (1999). *Estetica musicale. La storia e le fonti*. La Nuova Italia.

Guerra, C., & Masó, J. (Eds.). (2021). *La Déconniatrie: art, exil et psychiatrie autour de François Tosquelles*. Arcàdia.

Guide to the use of yoga for stress-related illnesses for medical professionals [in Japanese]. (2025). Evidence-based Japanese Integrative Medicine Information Site. https://www.ejim.mhlw.go.jp/doc/pdf/y01.pdf

Guillemin, M. (2004). Understanding illness: Using drawings as a research method. *Qualitative Health Research*, *15*(2), 272–289. DOI: 10.1177/1049732303260445 PMID: 14768462

Hadot, P. (1987). *Spiritual exercises and ancient philosophy*. Études Augustiniennes.

Haibloom, S. (2012). *Taijin kyofusho: what clinicians need to know* [Doctoral dissertation, Alliant International University–Los Angeles]. DOI: 10.13140/2.1.4420.2249

Hair, J. F., Risher, J. J., Sarstedt, M., & Ringle, C. M. (2019). When to use and how to report the results of PLS-SEM. In *European Business Review* (Vol. 31, Issue 1). DOI: 10.1108/EBR-11-2018-0203

Hair, J. F.Jr, Hult, G. T. M., Ringle, C. M., & Sarstedt, M. (2021). A primer on partial least squares structural equations modeling (PLS-SEM). Sage Publications. *Journal of Tourism Research*, *6*(2).

Han, B-C. (2024, March 20). The disenchantment of the world. *The Paris Review*. https://www.theparisreview.org/blog/2024/03/20/the-disenchantment-of-the-world/

Han, Y. Y., Yan, Q., Forno, E., Cortez, M., & Celedón, J. C. (2022). Child maltreatment, anxiety and depression, and asthma among British adults in the UK Biobank. *The European Respiratory Journal*, *60*(4), 2103160. Advance online publication. DOI: 10.1183/13993003.03160-2021 PMID: 35301250

Hao, Y., Zhao, H., Bai, R., Xu, Z., Feng, Y., & Gu, H. (2025). Thirty–year trends in anxiety disorders incidence across China, Japan, and Republic of Korea: An age–period–cohort analysis based on GBD 2021. *Health Care*, *13*(12), 1376. DOI: 10.3390/healthcare13121376 PMID: 40565403

Haraway, D. (1988). Situated Knowledges: The Science Question in Feminism and the Privilege of Partial Perspective. *Feminist Studies*, *14*(3), 575–599. DOI: 10.2307/3178066

Harding, S. (1986). *The Science Question in Feminism*. Cornell University Press.

Harding, S. (1991). *Whose Science? Whose Knowledge? Thinking from Women's Lives*. Cornell University Press.

Harding, S. (2015). *Objectivity and Diversity. Another Logic of Scientific Research*. The University of Chicago Press.

Harper, A. R., & Pargament, K. I. (2015). Trauma, religion, and spirituality: Pathways to healing. In Pargament, K. I. (Ed.), Vol. 2, pp. 349–367). APA handbook of psychology, religion, and spirituality. Springer., DOI: 10.1007/978-3-319-18866-9_19

Harré, R. (2003). Grammaire et lexiques, vecteurs des représentations sociales. [Grammar and lexicons, media of social representations] In Jodelet, D. (Ed.), *Les représentations sociales* [*Social representations*]. (pp. 149–169). Presses Universitaires de France. DOI: 10.3917/puf.jodel.2003.01.0149

Hashimoto, A. (2015). *The Long Defeat. Cultural Trauma, Memory, and Identity in Japan*. Oxford University Press.

Hashimoto, A. (2015). *The long defeat: Cultural trauma, memory, and identity in Japan*. Oxford University Press.

Hass-Cohen, N. (2003). Art Therapy Mind Body Approaches: Some Applications of Relational Neuroscience to Art Therapy. *Progress: Family Systems Research and Therapy*, *12*, 24–38.

Havelange, C. (2014). *Plaidoyer pour une recherche-compagne* [conference presentation]. 9e édition des Ateliers de la Recherche en Design (ARD), Liège, Belgium. https://hdl.handle.net/2268/175916

Havelange, C. (2018). *Gaspard – Une écriture ouvrière au XIXe siècle*. Les presses du réel.

Havelange, C. (2022). *La recherche-création: remarques rétrospectives sur le doctorat en art et sciences de l'art* [Conference presentation]. La recherche-création avec Yves Citton, Louvain-la-Neuve, Belgium. https://hdl.handle.net/2268/297848

Heart, M. Y. H. B. (2003). The historical trauma response among natives and its relationship with substance abuse: A Lakota illustration. *Journal of Psychoactive Drugs*, *35*(1), 7–13. DOI: 10.1080/02791072.2003.10399988 PMID: 12733753

Hebdige, D. (1994). *Subculture, the meaning of style*. Routlege.

Heeren, , AMcNally, , R. J. (2016). An integrative network approach to social anxiety disorder: the complex dynamic interplay among attentional bias for threat, attentional control, and symptoms. *Journal of Anxiety Disorders, 42*, 95–104. https://doi.org/10.1016/j.janxdis.2016.06.009

Heffernan, J. A. W. (1993). *Museum of words: The poetics of ekphrasis from Homer to Ashbery*. University of Chicago Press.

Heffernan, J. A. W. (2015). Ekphrasis: Theory. In Rippl, G. (Ed.), *Handbook of Intermediality: Literature—Image—Sound—Music* (pp. 35–49). De Gruyter.

Heiman, M., Strnad, D., Weiland, W., & Wise, T. N. (1994). Art Therapy and Alexithymia. *Art Therapy: Journal of the American Art Therapy Association, 11*(2), 143–146. DOI: 10.1080/07421656.1994.10759067

Henson, C., Truchot, D., & Canevello, A. (2021). What promotes post traumatic growth? A systematic review. In *European Journal of Trauma and Dissociation* (Vol. 5, Issue 4). DOI: 10.1016/j.ejtd.2020.100195

Heraclitus, . (1987). *Fragments*. University of Toronto Press.

Herrera, B.M., & Vargas, P.C. (2019). Benefits of Mental Practice in Sport Practice. *Apunts. Educació Física i Esports*, 35 (135), 82–99. DOI: 10.5672/apunts.2014-0983.es

Higgins, K. (2003). Comparative aesthetics. In Levinson, J. (Ed.), *The Oxford handbook of aesthetics* (pp. 679–692). Oxford University Press. DOI: 10.1093/oxfordhb/9780199279456.003.0040

Hirsch, J.-P. (26th October 2018). *Ryoko Sekiguchi Nagori* [Video]. YouTube. https://www.youtube.com/watch?v=4WT2K9jJadM

Hirsch, M. (1997). *Family frames: Photography, narrative, and postmemory*. Harvard University Press.

Hirsch, M. (2008). The Generation of Postmemory. *Poetics Today*, *29*(1), 103–128. DOI: 10.1215/03335372-2007-019

Hirsch, M. (2012). *The generation of postmemory: Writing and visual culture after the Holocaust*. Columbia University Press.

Hofmann, S. G., Asnaani, A., & Hinton, D. E. (2010). Cultural aspects in social anxiety and social anxiety disorder. *Depression and Anxiety*, *27*(12), 1117–1127. DOI: 10.1002/da.20759 PMID: 21132847

Hofstede, G. (2001). *Culture's consequences: comparing values, behaviors, institutions, and organizations across nations*. SAGE Publications.

Hubaut, J. (2006). *Joël Hubaut, Re–mix épidémik—Esthétique de la dispersion*. Les Presses du Réel.

Hunt, W. A. (1941). Recent Developments in the Field of Emotions. *Psychological Bulletin*, *38*(5), 249–276. DOI: 10.1037/h0054615

Incardona, F. (2018). Presentazione (1989). In F. Incardona, *Scritti critici e di poetica* (S. Lombardi Vallauri, Ed.; with the collaboration of M. Crescimanno & M. Spagnolo; pp. 119–125). Aracne.

Information, M., & Chin, W. W. (2013). Commentary Issues and Opinion on Structural Equation Modeling. *Management Information Systems Quarterly*, *22*(1).

Ingemark, C. A. (Ed.). (2013). *Therapeutic uses of storytelling: An interdisciplinary approach*. Nordic Academic Press.

Ishikawa, H., Kawakami, N., & Kessler, R. C. (2016). Lifetime and 12-month prevalence, severity and unmet need for treatment of common mental disorders in Japan: Results from the final dataset of world mental health Japan survey. *Epidemiology and Psychiatric Sciences*, *25*(3), 217–229. DOI: 10.1017/S2045796015000566 PMID: 26148821

Iwabuchi, K. (2002). *Recentering Globalization: Popular Culture and Japanese Transnationalism*. Duke University Press.

Iwata, Y., Suzuki, K., Takei, N., Toulopoulou, T., Tsuchiya, K. J., Matsumoto, K., Takagai, S., Oshiro, M., Nakamura, K., & Mori, N. (2011). Jiko-shisen-kyofu (Fear of One's Own Glance), but not taijin-kyofusho (Fear of Interpersonal Relations), is an east Asian culture-related specific syndrome. *The Australian and New Zealand Journal of Psychiatry*, *45*(2), 148–152. DOI: 10.3109/00048674.2010.534068 PMID: 21091156

Jackson, J. C., & Lindquist, K. (in press). Origins and Consequences of Cultural Variation in Emotion Vocabulary. In Yik, M. (Ed.), *The Oxford Handbook of Emotion and Culture*. Oxford University Press.

Jankélévitch, V. (1963). La méconnaissance. *Revue de Metaphysique et de Morale*, *68*(4), 389–406. https://www.jstor.org/stable/40900772

Jans-Beken, L., Jacobs, N., Janssens, M., Peeters, S., Reijnders, J., Lechner, L., & Lataster, J. (2020). Gratitude and health: An updated review. *The Journal of Positive Psychology*, *15*(6). Advance online publication. DOI: 10.1080/17439760.2019.1651888

Jans-Beken, L., & Wong, P. T. P. (2021). Development and preliminary validation of the Existential Gratitude Scale (EGS). *Counselling Psychology Quarterly*, *34*(1). Advance online publication. DOI: 10.1080/09515070.2019.1656054

Jansson, M. (2018). Ekphrasis and Digital Media. *Poetics Today*, *39*(2), 299–318. DOI: 10.1215/03335372-4324468

Japan Mindfulness Association [in Japanese]. (2025). https://mindfulness.smoosy.atlas.jp/ja

Jenkins, R. (2000). Disenchantment, enchantment and re-enchantment. *Max Weber Studies*, *1*(1), 11–32.

Jolly, J. (2010). Florence L. Goodenough: Portrait of a psychologist. *Roeper Review*, *32*, 98–105. DOI: 10.1080/02783191003587884

Jones, M. P., & Creed, E. (2013). A multidimensional model of psychobiological interactions in functional dyspepsia: A structural equation modelling approach. *Gut*, *62*(11), 1573–1580. DOI: 10.1136/gutjnl-2012-302741 PMID: 22917658

Jöreskog, K. G. (1971). Simultaneous factor analysis in several populations. *Psychometrika*, *36*(4). Advance online publication. DOI: 10.1007/BF02291366

Joseph, S., & Linley, P. A. (2006). Growth following adversity: Theoretical perspectives and implications for clinical practice. *Clinical Psychology Review*, *26*(8). Advance online publication. DOI: 10.1016/j.cpr.2005.12.006 PMID: 16473442

Kabat-Zinn, J. (2016). *Mindfulness for Beginners*. Sounds True Editions.

Kadri, R. (2024, June 30). Repetition of spiritual mantra meditation: A review. *Jurnal Kajian Islam dan Turath Antara, 1*(1), Article 5204. https://doi.org/DOI: 10.51200/kitab.v1i1.5204

Kalland, A. (2002). Holism and Sustainability: Lessons from Japan. *Worldviews: Global Religions, Culture, and Ecology*, *6*(2), 145–158.

Kanesaki, H., Watanabe, K., Osugi, K., Ohara, H., Takada, K., & Kinoshita, M. (2023). Utility of scratch art therapy in adult epilepsy patients with difficulties in social adaptation. *Epileptic Disorders: International Epilepsy Journal with Videotape*, *25*(5), 702–711. DOI: 10.1002/epd2.20127 PMID: 37518932

Kaplan, J., Somohano, V. C., Zaccari, B., & O'Neil, M. E. (2024). Randomized controlled trials of mind–body interventions for post-traumatic stress disorder: A systematic review. *Frontiers in Psychology*, *14*, 1219296. DOI: 10.3389/fpsyg.2023.1219296 PMID: 38327501

Karjus, A., Blythe, R. A., Kirby, S., Wang, T., & Smith, K. (2021). Conceptual Similarity and Communicative Need Shape Colexification: An Experimental Study. *Cognitive Science*, *45*. Advance online publication. DOI: 10.1111/cogs.13035 PMID: 34491584

Kasahara-Kiritani, M., Matoba, T., Kikuzawa, S., Sakano, J., Sugiyama, K., Yamaki, C., Mochizuki, M., & Yamazaki, Y. (2018). Public perceptions toward mental illness in Japan. *Asian Journal of Psychiatry*, *35*, 55–60. DOI: 10.1016/j.ajp.2018.05.021 PMID: 29787953

Kasperek-Zimowska, B. J., Bednarek, A., Giguere, M., Orłowski, W., & Sawicka, M. (2021). The specificity of the use of bibliotherapy as an element of psychiatric rehabilitation in a group of patients suffering from schizophrenia. *Advances in Psychiatry and Neurology/Postępy Psychiatrii i Neurologii, 30*(4), 278–286. DOI: 10.5114/ppn.2021.111946

Katon, W. J., Richardson, L., Lozano, P., & McCauley, E. (2004). The relationship of asthma and anxiety disorders. *Psychosomatic Medicine*, *66*(3), 349–355. DOI: 10.1097/01.psy.0000126202.89941.2c PMID: 15184694

Kawai, K., Yamada, H., Tomioka, H., Iwanami, A., & Inamoto, A. (2023). Factors associated with physical restraints in a psychiatric unit in Japan: A retrospective study. *East Asian Archives of Psychiatry: Official Journal of the Hong Kong College of Psychiatrists*, *33*(4), 120–125. DOI: 10.12809/eaap2334 PMID: 38955784

Kawamichi, H., Yoshihara, K., Sasaki, A. T., Sugawara, S. K., Tanabe, H. C., Shinohara, R., Sugisawa, Y., Tokutake, K., Mochizuki, Y., Anme, T., & Sadato, N. (2015). Perceiving active listening activates the reward system and improves the impression of relevant experiences. *Social Neuroscience, 10*(1), 16–26. DOI: 10.1080/17470919.2014.954732 PMID: 25188354

Kearney, K., & Hyle, A. E. (2004). Drawing out emotions in organizations: The use of participant-produced drawings in qualitative inquiry. *Qualitative Research, 43*, 361–383. DOI: 10.1177/1468794104047234

Kennedy, D. (2016). *The Ekphrastic Encounter in Contemporary British Poetry and Elsewhere*. Routledge.

Kennedy, D., & Meek, R. (2018). Introduction: From paragone to encounter. In Kennedy, D., & Meek, R. (Eds.), *Ekphrastic encounters: New interdisciplinary essays on literature and the visual arts* (pp. 1–24). Manchester University Press.

Khalfa, J. (2009). Naissance de la négritude. *Les Temps Modernes, 656*(5), 38–63. DOI: 10.3917/ltm.656.0038

Kick, L., Stegmann, S., Diedrich, A., & Galatzer-Levy, I. (2024). Alexithymia as a mediator between adverse childhood events and the development of psychopathology: A meta-analysis. *Frontiers in Psychiatry, 15*, 1412229. https://www.frontiersin.org/journals/psychiatry/articles/10.3389/fpsyt.2024.1412229 PMID: 39011338

Kim, E., & Bae, S. (2019). Gratitude Moderates the Mediating Effect of Deliberate Rumination on the Relationship Between Intrusive Rumination and Post-traumatic Growth. *Frontiers in Psychology, 10*. Advance online publication. DOI: 10.3389/fpsyg.2019.02665 PMID: 31849774

Kim, S. H., Schneider, S. M., Kravitz, L., Mermier, C., & Burge, M. R. (2013). Mind-body practices for post-traumatic stress disorder. *Journal of Investigative Medicine, 61*(5), 827–834. DOI: 10.2310/JIM.0b013e3182906862 PMID: 23609463

King, A., Erickson, T., Giardino, N., Favorite, T., Rauch, S., Robinson, E., Kulkarni, M., & Liberzon, I. (2013). A Pilot Study of Group Mindfulness-Based Cognitive Therapy (MBCT) for Combat Veterans with Posttraumatic Stress Disorder (PTSD). *Depression and Anxiety, 30*, 638–645. PMID: 23596092

Kistler, A., Mariauzouls, C., & von Berlepsch, K. (1998). Fingertip temperature as an indicator for sympathetic responses. *International Journal of Psychophysiology, 29*(1), 35–41. DOI: 10.1016/S0167-8760(97)00087-1 PMID: 9641246

Kitayama, O. (2004). Cross-Cultural Varieties in Experiencing Affect. In Akhtar, S., & Blum, H. (Eds.), *The language of emotions: development, psychopathology, and technique* (pp. 155–174). Jason Aronson.

Kleim, B., & Ehlers, A. (2009). Evidence for a curvilinear relationship between posttraumatic growth and posttrauma depression and PTSD in assault survivors. *Journal of Traumatic Stress, 22*(1). Advance online publication. DOI: 10.1002/jts.20378 PMID: 19230007

Klein, C. (2024, January). *Mental health in Japan - statistics and facts.* Statista Japan Research Department. https://www.statista.com/topics/8609/mental-health-in-japan/#topicOverview

Klein, M. (1984). *Envy and gratitude, and other works, 1946-1963* (Free Press ed, Vol. 3). Free Press.

Klein, M. (1946). Notes on Some Schizoid Mechanisms. *The International Journal of Psycho-Analysis, XXVII*(3 & 4), 99–110. PMID: 20261821

Koch, S. C., & Fuchs, T. (2011). Embodied arts therapies. *The Arts in Psychotherapy, 38*(4), 276–280. DOI: 10.1016/j.aip.2011.08.007

Koike, S., Yamaguchi, S., Ohta, K., Ojio, Y., Watanabe, K., & Ando, S. (2017). Mental-health-related stigma among Japanese children and their parents and impact of renaming of schizophrenia. *Psychiatry and Clinical Neurosciences, 71*, 170–179. DOI: 10.1111/pcn.12423 PMID: 27470981

Koyama, A., Miyake, Y., Kawakami, N., Tsuchiya, M., Tachimori, H., & Takeshima, T.World Mental Health Japan Survey Group, 2002-2006. (2010). Lifetime prevalence, psychiatric comorbidity and demographic correlates of "hikikomori" in a community population in Japan. *Psychiatry Research, 176*(1), 69–74. DOI: 10.1016/j.psychres.2008.10.019 PMID: 20074814

Kramer, E. (1971). *Art as therapy with children.* Schocken Books.

Kreibig, S. D., Wilhelm, F. H., Roth, W. T., & Gross, J. J. (2007). Cardiovascular, electrodermal, and respiratory response patterns to fear- and sadness-inducing films. *Psychophysiology, 44*(5), 787–806. DOI: 10.1111/j.1469-8986.2007.00550.x PMID: 17598878

Krumhansl, C. L. (1997). An exploratory study of musical emotions and psychophysiology. *Canadian Journal of Experimental Psychology, 51*(4), 336–353. DOI: 10.1037/1196-1961.51.4.336 PMID: 9606949

Kundnani, H. (2011). Perpetrators and victims. *German Life and Letters, 64*(2), 272–282.

Kutty, N. (2022, October 17). Why making mental health care more accessible is particularly challenging in Japan. *World Economic Forum.* https://www.weforum.org/agenda/2022/10/japans-challenges-in-making-mental-health-more-accessible/

Lacan, J. (2001). *Autres écrits.* Le Seuil.

LaCapra, D. (1994). *Representing the Holocaust: History, theory, trauma.* Cornell University Press.

Lakoff, G., & Johnson, M. (1980). *Metaphors We Live By.* University of Chicago Press.

Lakoff, G., & Johnson, M. (1999). *Philosophy in the Flesh. The Embodied Mind and its Challenge to Western Thought.* Basic Books.

Lakoff, G., & Turner, M. (1989). *More Than Cool Reason. A Field Guide to Poetic Metaphor.* University of Chicago Press.

Lambert, N. M., Graham, S. M., Fincham, F. D., & Stillman, T. F. (2009). A changed perspective: How gratitude can affect sense of coherence through positive reframing. *The Journal of Positive Psychology, 4*(6). Advance online publication. DOI: 10.1080/17439760903157182

Langer, E. J. (2014). *Mindfulness.* Da Capo Press.

Larsen, S. E., Hopkins, S., & Harris, I. (2025). Addressing religious or spiritual dimensions of trauma and PTSD. *U.S. Department of Veterans Affairs.* https://www.ptsd.va.gov/professional/treat/txessentials/spirituality_trauma.asp

Lauche, R., Cramer, H., Häuser, W., Dobos, G., & Langhorst, J. (2013). A systematic review and meta-analysis of qigong for the fibromyalgia syndrome. *Evidence-Based Complementary and Alternative Medicine : eCAM, 2013*, 635182. Advance online publication. DOI: 10.1155/2013/635182 PMID: 24288564

Lebow, H. I. (2023, January 21). How your body remembers trauma. *Psych Central.* https://psychcentral.com/health/how-your-body-remembers-trauma

Leddy, T., & Puolakka, K. (2023). Dewey's aesthetics. In Zalta, E. N., & Nodelman, U. (Eds.), *The Stanford Encyclopedia of Philosophy* (Winter 2023 ed.). https://plato.stanford.edu/archives/win2023/entries/dewey-aesthetics/

Ledesma Pedraz, M. (2008). Alexandra David-Néel ou l'art de la fugue et du déguisement. *Clio. Histoire, femmes et sociétés, 28*, 213-22. DOI: 10.4000/clio.8712

Lee, K. M., & Satpute, A. B. (2024). More than labels: Neural representations of emotion words are widely distributed across the brain. *Social Cognitive and Affective Neuroscience*, *19*(1), 1–11. DOI: 10.1093/scan/nsae043 PMID: 38903026

Lee, R. T., & Moore, J. A. (2017). Integrative oncology and ethics. In *Integrative oncology* (pp. 101–119). Elsevier., DOI: 10.1016/B978-0-12-803831-4.00006-3

Leguina, A. (2015). A primer on partial least squares structural equation modeling (PLS-SEM). *International Journal of Research & Method in Education*, *38*(2). Advance online publication. DOI: 10.1080/1743727x.2015.1005806

Leibovici, F. (2007). *Des Documents poétiques.* Al Dante / Questions théoriques.

Lessing, G. E. (2012). *Laokoon, oder, Über die Grenzen der Malerei und Poesie: Studienausgabe* (Vollhardt, F., Ed.). Reclam.

Lévi–Strauss, C. (1962). *La Pensée sauvage*. Plon.

Lewis, R. (1995). *Gendering Orientalism: Race, femininity and representation.* Routledge.

Librairie mollat (Director). (2013, January 31). *Philippe Artières—Vie et mort de Paul Gény* [Video]. *YouTube*. https://www.youtube.com/watch?v=-cHibcs3lrY

Lindhé, C. (2013). "A Visual Sense is Born in the Fingertips": Towards a Digital Ekphrasis. *Digital Humanities Quarterly*, 7(1).

Lindquist, K. A., & Barrett, L. F. (2008). Constructing Emotion: The Experience of Fear as a Conceptual Act. *Psychological Science*, *19*(9), 898–903. DOI: 10.1111/j.1467-9280.2008.02174.x PMID: 18947355

Linley, P. A., & Joseph, S. (2004). Positive Change Following Trauma and Adversity: A Review. In *Journal of Traumatic Stress* (Vol. 17, Issue 1). DOI: 10.1023/B:-JOTS.0000014671.27856.7e

Litz, B., & Carney, J. (2018). Employing Loving-Kindness Meditation to Promote Self- and Other-Compassion Among War Veterans With Posttraumatic Stress Disorder. *Spirituality in Clinical Practice*, *5*(3), 201–211. DOI: 10.1037/scp0000174

Locatelli, F. (2021). Quand la marche se fait écriture: Le voyageur-penseur au milieu des sommets (XVIIIe-XIXe siècles). *Seminario di filologia francese, revue italienne d'études françaises, 11*. DOI: 10.4000/rief.8022

Lombardi Vallauri, S. (2012). Azione fisica ed empatia nell'opera musicale-performativa di Dario Buccino. In C. Falletti & G. Sofia (Eds.), *Prospettive su teatro e neuroscienze: Dialoghi e sperimentazioni* (pp. 205–209). Bulzoni.

Lombardi Vallauri, S. (2016a). The composition of experience in the musical-holistic art of Dario Buccino. In A. Bratus & M. Lutzu (Eds.), *Dossier: "Analysis beyond notation in XXth and XXIst century music"* [Special issue]. *El Oído Pensante, 4*(1), 1–27. https://revistascientificas.filo.uba.ar/index.php/oidopensante/article/view/7531/6740

Lombardi Vallauri, S. (2017b). Lo spazio teatrale-musicale come ambito di azione etica: *Rappresentazione et Esercizio* di Domenico Guaccero e *La Passion selon Sade* di Sylvano Bussotti. In G. Borio, G. Ferrari, & D. Tortora (a cura di), *Teatro di avanguardia e composizione sperimentale per la scena in Italia: 1950–1975* (pp. 187–209). Fondazione Giorgio Cini Onlus. https://www.cini.it/publications/teatro-avanguardia-composizione-sperimentale-la-scena-italia-1950-1975

Lombardi Vallauri, S. (2011). Perfetta effimera accensione di vita: Formalizzazione sonora, performativa ed esperienziale nella musica di Dario Buccino. *Poli-Femo: Nuova serie di Lingua e Letteratura, 2*, 123–140.

Lombardi Vallauri, S. (2013). Fedeli tradimenti: la ricezione cageana di tre compositori italiani nel Duemila. In Cuomo, V., & Distaso, L. V. (Eds.), *Il caso, il silenzio, la natura. La ricerca di John Cage* (pp. 41–59). Mimesis.

Lombardi Vallauri, S. (2015). L'*anti-opera* come veicolo: il teatro musicale come pratica autotrasformativa per il *performer*. In Ramerino, A. (Ed.), *Teatro e musica* (pp. 131–146). Bulzoni.

Lombardi Vallauri, S. (2016b). Sull'accompagnamento musicale del discorso filosofico. Sull'ascolto musicale come pratica sapienziale. In Bianchi, A. (Eds.), *Scritti per Luigi Lombardi Vallauri* (Vol. 1, pp. 793–807). Wolters Kluwer – CEDAM.

Lombardi Vallauri, S. (2017a). Interaction between noisy instrumental timbre and traditional intervallic systems in composers from Sicily, 1960–1985. In *Proceedings of the 9th European Music Analysis Conference*. In *EuroMAC 2017*. Université de Strasbourg., Retrieved from http://euromac2017.unistra.fr/wp-content/uploads/2017/05/Ext-lombardi-vallauri-stefano.pdf

Lombardi Vallauri, S. (2024). Liminal music: Sciarrino, Mundry, Momi. In Bossini, O. (Ed.), *Absolute music* [Program booklet of the Venice Biennale Musica 2024]. (pp. 103–111). La Biennale di Venezia.

Louvel, L. (2018). Types of Ekphrasis. *Poetics Today*, *39*(2), 245–263. DOI: 10.1215/03335372-4324432

Luca, G. (2001). Le Tangage de ma langue. In *Gherasim Luca by Gherasim Luca*. José Corti / Rien de Commun, 2 CDs.

Luca, G. (2008). *Série Brésil*. CipM, sixteen plates.

Luca, G., & Catti, M. (post–1953). *Le Tangage de ma langue*. Ghérasim Luca Archives, Bibliothèque Littéraire Doucet.

Luca, G. (1962). *Ghérasim Luca*. Ghérasim Luca Archives, Bibliothèque Littéraire Doucet.

Luca, G. (2001). *Le Vampire passif*. José Corti. (Original work published 1945)

Luca, G., & Hérold, J. (1953). *Héros–limite*. Le Soleil Noir.

Luca, G., & Hubaut, J. (1987). *Satyr and Satrap—Rebus Super 8*. Éditions de la C.R.E.M.

Luca, G., & Lam, W. (1967). *Apostroph'apocalypse*. Giorgio Upiglio.

Luca, G., & Trost, D. (1945). *Présentation de Graphies Colorées, Cubomanies et Objets*. Brezoianu Hall Exhibition.

Luchetta, S. (2020). Dalla Baita al Ciliegio. La montagna nella narrativa di Mario Rigoni Stern [*From the Baita to the Cherry-Tree. Mountain in Mario Rigoni Stern's narrative*]. *Mimesis*.

Lynch, J., Prihodova, L., Dunne, P. J., Carroll, Á., Walsh, C., McMahon, G., & White, B. (2018). Mantra meditation for mental health in the general population: A systematic review. *European Journal of Integrative Medicine*, *23*, 44–49. DOI: 10.1016/j.eujim.2018.09.010

Lyotard, J.-F. (1971). *Discours, Figure*. Klincksieck.

MacAskill, W., Chua, W. J., Woodall, H., & Pinidiyapathirage, J. (2023). Beyond the Written Reflection: A Systematic Review and Qualitative Synthesis of Creative Approaches to Reflective Learning Amongst Medical Students. *Perspectives on Medical Education*, *12*(1), 361–371. DOI: 10.5334/pme.914 PMID: 37720690

Macey, D. (2012). *Frantz Fanon: A Life*. Verso.

Macioti, M. (1995). *Oralità e vissuto. L'uso delle storie di vita nelle scienze sociali* (2nd ed.). Liguori.

Magno, E. (2009). Introduzione all'estetica indiana. Arte e liberazione del sé. *Mimesis*.

Ma, J., & Akira, K. (1990). *Chinese qigong studies*. Toyo Gakujutsu Shuppansha.

Malchiodi, C. A. (2020). *Trauma and expressive arts therapy: brain, body, and imagination in the healing process*. The Guilford Press.

Malesu, V. K. (2025). The science behind breathwork and stress reduction. *News Medical Life Sciences*. https://www.news-medical.net/health/The-Science-Behind-Breathwork-and-Stress-Reduction.aspx

Manuello, J., Vercelli, U., Nani, A., Costa, T., & Cauda, F. (2016). Mindfulness meditation and consciousness: An integrative neuroscientific perspective. *Consciousness and Cognition*, *40*, 67–78. DOI: 10.1016/j.concog.2015.12.005 PMID: 26752605

Marconi, L. (2001). *Musica espressione emozione*. Clueb.

Marcus Aurelius. (1906). *Meditations*. Dent.

Marcus Aurelius. (1907). *To Himself*. MacMillan.

Markus, H. R., & Kitayama, S. (1991). Culture and the self: Implications for cognition, emotion, and motivation. *Psychological Review*, *98*(2), 224–253. DOI: 10.1037/0033-295X.98.2.224

Marsilio, M. (2021, May 19). Arboreto salvatico: lo sguardo "ecocritico" di Mario Rigoni Stern [Wild thicket. Mario Rigoni Stern's "ecocritical" glance]. *La letteratura e noi* [Literature and us]. Retrieved September 5, 2025, from https://laletteraturaenoi.it/2021/05/19/arboreto-salvatico-lo-sguardo-ecocritico-di-mario-rigoni-stern/

Martins, L. A., Schiavo, A., Paz, L. V., Xavier, L. L., & Mestriner, R. G. (2024). Neural underpinnings of fine motor skills under stress and anxiety: A review. *Physiology & Behavior*, *282*, 114593. DOI: 10.1016/j.physbeh.2024.114593 PMID: 38782244

Mastropietro, A. (2020). *Nuovo teatro musicale fra Roma e Palermo, 1961–1973*. Libreria Musicale Italiana (LIM).

Maturana, H. R., & Varela, F. J. (with Beer, S.). (1980). *Autopoiesis and Cognition: The Realization of the Living*. D. Reidel Publishing Company.

Maturana, H. R. (1970). *Biology of Cognition. Biological Computer Laboratory Research Report BCL 9.0*. University of Illinois.

Maturana, H., & Varela, F. (1980). *Autopoiesis and Cognition*. D. Reidel Publishing Company.

Mazza, A., Davis, P., Johnson, L., Larkin, F., & Cole, S. N. (2026). Identifying therapies to effectively reduce alexithymia: A systematic review and meta-analysis. *Journal of Affective Disorders*, *400*, 1–13. DOI: 10.1016/j.jad.2026.121167 PMID: 41525940

Mazzacurati, C., & Paolini, M. (2006). *Ritratti. Mario Rigoni Stern* [Portraits. Mario Rigoni Stern]. Biblioteca dell'immagine.

McBride, O., Schroevers, M. J., & Ranchor, A. V. (2009). The structure of adversarial growth in a sample of cancer patients 8 years post-diagnosis: A revision of the SLQ-38. *Psychology & Health, 24*(10). Advance online publication. DOI: 10.1080/08870440802108900 PMID: 20204988

McCullough, M. E., Emmons, R. A., & Tsang, J. A. (2002). The grateful disposition: A conceptual and empirical topography. *Journal of Personality and Social Psychology, 82*(1). Advance online publication. DOI: 10.1037/0022-3514.82.1.112 PMID: 11811629

McCullough, M. E., Tsang, J. A., & Emmons, R. A. (2004). Gratitude in Intermediate Affective Terrain: Links of Grateful Moods to Individual Differences and Daily Emotional Experience. *Journal of Personality and Social Psychology, 86*(2). Advance online publication. DOI: 10.1037/0022-3514.86.2.295 PMID: 14769085

McNiff, S. (2004). *Art heals: how creativity cures the soul.* Shambhala Publications.

Meijer-Degen, F., & Lansen, J. (2006). Alexithymia—A challenge to art therapy: The story of Rita. *The Arts in Psychotherapy, 33*(3), 167–179. DOI: 10.1016/j.aip.2005.10.002

Menary, R. (2008). Embodied Narratives. *Journal of Consciousness Studies, 15*(6), 63–84.

Menhinick, K. A., & Sanders, C. J. (2023). LGBTQ+ Stress, Trauma, Time, and Care. *Pastoral Psychology, 72*(3), 367–384. DOI: 10.1007/s11089-023-01073-z PMID: 37313005

Meschonnic, H. (1982). *Critique du rythme—Anthropologie historique du langage.* Verdier/poche.

Michell, H. (2015). *Bush Cree Storytelling Methodology: Northern Stories that Teach, Heal, and Transform.* In Education, 21(2), Article 2. https://doi.org/DOI: 10.37119/ojs2015.v21i2.213

Miike, Y. (2003). Japanese enryo-sasshi communication and the psychology of amae: Reconsideration and reconceptualization. *Keio Communication Review, 25*, 93–115.

Mikles, N., & Joseph, L. (2015). Tracking the Tulpa: Exploring the Tibetan origins of a contemporary paranormal idea. *Nova Religio, 19*(1), 87–97.

Milani, G., & Rigoni Stern, M. (2008). Intervista a Mario Rigoni Stern. [Interview with Mario Rigoni Stern] In Milani, G. (Ed.), *Mario Rigoni Stern, Hermann Heidegger. Ritorno sul fronte* (pp. 9–38). Transeuropa.

Milkova, S. (2016). Elena Ferrante's Visual Poetics: Ekphrasis in Troubling Love, My Brilliant Friend, and The Story of a New Name. In G. Russo Bullaro & S. V. Love (Eds.), *The Works of Elena Ferrante. Reconfiguring the Margins* (pp. 159–182). Palgrave Macmillan US.

Milkova, S. (2021). *Elena Ferrante as world literature*. Bloomsbury Academic.

Mills, S. (1993). *Discourses of difference: An Analysis of women's travel writing and colonialism*. Routledge.

Ministry of Health, Labour and Welfare of Japan. (2003). *Seishin hoken ni okeru shakaiteki iryō-teki kea ni kansuru hōkokusho* [Report on social and health care in mental health]. https://www.mhlw.go.jp/topics/2003/bukyoku/syougai/dl/j4a.pdf

Ministry of Health, Labour and Welfare of Japan. (2010). *Minna no mentaru herusu: Seishin shōgai, sābisu, seisaku ni kansuru sōgō saito* [Minna no mental health: comprehensive website on mental illness, services, and policies]. https://www.mhlw.go.jp/kokoro/

Ministry of Health, Labour and Welfare of Japan. (2024a, August 26). *Global health vision of the Ministry of Health, Labour and Welfare of Japan*. https://www.mhlw.go.jp/content/10501000/001295190.pdf

Ministry of Health, Labour and Welfare of Japan. (2024b). *Seishin shōgaisha no hoken fukushi ni kansuru hōritsu* [Act on mental health and welfare for persons with mental disorders or disabilities]. https://www.mhlw.go.jp/english/wp/wp-hw3/dl/Part02-06.pdf

Misawa, F. (2020). Yamanashi Kenritsu Kita Byoin ni okeru shintai kousoku (Physical restraint in Yamanashi Prefectural Kita Hospital). *Seishin Shinkeigaku Zasshi. Psychiatria et Neurologia Japonica*, *122*(12), 955–961.

Mitchell, W. J. T. (1986). *Iconology: Image, text, ideology*. University of Chicago Press.

Mitchell, W. J. T. (1994). *Picture Theory*. University of Chicago Press.

Miyahara, K., & Tanaka, S. (2023). Narrative Self-Constitution as Embodied Practice. *Philosophical Psychology*, *38*(4), 1731–1755. DOI: 10.1080/09515089.2023.2286281

Miyamoto, I. (1974). The Real Value of Tied Aid: The Case of Indonesia in 1967-69. *Economic Development and Cultural Change*, *22*(3), 436–452.

Moldovan, R., Cobeanu, O., & David, D. (2013). Cognitive bibliotherapy for mild depressive symptomatology: Randomized clinical trial of efficacy and mechanisms of change. *Clinical Psychology & Psychotherapy*, *20*(6), 482–493. DOI: 10.1002/cpp.1814 PMID: 22941790

Montaigne, M. (de) (1965). *Les Essais. Livre III*. Gallimard.

Morante, E. (1990). *Alibi* (1. ed). Garzanti.

Morgan, N., Irwin, M. R., Chung, M., & Wang, C. (2014). The effects of mind–body therapies on the immune system: Meta-analysis. *PLoS One*, *9*(7), e100903. Advance online publication. DOI: 10.1371/journal.pone.0100903 PMID: 24988414

Mosher, L. R., & Hendrix, V. (2004). *Soteria. Through madness to deliverance*. Xlibris.

Motta, A. (1982). *Mario Rigoni Stern*. La Nuova Italia.

Munenori, Y. (2012). *The Life-Giving Sword. Secret Teachings From the House of the Shogun*. Shambahla.

Muñoz, J. E. (2006). Feeling Brown, Feeling Down: Latina Affect, the Performativity of Race, and the Depressive Position. *Signs (Chicago, Ill.)*, *31*(3), 675–688. DOI: 10.1086/499080

Muxel, A. (2007). *Individu et mémoire familiale*. Hachette.

Nagano, J., Kakuta, C., Motomura, C., Odajima, H., Sudo, N., Nishima, S., & Kubo, C. (2010). The parenting attitudes and the stress of mothers predict the asthmatic severity of their children: A prospective study. *BioPsychoSocial Medicine*, *4*, 12. Advance online publication. DOI: 10.1186/1751-0759-4-12 PMID: 20929533

Nakamura, E. (2016). "Invisible" War Trauma in Japan: Medicine, Society and Military Psychiatric Casualties. *Historia Scientiarum*, *25*(2), 140–160.

Nancy, J.-L. (2000). *Corpus*. Métailié.

Napolitano Valditara, L. (2003). Alle origini del "gnōthi sautòn". Da Delfi al sapere socratico di non sapere. *Esercizi Filosofici*, *2*, 110–125.

Naylor, E. V., Antonuccio, D. O., Litt, M., Johnson, G. E., Spogen, D. R., Williams, R., McCarthy, C., Lu, M. M., Fiore, D. C., & Higgins, D. L. (2010). Bibliotherapy as a Treatment for Depression in Primary Care. *Journal of Clinical Psychology in Medical Settings*, *17*, 258–271. DOI: 10.1007/s10880-010-9207-2 PMID: 20803165

Nelson, J. (2003). Social Memory as Ritual Practice: Commemorating Spirits of the Military Dead at Yasukuni Shinto Shrine. *The Journal of Asian Studies*, *62*(2), 443–467.

Nerval, G. (2005). *Les Chimères, La Bohème galante, Petits Châteaux de Bohème*. Poésie/Gallimard. (Original work published 1854)

Ning, J., Tang, X., Shi, H., Yao, D., Zhao, Z., & Li, J. (2023). Social support and posttraumatic growth: A meta-analysis. In *Journal of Affective Disorders* (Vol. 320). DOI: 10.1016/j.jad.2022.09.114

Nippoda, Y. (2012). Japanese culture and therapeutic relationship. *Online Readings in Psychology and Culture*, *10*(3). DOI: 10.9707/2307-0919.1094

Nishi, D., Ishikawa, H., & Kawakami, N. (2019). Prevalence of mental disorders and mental health service use in Japan. *Psychiatry and Clinical Neurosciences*, *73*(8), 458–465. DOI: 10.1111/pcn.12894 PMID: 31141260

Nishi, D., Matsuoka, Y., & Kim, Y. (2010). Posttraumatic growth, posttraumatic stress disorder and resilience of motor vehicle accident survivors. *BioPsychoSocial Medicine*, *4*. Advance online publication. DOI: 10.1186/1751-0759-4-7 PMID: 20573276

Nishihara, D. (2005). Said, Orientalism, and Japan. *Alif: Journal of Comparative Poetics*, *25*, 241–253.

Niti, M., Ng, T. P., Mahendran, R., & Kua, E. H. (2007). Depressive disorder in older adults: The role of sub-threshold depression and neuroticism. *International Journal of Geriatric Psychiatry*, *22*, 1040–1047. DOI: 10.1002/gps.1790

Nitobé, I. (1908). *Bushido. The Soul of Japan*. The Project Gutenberg eBook (13th ed.) https://www.holybooks.com/ (original work published 1904)

Nolte, J. (2009). *The human brain: An introduction to its functional anatomy* (6th ed.). Mosby/Elsevier.

Nono, L. (2001b). *Il potere musicale* (1969). In De Benedictis, A. I., & Rizzardi, V. (Eds.), *L. Nono, Scritti e colloqui* (Vol. 1, pp. 261–271). Ricordi-LIM.

Nwokah, E. E., & Graves, K. N. (2009). Word Play: The Creation and Function of Novel Words in the Pretend Play of Two Siblings. *American Journal of Play*, *1*(4), 429–450.

OECD. (2013). *OECD Guidelines on Measuring Subjective Well-Being*. OECD Publishing., DOI: 10.1787/9789264191655-

Ohio Department of Job and Family Services, Office of Families and Children. (2024). *QRTP infosheet issue four: Culturally responsive trauma-informed approach* [PDF]. https://dam.assets.ohio.gov/image/upload/jfs.ohio.gov/ofam/QRTP-InfosheetIssueFour-CulturallyResponsiveTrauma-InformedApproachFinal.pdf

Okakura, K. (1906). *The Book of Tea*. Putnam.

Oka, T., Tanahashi, T., Chijiwa, T., Lkhagvasuren, B., Sudo, N., & Oka, K. (2018). Changes in fatigue, autonomic functions, and blood biomarkers due to sitting isometric yoga in patients with chronic fatigue syndrome. *BioPsychoSocial Medicine*, *12*, 3. Advance online publication. DOI: 10.1186/s13030-018-0123-0 PMID: 29643935

Okuzono, S. S., Cowden, R. G., Padgett, R. N., Yancey, G., Johnson, B. R., & VanderWeele, T. J. (n.d.) Sociodemographic Variation in Gratitude Using a Cross-National Analysis with 22 Countries. *International Journal of Applied Positive Psychology*, *10*, 60.

Öngür, D., An, X., & Price, J. L. (1998). Prefrontal cortical projections to the hypothalamus in macaque monkeys. *The Journal of Comparative Neurology*, *401*, 480–505. PMID: 9826274

Ong, W. J. (1982). *Orality and literacy: The technologizing of the word*. Routledge.

Ono, A. (2001). *Japonisme in Britain: A Source of Inspiration: J. McN. Whistler, Mortimer Menpes, George Henry, E. A. Hornel and Nineteenth Century Japan* [Doctoral dissertation, University of Glasgow]. Enlighten Team.

Ono, K. (2024). *Genba de katsuyō suru hyōgen ātoserapi no jissai* [Expressive art therapy in the field]. Seishin Shobo.

Ono, S. (1962). *Shinto. The Kami Way*. Tuttle.

ONS. (2011). *ONS Opinions and Lifestyle Survey—Well-Being Module*. ESDS UK Government Publishing.

Oosterbroek, T., & Dirk, B. (2021). The experience of Trauma Center–Trauma Sensitive Yoga training on professional practice of mental health professionals and yoga instructors. *Complementary Therapies in Clinical Practice*, *43*, 101365. DOI: 10.1016/j.ctcp.2021.101365 PMID: 33819832

Orme-Johnson, D. W., Barnes, V. A., Rees, B., Tobin, J., & Walton, K. G. (2024). Effectiveness of meditation techniques in treating post-traumatic stress disorder: A systematic review and meta-analysis. *Medicina*, *60*(12), 2050. DOI: 10.3390/medicina60122050 PMID: 39768929

Orvell, M. (1992). Writing Posthistorically: Krazy Kat, Maus, and the Contemporary Fiction Cartoon. *American Literary History*, *4*(1), 110–128. https://www.jstor.org/stable/489940

Overview of yoga. (2025). UpToDate. https://www.uptodate.com/contents/overview-of-yoga

Parikh, D., De Ieso, P., Garvey, G., Thachil, T., Ramamoorthi, R., Penniment, M., & Jayaraj, R. (2015). Post-traumatic stress disorder and post-traumatic growth in breast cancer patients - A systematic review. *Asian Pacific Journal of Cancer Prevention : APJCP*, *16*(2). Advance online publication. DOI: 10.7314/APJCP.2015.16.2.641 PMID: 25684500

Park, C. L., Cohen, L. H., & Murch, R. L. (1996). Assessment and Prediction of Stress-Related Growth. *Journal of Personality*, *64*(1). Advance online publication. DOI: 10.1111/j.1467-6494.1996.tb00815.x PMID: 8656319

Park, S. H., Han, K. S., & Kang, C. B. (2017). Blood pressure response to meditation and yoga: A systematic review and meta-analysis. *Journal of Alternative and Complementary Medicine (New York, N.Y.)*, *23*(9), 685–695. DOI: 10.1089/acm.2016.0217 PMID: 28384004

Park, S., & Gupta, S. (2012). Handling endogenous regressors by joint estimation using copulas. *Marketing Science*, *31*(4). Advance online publication. DOI: 10.1287/mksc.1120.0718

Peck, R. (Director). (2024b). *Ernest Cole, photographe*. Velvet Film.

Peck, R. (2024a). *Ernest Cole, photographe*. Denoël.

Perera, R. (2024). Mat to Clinic: A Systematic Review on Role of Therapeutic Yoga in Clinical Management of Mental Disorders and Wellbeing Promotion in Integrative Health Care. SICASH 2024, SLIIT International Conference on Advancements in Sciences and Humanities Proceedings, 420-225.

Perret, C. (2019). *Le Temps de l'œuvre*. Éditions de la Sorbonne.

Perry, G., Polito, V., Sankaran, N., & Thompson, W. F. (2022). How chanting relates to cognitive function, altered states, and quality of life. *Brain Sciences*, *12*(11), 1456. DOI: 10.3390/brainsci12111456 PMID: 36358382

Pescosolido, B. A., Martin, J. K., Lang, A., & Olafsdottir, S. (2008). Rethinking theoretical approaches to stigma: A framework integrating normative influences on stigma (FINIS). *Social Science & Medicine*, *67*, 431–440. DOI: 10.1016/j.socscimed.2008.03.018 PMID: 18436358

Phan, K. L., Wager, T. D., Taylor, S. F., & Liberzon, I. (2004). Functional neuroimaging studies of human emotions. *CNS Spectrums*, *9*(4), 258–266. DOI: 10.1017/s1092852900009196 PMID: 15048050

Phan, K. L., Wager, T., Taylor, S. F., & Liberzon, I. (2002). Functional neuroanatomy of emotion: A meta-analysis of emotion activation studies in PET and fMRI. *NeuroImage*, *16*(2), 331–348. DOI: 10.1006/nimg.2002.1087 PMID: 12030820

Pigeot, J. (1983). Les Japonais peints par eux-mêmes: Esquisse d'un autoportrait [The Japanese painted by themselves: Sketch of a self-portrait]. *Le Debat*, *1*(23), 19–33. DOI: 10.3917/deba.023.0019

Plato. (1921). *Theaetetus*. In *Plato in twelve volumes* (Vol. 12). Harvard University Press. https://www.perseus.tufts.edu/hopper/text?doc=Perseus%3Atext%3A1999.01.0172

Plato. (1955). *Alcibiades I*. In *Plato in twelve volumes* (Vol. 8). Harvard University Press.

Plato. (1967a). *Meno*. In *Plato in twelve volumes* (Vol. 3). Harvard University Press.

Plato. (1967b). *Protagoras*. In *Plato in twelve volumes* (Vol. 3). Harvard University Press.

Pols, H., & Micale, M. S. (2021). History, Trauma, and Asia. In Micale, M. S., & Pols, H. (Eds.), *Traumatic Pasts in Asia. History, Psychiatry, and Trauma from the 1930s to the Present* (pp. 1–34). Berghahn.

Pool, J. L., & Ransohoff, J. (1949). Autonomic effects on stimulating rostral portion of cingulate gyri in man. *Journal of Neurophysiology*, *12*(6), 385–392. DOI: 10.1152/jn.1949.12.6.385 PMID: 15408005

Portelli, A. (2014). Un lavoro di relazione. Osservazioni sulla storia orale. https://www.aisoitalia.org/wp-content/uploads/2014/04/Alessandro-Portelli-Storia-orale-un-lavoro-di-relazione.pdf

Portelli, A. (2019). *L'ordine è già stato eseguito. Roma, le Fosse Ardeatine, la memoria*. Donzelli.

Potash, J. S. (2020). We the art therapists: Democracy through creative action. *Art Therapy: Journal of the American Art Therapy Association*, *37*(1), 3–5. DOI: 10.1080/07421656.2020.1724592

Prins, J. B., van der Meer, J. W. M., & Bleijenberg, G. (2006). Chronic fatigue syndrome. *Lancet*, *367*(9507), 346–355. DOI: 10.1016/S0140-6736(06)68073-2 PMID: 16443043

Psychological factors affecting other medical conditions: Clinical features, assessment, and diagnosis. (2025). UpToDate. https://www.uptodate.com/contents/psychological-factors-affecting-other-medical-conditions-clinical-features-assessment-and-diagnosis

Puolakka, K. (2014). Dewey and everyday aesthetics. *Contemporary Aesthetics*, *12*, 1–15.

Quatremare Martín, F. (2022). Identités plurielles au cours des voyages d'Alexandra David-Néel. *HYBRIDA*, *4*, 195–216.

Rafiei, A., Noruzi, A., & Ferdousi, T. (2023). Cognitive bibliotherapy for delinquent adolescents with psychopathic disorder: A quasi-experimental study. *Journal of Poetry Therapy*, *36*(4), 259–272. DOI: 10.1080/08893675.2023.2179437

Raikar, S. (n.d.). Limbic System. In *Encyclopedia Britannica*. Retrieved September 3, from https://www.britannica.com/science/limbic-system

Rangasamy, V., Susheela, A.T., Mueller, A., Chang, T.F.H., & Sadhasivam, S., & Subramaniam*, B. (2019). The effect of a one-time 15-minute guided meditation (Isha Kriya) on stress and mood disturbances among operating room professionals: A prospective interventional pilot study. *F1000 Research*, *8*, 335. DOI: 10.12688/f1000research.18446.1 PMID: 32665843

Ranisha, K., & Kumari, S. (2024). Effect of a yogic stress management technique (cyclic meditation) on stress, mindfulness, and well-being: A systematic review. *Yoga Mimamsa*, *56*(2), 129–140. DOI: 10.4103/ym.ym_51_24

Ranisha, K., Kumari, S., & Dwivedi, U. (2024). Human Development Model Based on Yogic Wisdom for Well-being and Self-actualization: A Conceptual Framework. *Journal of Human Values*, *30*(2), 202–213. DOI: 10.1177/09716858231210598

Rao, P. D. (2024). Mantra-based cognitive resilience: Evaluating the viability of ancient sound practices as a culturally embedded mental health intervention. *Frontiers in Health Informatics*, *13*(7), 805–823.

Rastogi, R., Rao, P. D., & Mehta, S. (2020). Mantra-based cognitive resilience: Evaluating the viability of ancient sound practices as culturally embedded mental health intervention. *Health Informatics Journal*, *26*(4), 2792–2804. DOI: 10.1177/1460458220948748 PMID: 32691659

Regev, D., & Cohen-Yatziv, L. (2018). Effectiveness of art therapy with adult clients in 2018 – What progress has been made? *Frontiers in Psychology*, *9*, 1531. DOI: 10.3389/fpsyg.2018.01531 PMID: 30210388

Renault, L. (2020). L'approche énactive et la place de l'altérité – Dialogue entre Varela et Buber. *Journal of French and Francophone Philosophy—Revue de la philosophie française et de langue française*, vol. XXVIII, n° 1/2020, 143-166.

Revelli, N. (1966). *La strada del davai*. Einaudi.

Revelli, N. (1977). *Il mondo dei vinti. Storie di vita contadina* (Vol. 1–2). Einaudi.

Richardson, L. (2005). Writing: A Method of Inquiry. In E. A. St. Pierre (Ed.), *The Sage handbook of qualitative research, 3rd ed* (pp. 959–978). Sage Publications Ltd.

Richter, M., Eck, J., Straube, T., Miltner, W. H. R., & Weiss, T. (2010). Do words hurt? Brain activation during the processing of pain-related words. *Pain, 148*(2), 198–205. DOI: 10.1016/j.pain.2009.08.009 PMID: 19846255

Ricoeur, P. (2000). *La mémoire, l'histoire, l'oubli*. Seuil.

Rigoni Stern, M. (2003a). [...]. In *Sentieri sotto la neve* [Pathways under the snow] (3rd ed., 67–72). ed. Einaudi.

Rigoni Stern, M. (2004b). Ritorno sul Don [Return to the Don river]. In *Il sergente nella neve – Ritorno sul Don* (17th ed. 277–317). Einaudi.

Rigoni Stern, M. (2004c). La scure [The axe]. In *Il sergente nella neve – Ritorno sul Don* (17th ed. 269–275). Einaudi.

Rigoni Stern, M. (1967). The Sergeant in the Snow. In *R. Biason, M. Tobino, & M. Rigoni Stern, The Lost Legions. Three Italian War Novels by Renzo Biason, Mario Tobino, and Mario Rigoni Stern* (Colquhoun, A., & Cowan, A., Trans.; pp. 303–412). Knopf.

Rigoni Stern, M. (2004a). Un ragazzo delle nostre contrade. [*A boy from our hamlet*] In *Il sergente nella neve – Ritorno sul Don* [*The sergeant in the snow – Return to the Don river*]. 17th ed., pp. 249–268). Einaudi.

Rigoni Stern, M. (2004e). Il cane che vidi piangere. [The dog I saw cry] In *Aspettando l'alba e altri racconti* (pp. 120–125). Einaudi.

Rigoni Stern, M. (2014). *Il coraggio di dire no. Conversazioni e interviste 1963–2007* [The courage of saying no. Coversations and interviews]. Einaudi.

Rimm-Kaufman, S. E., & Kagan, J. (1996). The psychological significance of changes in skin temperature. *Motivation and Emotion*, *20*, 63–78. 10.1007/BF02251007

Rodrigues, S. M., LeDoux, J. E., & Sapolsky, R. M. (2009). The influence of stress hormones on fear circuitry. *Annual Review of Neuroscience*, *32*, 289–313. DOI: 10.1146/annurev.neuro.051508.135620 PMID: 19400714

Rodríguez-Jiménez, R.-M., Carmona, M., García-Merino, S., Díaz-Rivas, B., & Thuissard-Vasallo, I. J. (2022). Stress, subjective well-being and selfknowledge in higher education teachers: A pilot study through bodyfulness approaches. *PLoS One*, *17*(12), 1–34. DOI: 10.1371/journal.pone.0278372 PMID: 36520842

Rogers, C. (1959). A theory of therapy, personality and interpersonal relationships as developed in the client-centered framework. In Koch, S. (Ed.), *Psychology: A study of a science* (Vol. 3). McGraw-Hill.

Rogers, C. R. (1957). The necessary and sufficient conditions of therapeutic personality change. *Journal of Consulting Psychology*, *21*(2), 95–103. DOI: 10.1037/h0045357 PMID: 13416422

Rogers, C. R. (1961). *On becoming a person: a therapist's view of psychotherapy*. Houghton Mifflin.

Rojcewicz, S. (2004). Poetry therapy in ancient Greek literature. *Journal of Poetry Therapy*, *17*(4), 209–213.

Rosenthal, R., Rosnow, R. L., & Alan, E. Kazdin. (2009). *Artifacts in Behavioral Research: Robert Rosenthal and Ralph L. Rosnow's Classic Books*. Oxford University Press. https://doi.org/DOI: 10.1093/acprof:oso/9780195385540.001.0001

Rots, A. (2013). *Forests of the Gods. Shinto, Nature, and Sacred Space in Contemporary Japan*. Doctoral Thesis. University of Oslo.

Ruini, C., & Vescovelli, F. (2013). The Role of Gratitude in Breast Cancer: Its Relationships with Post-traumatic Growth, Psychological Well-Being and Distress. *Journal of Happiness Studies*, *14*(1). Advance online publication. DOI: 10.1007/s10902-012-9330-x

Rule, P. (2015). *Dialogue and boundary learning*. Sense Publishers.

Rusk, R. D., Vella-Brodrick, D. A., & Waters, L. (2016). Gratitude or Gratefulness? A Conceptual Review and Proposal of the System of Appreciative Functioning. In *Journal of Happiness Studies* (Vol. 17, Issue 5). DOI: 10.1007/s10902-015-9675-z

Said, E. (1978). *Orientalism*. Pantheon Books.

Saillant, F., & Araujo, A. L. (2007). Slavery in Brazil: The work of the black movement. *Ethnologie française*. *Presses Universitaires de France*, *37*(3), 457–466.

Saito, H. (2017). *The History Problem. The Politics of War Commemoration in East Asia*. University of Hawai'i Press.

Saito, H. (2017). *The history problem*. University of Hawai'i Press.

Salzberg, S., & Kabat-Zinn, J. (1997). Mindfulness as Medicine. In Goleman, D. (Ed.), *Healing Emotions. Conversations with the Dalai Lama on Mindfulness, Emotions, and Health* (pp. 107–144). Shambhala Publications.

Sandelowski, M. (2004). Using qualitative research. *Qualitative Health Research, 14*(10), 1366–1386. DOI: 10.1177/1049732304269672 PMID: 15538005

Sato, S. (1981). *Two Moons. Short Zen Stories*. Dai Nihon.

Savage, M. K., Lepping, P., Newton-Howes, G., Arnold, R., Staggs, V. S., Kisely, S., Hasegawa, T., Reid, K. S., & Noorthoorn, E. O. (2024). Comparison of coercive practices in worldwide mental healthcare: Overcoming difficulties resulting from variations in monitoring strategies. *British Journal of Psychiatry Open, 10*(1), e26. DOI: 10.1192/bjo.2023.613 PMID: 38205597

Saxena, R. (2023). Significance of religious chanting in various religions. *International Journal of Creative Research and Thoughts, 11*(12). https://ijcrt.org/papers/IJCRT2312100.pdf

Saygideger, Y., Özdemir, H., Ekinci, R. M. K., & Yücel, G. Y. (2022). Adulthood asthma as a consequence of childhood adversity: A systematic review of epigenetically affected genes. *Journal of Developmental Origins of Health and Disease, 13*(6), 674–682. DOI: 10.1017/S2040174422000058 PMID: 35256035

Scarlet, J. (2017). *Superhero therapy: mindfulness skills to help teens and young adults deal with anxiety, depression, and trauma*. New Harbinger Publications.

Scelsi, G. (2010). *Il sogno 101* (Martinis, L., & Pellegrini, A. C., Eds.). Quodlibet.

Schwab, G. (2010). *Haunting legacies: Violent histories and transgenerational trauma*. Columbia University Press.

Scott, K. M., Von Korff, M., Alonso, J., Angermeyer, M. C., Bromet, E., Fayyad, J., de Girolamo, G., Demyttenaere, K., Gasquet, I., Gureje, O., Haro, J. M., He, Y., Kessler, R. C., Levinson, D., Medina Mora, M. E., Oakley Browne, M., Posada-Villa, J., Watanabe, M., Williams, D., & Karam, A. N. (2007). Mental disorders among adults with asthma: Results from the World Mental Health Survey. *General Hospital Psychiatry, 29*(2), 123–133. DOI: 10.1016/j.genhosppsych.2006.12.006 PMID: 17336661

Sedgwick, E. K. (with Frank, A.). (2003). *Touching Feeling: Affect, Pedagogy, Performativity*. Duke University Press.

Sedgwick, E. K. (2011). *The weather in Proust* (Goldberg, J., Ed.). Duke University Press.

Sedgwick, E. K., & Frank, A. (1995). Shame in the Cybernetic Fold: Reading Silvan Tomkins. *Critical Inquiry, 21*(2), 496–522. DOI: 10.1086/448761

Sekiguchi, R. (2023). *Nagori*. P.O.L. (Original work published 2018)

Senzaki, N., & Reps, P. (1957). *101 Zen Stories*. Charles Tuttle.

Seppälä, E., Nitschke, J., Tudorascu, D., Hayes, A., Goldstein, M., Nguyen, D., Perlman, D., & Davidson, R. (2014). Breathing-Based Meditation Decreases Posttraumatic Stress Disorder Symptoms in U.S. Military Veterans: A Randomized Controlled Longitudinal Study. *Journal of Traumatic Stress, 27*, 397–405. PMID: 25158633

Sherin, J. E., & Nemeroff, C. B. (2011). Post-traumatic stress disorder: The neurobiological impact of psychological trauma. *Dialogues in Clinical Neuroscience, 13*(3), 263–278. DOI: 10.31887/dcns.2011.13.2.jsherin PMID: 22034143

Shiner, R. A., & Jost, L. (2003). *Eudaimonia and well-being*. Academic Printing and Publishing.

Shusterman, R. (2008). *Body Consciousness. A philosophy of Mindfulness and somaesthetics*. Cambridge University Press.

Shusterman, R. (2012). *Thinking through the body. Essays in Somaeasthetics*. Cambridge University Press.

Sifneos, P. E. (1973). The prevalence of "alexithymic" characteristics in psychosomatic patients. *Psychotherapy and Psychosomatics, 22*(2), 255–262. DOI: 10.1159/000286529 PMID: 4770536

Silvestro, O., Raffaele, L., & Vicario, C. M. (2023). Alexithymia and asthma: A systematic review. *Frontiers in Psychology, 14*, 1221648. Advance online publication. DOI: 10.3389/fpsyg.2023.1221648 PMID: 37609491

Singhdeo, A. (2023, August 28). *What are the benefits of mantra chanting?* Shvasa Yoga Blog. https://www.shvasa.com/yoga-blog/what-are-the-benefits-of-mantra-chanting

Singh, S., Gupta, K. V., Behera, L., & Bhushan, B. (2025). Elevated correlations in cardiac–neural dynamics: An impact of mantra meditation on stress alleviation. *Biomedical Signal Processing and Control, 99*, 106813. DOI: 10.1016/j.bspc.2024.106813

Slivinske, J., & Slivinske, L. (2013). *Therapeutic storytelling for adolescents and young adults*. Oxford University Press.

Smith, C., Hancock, H., Blake-Mortimer, J., & Eckert, K. (2007). A randomised comparative trial of yoga and relaxation to reduce stress and anxiety. *Complementary Therapies in Medicine*, *15*(2), 77–83. DOI: 10.1016/j.ctim.2006.05.001 PMID: 17544857

Sodergren, S. C., & Hyland, M. E. (2000). What are the positive consequences of illness? *Psychology & Health*, *15*(1). Advance online publication. DOI: 10.1080/08870440008400290

Sorrells, S. F., Caso, J. R., Munhoz, C. D., & Sapolsky, R. M. (2009). The stressed CNS: When glucocorticoids aggravate inflammation. *Neuron*, *64*(1), 33–39. DOI: 10.1016/j.neuron.2009.09.032 PMID: 19840546

Soulé, I., Littzen-Brown, C., Vermeesch, A.L.*, & Garrigues, L. (2022). Expanding the Mind–Body–Environment Connection to Enhance the Development of Cultural Humility. International Journal of Environmental Research and Public Health, 19 (20): 13641, 1-8. DOI: 10.3390/ijerph192013641

Spatz, B. (2017). Embodied research: A methodology. *Liminalities: A Journal of Performance Studies, 13*(2). http://liminalities.net/13-2/embodied.pdf

Spillius, E. B., & Hinshelwood, R. D. (2011). *The new dictionary of Kleinian thought*. Routledge.

Spivak, G. C. (2007). Can the Subaltern Speak? In C. Nelson & L. Grossberg (Eds.), *Marxism and the interpretation of culture* (pp. 271–313). University of Illinois Press.

Spry, T. (2001). Performing Autoethnography: An Embodied Methodological Praxis. *Qualitative Inquiry*, *7*(6), 706–732. DOI: 10.1177/107780040100700605

Srirangarajan, , TOshio, , AYamaguchi, , AAkutsu, , S. (2020). Cross-Cultural Nomological Network of Gratitude: Findings From Midlife in the United States and Japan. *Frontiers in Psychology*, *11*, 571. https://doi.org/10.3389/fpsyg.2020.00571

Stavru, A. (2021). Eudaimonia e protrettica socratica in Platone, Senofonte ed Eschine: Rendere migliori gli altri per essere felici? *Thaumàzein, 9*(1), 363–367. https://rivista.thaumazein.it/index.php/thaum/article/view/170

Stein, J. (2017). The Meaning of "Loneliness" for Traumatized Veterans: A Semiotic Investigation of Veterans' Written Narratives. *Journal of Veterans Studies*, *2*(2), 121–139. DOI: 10.21061/jvs.v2i2.19

Stiglitz, J., Sen, A., & Fitoussi, J.-P. (2009). The Measurement of Economic Performance and Social Progress Revisited. French State commissioned report from the CMEPSP, 1-63.

Stoloff, J-C. (2020). Identifier, s'identifier, croire [Identifying, self-identifying, believing]. *Le présent de la psychanalyse, 4*(2), 115–129.

Straube, T., Sauer, A., & Miltner, W. H. R. (2011). Brain activation during direct and indirect processing of positive and negative words. *Behavioural Brain Research, 222*, 66–72. DOI: 10.1016/j.bbr.2011.03.037 PMID: 21440008

Suchet, M. (2014). *L'Imaginaire hétérolingue* [*The Heterolingual Imagination*]. Classiques Garnier.

Sugimoto, Y. (2020). *An introduction to Japanese society*. Cambridge University Press.

Surmitis, K. A., Fox, J., & Gutierrez, D. (2018). Meditation and appropriation: Best practices for counselors who utilize meditation. *Counseling and Values, 63*(1), 4–16. DOI: 10.1002/cvj.12069

Suzuki, D. (1993). *Zen and Japanese Culture*. Charles Tuttle. (Original work published 1959)

Suzuki, D. T. (1993). *Zen and Japanese culture*. Charles E. Tuttle. (Original work published 1959)

Swain, T. A., & McGwin, G. (2016). Yoga-related injuries in the United States from 2001 to 2014. *Orthopaedic Journal of Sports Medicine, 4*(11), 2325967116671703. Advance online publication. DOI: 10.1177/2325967116671703 PMID: 27896293

Swami Vivekananda. (2018). *Raja Yoga: Being Lectures by the Swami Vivekananda, with Patanjali's Aphorisms, Commentaries and a Glossary of Terms*. Routledge.

Tagg, J. (2009). *The Disciplinary Frame: Photographic Truths and the Capture of Meaning*. Univ Of Minnesota Press.

Taishi, K. (2018). The Universality of Shintō, Clarified by Some Buddhist Concepts. *Japan Mission Journal*, 10–18.

Takahashi, T., Asano, S., Uchida, Y., Takemura, K., Fukushima, S., Matsushita, K., & Okuda, N. (2022). Effects of forests and forest-related activities on the subjective well-being of residents in a Japanese watershed: An economic analysis through the capability approach. *Forest Policy and Economics, 139*, 1–12. DOI: 10.1016/j.forpol.2022.102723

Taku, K., Calhoun, L. G., Cann, A., & Tedeschi, R. G. (2008). The role of rumination in the coexistence of distress and posttraumatic growth among bereaved Japanese university students. *Death Studies, 32*(5). Advance online publication. DOI: 10.1080/07481180801974745 PMID: 18767236

Talwar, S. (2007). Accessing Traumatic Memory through Art Making: An Art Therapy Trauma Protocol (ATTP). *The Arts in Psychotherapy, 34*, 22–35.

Tanji, F., Tomata, Y., Zhang, S., Otsuka, T., & Tsuji, I. (2018). Psychological distress and completed suicide in Japan: A comparison of the impact of moderate and severe psychological distress. *Preventive Medicine, 116*, 99–103. DOI: 10.1016/j.ypmed.2018.09.007 PMID: 30219687

Tawada, Y. (2003). の [*Exophony: Voyages Outside the Mother Tongue*]. Iwanami Shoten.

Tedeschi, R. G., & Calhoun, L. G. (2004). Posttraumatic Growth: Conceptual Foundations and Empirical Evidence. In *Psychological Inquiry* (Vol. 15, Issue 1). DOI: 10.1207/s15327965pli1501_01

Tedeschi, R. G., Shakespeare-Finch, J., Taku, K., Calhoun, L. G. (2018). *Posttraumatic growth: Theory, research, and applications*. Routledge.

Tedeschi, R. G., & Calhoun, L. G. (1996). The posttraumatic growth inventory: Measuring the positive legacy of trauma. *Journal of Traumatic Stress, 9*(3). Advance online publication. DOI: 10.1002/jts.2490090305 PMID: 8827649

Tedeschi, R. G., Calhoun, L. G., & Groleau, J. M. (2014). Clinical applications of post-traumatic growth. In Calhoun, L. G., & Tedeschi, R. G. (Eds.), *Handbook of post-traumatic growth* (pp. 291–310). Routledge., DOI: 10.4324/9781315805597

Tei, S., & Wu, H. Y.-J. (2021). Historical Reflection on Taijin-kyôfushô during Covid-19: A Global Phenomenon of Social Anxiety? *History and Philosophy of the Life Sciences, 43*(2), 60. DOI: 10.1007/s40656-021-00392-9 PMID: 33864152

Telles, S., Nagarathna, R., & Nagendra, H. R. (1995). Autonomic changes during "OM" meditation. *Indian Journal of Physiology and Pharmacology, 39*(4), 418–420. PMID: 8582759

Teo, A. R., & Gaw, A. C. (2010). Hikikomori, a Japanese culture-bound syndrome of social withdrawal? *The Journal of Nervous and Mental Disease, 198*(6), 444–449. DOI: 10.1097/NMD.0b013e3181e086b1 PMID: 20531124

Thévoz, S. (2024), Trainings for sorcery, magic, mystic philosophy—for that which is called "the great accomplishment": Alexandra David-Neel's written and unwritten Tibetan grimoires. In C. Bailey & A. Wenta (Eds.), *Tibetan magic. Past and present* (pp. 193–220). Bloomsbury..

Thévoz, S. (2016). On the Threshold of the "land of marvels": Alexandra David-Neel in Sikkim and the making of global Buddhism. *Transcultural studies, 7* (1), 149-186. DOI: 10.17885/heiup.ts.23541

Thiault, F. (2009). *Recherche indigène et familiarité avec l'objet de recherche.* Études de communication. langages, information, médiations, 32. https://doi.org/ DOI: 10.4000/edc.914

Thirion, Y. (1961). Le japonisme en France dans la seconde moitié du XIXe siècle à la faveur de la diffusion de l'estampe japonaise [Japonisme in France in the second half of the 19th century thanks to the spread of Japanese prints]. *Cahiers de l'Association internationale des études françaises, 13*, 117–130. DOI: 10.3406/caief.1961.2193

Thompson, P. (1984). Historians and oral history. In Puissant, J. (Ed.), *Collective memories* (pp. 281–295). Éditions de l'Université de Bruxelles.

Tick, E. (2014). *Warrior's Return. Restoring the Soul after War*. Sounds True.

Tisseron, S. (2011). *Les secrets de famille*. Presses Universitaires de France.

Tomkins, S. S. (1995). *Shame and its sisters: A Silvan Tomkins reader* (Sedgwick, E. K., Ed.). Duke University Press.

Tomkins, S. S. (2008). *Affect Imagery Consciousness*. Springer Pub.

Tosquelles, F. (1975a). Frantz Fanon à Saint-Alban. *Sud/Nord, 22*(1), 9–14. .DOI: 10.3917/sn.022.0009

Tosquelles, F. (1975b). *Trait d'union, journal de Saint-Alban: éditoriaux, articles, notes, 1950–1962*. Éditions d'une.

Tosquelles, F. (1986). *Le Vécu de la fin du monde dans la folie: le témoignage de Gérard de Nerval*. Éditions de l'AREFPPI.

Tosquelles, F. (2021). *Soigner les institutions*, textes choisis et présentés par Joana Masó. L'Arachnéen/Arcàdia.

Trefalt, B. (2017). Collecting Bones: Japanese Missions for the Repatriation of War Remains and the Unfinished Business of the Asia-Pacific War. *Australian Humanities Review 61*, 145–159.

Treisman, K. (2017). *Working with relational and developmental trauma in children and adolescents: The impact of complex trauma on children's sense of selves, relationships and development*. Routledge.

Troscianko, E. T. (2018). Literary reading and eating disorders: Survey evidence of therapeutic help and harm. *Journal of Eating Disorders*, *6*. Advance online publication. DOI: 10.1186/s40337-018-0191-5 PMID: 29692896

Tsai, C. C. (1994). *Zen Speaks*. Doubleday.

Tsutsui, K. (2009). The trajectory of perpetrators' trauma. *Social Forces*, *87*(3), 1389–1422.

Turner, M. (1996). *The Literary Mind. The Origins of Thought and Language*. Oxford University Press.

Unanue, , WGomez Mella, , M. ECortez, , D. ABravo, , DAraya-Véliz, , CUnanue, , JVan Den Broeck, , A. (2019). The Reciprocal Relationship Between Gratitude and Life Satisfaction: Evidence From Two Longitudinal Field Studies. *Frontiers in Psychology*, *10*, 2480. https://doi.org/10.3389/fpsyg.2019.02480

Ungvarsky, J. (2024). *Mere-exposure effect*. EBSCOhost. https://www.ebsco.com/research-starters/psychology/mere-exposure-effect

van Alphen, E. (1997). *Caught by history*. Stanford University Press.

Van Bael, K., Ball, M., Scarfo, J., & Suleyman, E. (2023). Assessment of the mind-body connection: Preliminary psychometric evidence for a new self-report questionnaire. *BMC Psychology*, *11*(309), 1–21. DOI: 10.1186/s40359-023-01302-3 PMID: 37803484

VanderWeele, T. J. (2017). On the promotion of human flourishing. *Proceedings of the National Academy of Sciences of the United States of America*, *114*(31), 8148–8156. DOI: 10.1073/pnas.1702996114 PMID: 28705870

Varela, F., Thompson, E., & Rosch, E. (2016). *The Embodied Mind—Cognitive Science and Human Experience*. MIT Press. Revised Edition [1991].

Varela, F., Thompson, E., & Rosch, E. (1993). *The Embodied Mind. Cognitive Science and Human Experience*. MIT Press.

Vernon, L. L., Dillon, J. M., & Steiner, A. R. W. (2009). Proactive coping, gratitude, and posttraumatic stress disorder in college women. *Anxiety, Stress, and Coping*, *22*(1). Advance online publication. DOI: 10.1080/10615800802203751 PMID: 18791902

Viart, D. (2019). *Les littératures de terrain*. Revue critique de fixxion française contemporaine, 18, Article 18. https://doi.org/DOI: 10.4000/fixxion.1275

Viart, D. (2009). Le silence des pères au principe du « récit de filiation ». *Etudes Francaises (Montreal, Quebec)*, *45*(3), 95–112. DOI: 10.7202/038860ar

Vieselmeyer, J., Holguin, J., & Mezulis, A. (2017). The role of resilience and gratitude in posttraumatic stress and growth following a campus shooting. *Psychological Trauma: Theory, Research, Practice, and Policy*, *9*(1). Advance online publication. DOI: 10.1037/tra0000149 PMID: 27548470

Visetti, G. P. (2003). Intervista a Mario Rigoni Stern [Interview with Mario Rigoni Stern]. *La Repubblica* (15 Dec.), 27.

Vlastos, G. (1991). *Socrates: Ironist and moral philosopher*. Cornell University Press.

Wang, C., & Xiao, R. (2021). Music and art therapy combined with cognitive behavioral therapy to treat adolescent anorexia patients. *American Journal of Translational Research*, *13*(6), 6534–6542. PMID: 34306394

Wastell, C. (2005). *Understanding Trauma and Emotion. Dealing with Trauma Using an Emotion-Focused Approach*. Allen & Unwin.

Watkins, P. C., Woodward, K., Stone, T., & Kolts, R. L. (2003). Gratitude and happiness: Development of a measure of gratitude, and relationships with subjective well-being. *Social Behavior and Personality*, *31*(5). Advance online publication. DOI: 10.2224/sbp.2003.31.5.431

Watts, A. (1989). *The way of Zen*. Vintage Books. (Original work published 1957)

Watts, A. (1989). *The Way of Zen*. Vintage.

Webb, R. (2009). *Ekphrasis, imagination and persuasion in ancient rhetorical theory and practice*. Ashgate.

Weber, M. (2004). Science as a vocation. In Owen, D., & Strong, T. (Eds.), *The vocation lectures* (pp. 1–33). Hackett.

Wehling-Giorgi, K. (2016). 'Ero separata da me': Memory, Selfhood and Mother-Tongue in Goliarda Sapienza and Elena Ferrante. In Bazzoni, A., Fortini, L., Bond, E., & Wehling-Giorgi, K. (Eds.), *Goliarda Sapienza in Context: Intertextual Relationships with Italian and European Culture* (pp. 288–311). Fairleigh Dickinson University Press.

Wehling-Giorgi, K. (2023). Unspeakable Things Spoken: Transgenerational Trauma, Fractured Bodies and Visual Tropes in Toni Morrison, Elsa Morante and Elena Ferrante's Works. *Romance Studies*, *41*(4), 248–266.

What is cognitive therapy? [in Japanese]. (2025). Japan Cognitive Therapy Association. https://jact.jp/introduction/

What is transactional analysis? [in Japanese]. (2025). Japan Transactional Analysis Association. http://www.js-ta.jp/analysis.html

Wheatley, D., & Bickerton, C. (2017). Subjective well-being and engagement in arts, culture, and sport. *Journal of Cultural Economics, 41*, 23–45. DOI: 10.1007/s10824-016-9270-0

Whitfield-Gabrieli, S., & Ford, J. M. (2012). Default mode network activity and connectivity in psychopathology. *Annual Review of Clinical Psychology, 8*, 49–76. DOI: 10.1146/annurev-clinpsy-032511-143049 PMID: 22224834

WHO. (2021). *Health Promotion Glossary of Terms 2021*. WHO Publishing.

Wierzbicka, A. (2009). Language and Metalanguage: Key Issues in Emotion Research. *Emotion Review, 1*(1), 3–14. DOI: 10.1177/1754073908097175

Wilde, L. (2020). Trauma Across Cultures: Cultural Dimensions of the Phenomenology of Post-Traumatic Experiences. *Phenomenology and Mind, 18*, 222–229. DOI: 10.17454/pam-1816

Wilkins, E. G. (1927). ΕΓΓΥΑ, ΠΑΡΑ ΔΑΤΗ. *Classical Philology, 22*(2), 121–135.

Williams, P. (1993). *Nous, on n'en parle pas, les vivants et les morts chez les Manouches*. Editions de la Maison des sciences de l'homme.

Winnicott, D. W. (1971). *Playing and reality*. Routledge.

Wood, A. M., Froh, J. J., & Geraghty, A. W. A. (2010). Gratitude and well-being: A review and theoretical integration. In *Clinical Psychology Review* (Vol. 30, Issue 7). DOI: 10.1016/j.cpr.2010.03.005

Wu, X., Kaminga, A. C., Dai, W., Deng, J., Wang, Z., Pan, X., & Liu, A. (2019). The prevalence of moderate-to-high posttraumatic growth: A systematic review and meta-analysis. In *Journal of Affective Disorders* (Vol. 243). DOI: 10.1016/j.jad.2018.09.023

Yang, Q., Cao, X., & Jiang, X. (2022). The Role of Multilingual Script Systems in Face Processing. In Jiang, X. (Ed.), *Multilingualism–Interdisciplinary Topics* (pp. 85–100). IntechOpen.

Yasui, Y., Breder, C. D., Saper, C. B., & Cechetto, D. F. (1991). Autonomic responses and efferent pathways from the insular cortex in the rat. *The Journal of Comparative Neurology, 303*(3), 355–374. DOI: 10.1002/cne.903030303 PMID: 2007654

Ye, G., Baldwin, D. S., & Hou, R. (2021). Anxiety in asthma: A systematic review and meta-analysis. *Psychological Medicine, 51*(1), 11–20. DOI: 10.1017/S0033291720003037 PMID: 33431086

Yi, C., Naixin, L., Onosahwo Iyendo, T., & Apuke, O. D. (2024). Cognitive behavior, art, and music therapies intervention for treating the depression of children: A randomized control trial. *Psychiatry Research, 333*. Advance online publication. DOI: 10.1016/j.psychres.2024.115716 PMID: 38244284

Yoshida, K., & Ito, J. (2012). Recovery-oriented community-based mental health service in Japan: The development of outreach services. *International Journal of Mental Health, 41*(2), 29–37. DOI: 10.2753/IMH0020-7411410203

Yoshihara, K. (2009). Naikan therapy [in Japanese]. In K. C. (Ed.), *Standard textbook of psychosomatic medicine* (3rd ed., pp. 339–343). Igaku-Shoin.

Yoshihara, K. (2015). Psychosomatic treatment for allergic diseases. *BioPsychoSocial Medicine, 9*, 8. Advance online publication. DOI: 10.1186/s13030-015-0036-8 PMID: 25844089

Yoshihara, K., Hiramoto, T., Oka, T., Kubo, C., & Sudo, N. (2014). Effect of 12 weeks of yoga training on the somatization, psychological symptoms, and stress-related biomarkers of healthy women. *BioPsychoSocial Medicine, 8*(1), 1. Advance online publication. DOI: 10.1186/1751-0759-8-1 PMID: 24383884

Yoshihara, K., Hiramoto, T., Oka, T., & Sudo, N. (2011). Profile of mood states and stress-related biochemical indices in long-term yoga practitioners. *BioPsychoSocial Medicine, 5*(1), 6. Advance online publication. DOI: 10.1186/1751-0759-5-6 PMID: 21635790

Yoshihara, K., & Kubo, C. (2008). Stress, fatigue, and psychosomatic illnesses [in Japanese]. *Psychiatry, 50*, 597–602.

Yoshihara, K., & Sudo, N. (2016). Mental health related diseases and treatment: Psychosomatic diseases [in Japanese]. *Clinical Research, 3*, 600–604.

Young, J. E. (2000). *At memory's edge*. Yale University Press.

Zaehner, R. C. (1979). *The Bhagavad Gita, with a commentary based on the original source*. Oxford University Press.

Zhou, X., & Wu, X. (2015). Longitudinal relationships between gratitude, deliberate rumination, and posttraumatic growth in adolescents following the Wenchuan earthquake in China. *Scandinavian Journal of Psychology, 56*(5). Advance online publication. DOI: 10.1111/sjop.12237 PMID: 26122407

Zwigenberg, R. (2018). Nuclear Minds: Japanese Psychiatry's Encounter with the Atom. *Jinbun*, *49*, 93–101.

About the Contributors

Charlène Clonts is Associate Professor (PhD.) (Maître de Conférences) at Kyushu University, Faculty of Humanities (Japan), where she teaches and performs research since March 2018. She is the Head of the international research-creation project "Well-Being with Arts" (WBA) funded by a grant from Q-AOS (KU Institute for Asian and Oceanian Studies). She studies the intersections of 20th-21st c. literatures (esp. Francophone), arts, and health humanities, with a particular focus on intermedia approaches and their transformative potential. She published numerous peer-review articles, chapters, and books, and presented in conferences (also keynotes, invited speeches...) about the performative effects of intermedia practices and the transpoetics related to East Asia and well-being. Recent publications: bilingual chapter "Wifredo Lam and Ghérasim Luca: Apostroph'Apocalypse", in "Wifredo Lam, Artist's Books", Jean-Michel Place, 2025; special issue ed. "Technotext", National University Taiwan, 2025; specialist book "Ghérasim Luca: Texte, Image, Son", Peter Lang, 2020; special issue ed. "Origami, le pli dans les littératures et les arts", Pau University, France, 2021. Within the ALTER research unit at the University of Pau (France), she participated actively as a member of French National Research Agency (ANR)-funded projects centred on the book as a space of creation (2011-2015) and on the European diaspora of the Romanian Avant-gardes (2016-2020), esp. Francophone. She taught as a lecturer at the University of Paris Panthéon-Sorbonne and the University of Paris Est-Créteil. She also worked during a decade for the French National Education. She obtained the French National Habilitation for Associate Professor (Maître de Conférences) in Aesthetics, Arts, Performance (Section 18) and French Literature and Linguistics (Section 9).

Lorenzo Cardilli is an Associate Professor in Contemporary Italian Literature at the University of Udine, Italy, within the Department of Humanities and Cultural Heritage (DIUM). His research interests include contemporary Italian literature, poetry, intermedia practices, the rhetoric of literary criticism, and the intersection of literature and digital humanities. Dr. Cardilli has been actively involved in various international research projects and has contributed to the academic community through his roles in organizing conferences and symposia. In 2019 he was invited by dr. Charlène Clonts to contribute to the organization of the international symposium "Body-mind interactions in arts, health, literatures & science: asian and indo-oceanian perspectives", held at Kyushu University. Dr. Cardilli has published in peer-reviewed journals and edited volumes, with notable works including his monograph "Figura e ripetizione in Dietro il paesaggio di Andrea Zanzotto" and numerous articles on contemporary Italian poetry and literary criticism. He is also a member of the scientific committee of the journal "L'Ulisse" and vice editor-in-chief of "Configurazioni. Ricerche sulla poesia contemporanea." In addition to his academic contributions, Dr. Cardilli has been involved in various teaching roles, including adjunct professorships at the Politecnico di Milano and visiting professorships at the Shanghai Publishing and Printing College. He has also delivered invited lectures at prestigious institutions such as Kyoto University and Osaka University.

Kazufumi Yoshihara, M.D., Ph.D., is a Professor of Center for Health Sciences and Counseling at the Kyushu University (Japan), while also maintaining clinical practice at the Department of Psychosomatic Medicine, Kyushu University Hospital. His research encompasses psychosomatic medicine, stress-related disorders, and the biopsychosocial mechanisms underlying mind–body interactions. Dr. Yoshihara has made substantial contributions to both clinical practice and academic research, with numerous publications in peer-reviewed journals aimed at bridging psychological well-being and physical health. He has been actively engaged in advancing integrated approaches to psychosomatic care and has played a pivotal role in fostering the next generation of clinicians and researchers in the field. A board-certified specialist in both General Internal Medicine and Psychosomatic Medicine, Dr. Yoshihara currently serves as a board member for the Japanese Society of Psychosomatic Internal Medicine, the Japanese Society for Fatigue Science, and the Japan Association of Oriental Psychosomatic Medicine, continuing to bridge the gap between research and clinical application.

***

Anna Bourges-Celaries holds a PhD from the University of Montreal (Canada). Her work focuses on exophony, and more specifically on exophonic Japanese writers: Shimazaki Aki (1954-), Tawada Yōko (1960-) and Sekiguchi Ryōko (1970-). She published the articles: « L'exophonie chez Sekiguchi Ryōko: transfert de saveurs [Sekiguchi Ryōko's exophony: transfer of flavours] » (journal Romanastica Comeniana), and « Des espaces japonais du français [The Japanese dimension of

French] » in the collective work Langue(s) et espaces dans les xénographies féminines en français (AMV Munich).

Oriane Chevalier is a PhD candidate in Comparative Literature at the Université Clermont Auvergne. Her thesis, supervised by Professor Yvan Daniel, is entitled "Go-betweens from East to West: the Far East seen through the prism of five female pioneers". Graduated from the École Normale Supérieure de Lyon, her research seeks to identify the characteristics of Feminine Orientalism by focusing on the relationship between Western women writers and the Far East. Her thesis looks at the diffusion of Chinese and Japanese literature by women in France, the United States, Northern Ireland and Spain at the turn of the nineteenth and twentieth centuries.

Deepika Chhikara is currently an Assistant Professor at the Vivekananda Institute of Professional Studies, Delhi, and a doctoral researcher at Guru Gobind Singh Indraprastha University. With over nine years in the academic sector, her work focuses on the intersections of consumer behavior, sustainability, and mindfulness. Her scholarly contributions include several book chapters and articles published in ABDC and Scopus-indexed journals. Prior to her career in education, she spent six years in marketing strategy, holding roles at luxury living brands like Jaguar Land Rover, Delhi Art Gallery, Hubert Burda Publishing. She is dedicated to synthesizing corporate insights with consumer research to foster a more nuanced and practical learning environment for her students.

Gianluca Cinelli, Ph.D., is an internationally published scholar in Italian Studies and Comparative Literature and an alumnus of the Alexander von Humboldt Foundation. His research interests include war literature, literature and ethics, the archetypal theory of storytelling, and the relationship between storytelling and cognition. He has published on Nuto Revelli, Primo Levi, Mario Rigoni Stern, Alessandro Manzoni, and Joseph Conrad. He is co-editor of the Close Encounters in War Journal (www.closeencountersinwar.org) and co-founder of the oral history project MemoGen (www.memogen3.wordpress.com).

Julie-Marie Duro Sasaki is a Ph.D. candidate in Arts and Art Science at the University of Liège (Belgium). With a background in photography and philosophy, her research explores embodied inquiry and the interplay between private life, academic experience, and artistic practice. Her work also engages with *kaiseki* cuisine, the sencha tea ceremony, and zen practices, in relation to pragmatic aesthetics and situated forms of knowledge.

Aira Dutta is currently a first-year master's student in Applied Psychology at O.P Jindal Global University, Haryana, India. She completed her B.A (Hons) in

Psychology at the same institution. Her academic journey is centered on the complexities of criminal behavior and correctional psychology, with a particular emphasis on how holistic framework can fundamentally reshape rehabilitative practices. Driven by an interest in intersection of spirituality and Heartfulness, Aira explores how contemplative practices centered on the heart, mind and body can foster profound personal growth and emotional well-being. Her goal is to bridge traditional psychological interventions with spiritual growth, contributing to a more compassionate and effective approach to offender reform

Renuka Kapoor is working as a Research Supervisor of undergraduate students at the University of Delhi (India). She completed her PhD in the field of Management (Human Resource Management) from Amity School of Business, Amity University, Noida. She has completed her graduation and master's in Commerce from the University of Delhi. She has also worked as a visiting faculty at the Amity School of Business and School of Open Learning (University of Delhi). Her research interests lie in the areas of emotional well-being, job satisfaction, and job performance. She has presented research papers at several national and international conferences and has published articles in UGC, ABDC, and SCOPUS-indexed journals. Dr. Kapoor actively engages in academic research and scholarly collaborations, contributing to the growing body of knowledge in the field of human resource management and workplace well-being. Through her academic and research contributions, she continues to support students and emerging scholars in developing research-oriented perspectives and critical thinking in the field of management.

Jean Khalfa, Emeritus Prof., Trinity College Cambridge, UK, specialises in the history of philosophy, modern literature (in particular contemporary poetry and writing in French from North Africa and the Caribbean), aesthetics and anthropology. He has published books and articles on Pascal, Rousseau, Deleuze, Sartre, Fanon, Césaire, St John Perse, Glissant, Michaux, Cavaillès, Maccheroni, Roche, on typographic forms and on the relationship between contemporary poetry and the image. In 2015 he published Fanon's collected writings, _*Écrits sur l'aliénation et la liberté*_ (Jean Khalfa and Robert Young, ed., La Découverte, 2015 and 2019 and Hibr, Algiers, 2015; English translation: Bloomsbury, 2018, 2020). His _*Poetics of the Antilles: Poetry, History and Philosophy in the Writings of Perse, Césaire, Fanon and Glissant*_ was published in 2017 by Peter Lang. His most recent book is _ *Wifredo LAM – Livres d'artiste/ Artist's Books*_ an edited volume on Wifredo Lam's books, published by Jean-Michel Place in 2025.

Poonam Khurana, Goldmedalist, PhD- Faculty of Management Studies, university of Delhi, Working as Professor (Management- HR and OB)and

Counsellor at Vivekananda Institute of Professional Studies, Delhi, India. Received Best Teachers Award for the year 2018- 2019 at Vivekananda Institute of Professional Studies for r Academic Excellence. Teaching experience of 19 years to BBA, MBA and B tech courses Publications in the area of Personal Ethics, Spirituality, Interpersonal behavior, cognitive mapping, emotional intelligence and teaching effectiveness in Journals of Repute. published 9 books including one text book titled "Work Psychology" and Edited book "Performance Management" by Taylor and Francis, CRC Press and 60 journal publications.

Stefano Lombardi Vallauri is associate professor of musicology at the IULM University of Milan, general editor of the scientific journal «Nuove Musiche», president (2024-2026) of the cultural association Athena Musica, coordinator of the IULM unit for the NextGenerationEU project "Sounding images - Screening sounds" funded by the European Union. His research focuses on the aesthetics and analysis of contemporary music, both classical and popular. Among his publications are the monograph *Dodecafonia postseriale. Gilberto Cappelli e Federico Incardona* (2013); the co-edited works *L'adattamento musicale* (2024), *L'arte orale. Poesia, musica, performance* (2020), *Jonathan Harvey* (2019), *La voce mediatizzata* (2019).

Patrizia Piredda, MA (Literature), MA (Philosophy), MLitt (Philosophy and Literature) and PhD (Philosophy and Literature). In 2018 and 2019 I received the Seal of Excellence Certificate from the European Commission (EU Framework Programme for Research and Innovation 2014-2020. I am an expert in Theory of Metaphor and my research interests include the philosophy of language, with particular attention to the epistemological role of metaphor, and the relationship between ethics and literature. I published scientific articles on Wittgenstein, Nietzsche, Pirandello, D'Annunzio, Savinio, Levi, Calvino, utopia and dystopia, on metaphors in the media and political discourse on Covid-19 and Quantum Mechanics. I am currently developing the MemoGen Project in collaboration with the Archivio Ligure della Scrittura Popolare (University of Genoa) and Centro Studi per la Pace "Sereno Regis".

Sofia Rossatelli is a postdoctoral researcher at the University of Milan, specialising in art therapies and psychosocial methodologies within contemporary Japanese sociocultural contexts. Her research focuses on non-pharmacological approaches to mental health and on the relationship between creativity, well-being and social participation. She conducts fieldwork particularly in Kyoto, collaborating with local arts therapy centres that integrate both Japanese and international perspectives on psychosocial care.

Alessandro Toma (they/them) is a PhD candidate at Durham University, UK. Their research investigates how post-World War II Italian women writers use affect as a tool to enact resistance to dominant cultural discourses. Alessandro has presented at international conferences on affect in literature, with a particular focus on Elena Ferrante, and co-chaired a panel on the political power of affect in nineteenth- and twentieth-century writing. They are a postgraduate fellow at Durham University's Institute of Medical Humanities and an early-career researcher of its Affective Experience Lab.

Kirti Tyagi is an assistant professor at Jindal School of Psychology and Counselling. She completed her Ph. D. from the Department of Humanities and Social Sciences, Indian Institute of Technology, Delhi, in the area of teens, risky decision-making, and domain-specific risk-taking. She completed her Bachelor of Arts (Hons) in Psychology from Jesus and Mary College, Delhi University, where she was laureled for being the college topper and university rank holder. She then pursued her master's in applied psychology from the Faculty of Arts, University of Delhi, and secured second rank in the master's program and received the South Campus Endowment Scholarship for meritorious students. She has also received several travel scholarships, summer school sponsorships, and academic awards. Her research interests lie in the area of adolescent risky decision-making, psychometric testing, risk perception, Habit formation, youth spirituality, existential anxiety, and games for social-emotional learning.

Index

Symbols

A

B

C

D

E

F

G

H

I

Y

Z

www.ingramcontent.com/pod-product-compliance
Lightning Source LLC
LaVergne TN
LVHW062331300926
849161LV00007B/1655